W9-AQB-282

Learning Disabilities
SOURCEBOOK

Fifth Edition

Health Reference Series

Fifth Edition

Learning Disabilities
SOURCEBOOK

*Basic Consumer Health Information about Dyslexia,
Dyscalculia, Dysgraphia, Speech and Communication
Disorders, Auditory and Visual Processing Disorders, and Other
Conditions That Make Learning Difficult, Including Attention
Deficit Hyperactivity Disorder, Down Syndrome and Other
Chromosomal Disorders, Fetal Alcohol Spectrum Disorders,
Hearing and Visual Impairment, Autism and Other Pervasive
Developmental Disorders, and Traumatic Brain Injury*

*Along with Facts about Diagnosing Learning Disabilities, Early
Intervention, the Special Education Process, Legal Protections,
Assistive Technology, and Accommodations, and Guidelines
for Life-Stage Transitions, Suggestions for Coping with Daily
Challenges, a Glossary of Related Terms, and a Directory of
Additional Resources*

OMNIGRAPHICS

615 Griswold, Ste. 901, Detroit, MI 48226

Bibliographic Note
Because this page cannot legibly accommodate all the copyright notices, the Bibliographic
Note portion of the Preface constitutes an extension of the copyright notice.

* * *

Health Reference Series
Keith Jones, *Managing Editor*
***

OMNIGRAPHICS
A PART OF RELEVANT INFORMATION
***

Copyright © 2016 Omnigraphics
ISBN 978-0-7808-1520-9
E-ISBN 978-0-7808-1521-6

Library of Congress Cataloging-in-Publication Data

Names: Omnigraphics, issuing body.

Title: Learning disabilities sourcebook: basic consumer health information about
dyslexia, dyscalculia, dysgraphia, speech and communication disorders, auditory
and visual processing disorders, and other conditions that make learning difficult,
including attention deficit hyperactivity disorder, down syndrome and other
chromosomal disorders, fetal alcohol spectrum disorders, hearing and visual
impairment, autism and other pervasive developmental disorders, and traumatic
brain injury; along with facts about diagnosing learning disabilities, early
intervention, the special education process, legal protections, assistive technology, and
accommodations, and guidelines for life-stage transitions, suggestions for coping with
daily challenges, a glossary of related terms, and a directory of additional resources.

Description: Fifth edition. | Detroit, MI: Omnigraphics, 2016. | Series: Health
reference series | Includes bibliographical references and index.

Identifiers: LCCN 2016015937 (print) | LCCN 2016022269 (ebook) | ISBN
9780780815209 (hardcover: alk. paper) | ISBN 9780780815216 (ebook) | ISBN
9780780815216 (eBook)

Subjects: LCSH: Learning disabilities--United States--Handbooks, manuals, etc.
| Learning disabled children--Education--United States--Handbooks, manuals,
etc. | Learning disabled--Education--United States--Handbooks, manuals, etc. |
Learning disabilities--United States--Diagnosis--Handbooks, manuals, etc.

Classification: LCC LC4705 .L434 2016 (print) | LCC LC4705 (ebook) | DDC
371.90973--dc23

LC record available at https://lccn.loc.gov/2016015937

Table of Contents

Part IV: Learning Disabilities and the Educational Process

Part V: Living with Learning Disabilities

Part VI: Additional Help and Information

Preface

About This Book

Learning disabilities are neurological disorders that affect the brain's ability to process, store, and communicate information. They are widespread, affecting as many as 4.6 million Americans according to the National Center for Learning Disabilities (NCLD). Recent statistics show that the number of children and youth ages 3–21 receiving special education services was 6.5 million, or about 13 percent of all public school students. Among students receiving special education services, 35 percent had specific learning disabilities. Learning disabilities directly impact many areas in the lives of those affected, making school difficult, making it hard to obtain and sustain employment, making daily tasks challenging, and even affecting relationships. Yet learning disabilities are invisible obstacles. For this reason they are often misunderstood, and their impact is often underestimated.

Learning Disabilities Sourcebook, Fifth Edition, provides information about dyslexia, dyscalculia, dysgraphia, speech and communication disorders, and auditory and visual processing disorders. It also provides details about other conditions that impact learning, including attention deficit hyperactivity disorder, autism, and other pervasive developmental disorders, hearing and visual impairment, and chromosomal disorders. The book offers facts about diagnosing learning disabilities, the special education process, and legal protections. Guidelines for life-stage transitions and coping with daily challenges, a glossary of related terms, and a directory of resources for additional help and information are also included.

How to Use This Book

This book is divided into parts and chapters. Parts focus on broad areas of interest. Chapters are devoted to single topics within a part.

Part I: Understanding and Identifying Learning Disabilities explains how the brain works, defines what learning disabilities are, and describes theories regarding their potential causes. It discusses early learning and language development milestones, the signs and symptoms of learning disabilities, and how learning disabilities are evaluated and diagnosed. Statistics on the prevalence of learning disabilities are also provided.

Part II: Types of Learning Disabilities describes the most common forms of learning disabilities, including problems with reading, writing, mathematics, speech, language, and communication. It explains what these disorders are, how they are diagnosed, and how they are treated. The part also discusses learning disabilities among gifted students, a fairly common—but often unrecognized—phenomenon.

Part III: Other Disorders That Make Learning Difficult discusses common disorders that have a component that affects a child's ability to learn, including attention deficit hyperactivity disorder, epilepsy, fetal alcohol spectrum disorders, pervasive developmental disorders, visual and hearing disabilities, and chromosomal disorders such as Down syndrome.

Part IV: Learning Disabilities and the Educational Process provides information about how learning disabilities are accommodated within the schools. It describes early intervention strategies, explains how the special education process works, and details the legal supports for students with learning disabilities. Specialized teaching techniques and alternative educational options, such as tutoring and home schooling, that are used to help learning-disabled students succeed are described. Guidelines for successfully negotiating the transitions to high school and to college are also provided.

Part V: Living with Learning Disabilities discusses how learning disabilities impact daily life. It includes tips for coping with a learning disability and for parenting a child with a learning disability. The impact of learning disabilities on self-esteem and social skills are discussed, as well as getting support for disability harassment. It offers suggestions to help those with learning disabilities deal with daily tasks, including meal preparation, money management, transportation, and learning to drive. It also provides detailed guidelines for handling the employment issues faced by those with learning disabilities.

Part VI: Additional Help and Information includes a glossary of terms related to learning disabilities, a list of sources of college funding for students with disabilities, and a directory of resources for further help and support.

Bibliographic Note

This volume contains documents and excerpts from publications issued by the following U.S. government agencies: Center for Parent Information and Resources (CPIR); Centers for Disease Control and Prevention (CDC); Committee on Science, Space, and Technology; Disability.gov; Early Childhood Learning and Knowledge Center (ECLKC); Education Resources Information Center (ERIC); *Eunice Kennedy Shriver* National Institute of Child Health and Human Development (NICHD); Genetic and Rare Diseases Information Center (GARD); Genetics Home Reference (GHR); Institute of Education Sciences (IES); Literacy Information and Communication System (LINCS); National Center for Education Statistics (NCES); National Council on Disability (NCD); National Human Genome Research Institute (NHGRI); National Institute of Mental Health (NIMH); National Institute of Neurological Disorders and Stroke (NINDS); National Institute on Deafness and Other Communication Disorders (NIDCD); Office of Disability Employment Policy (ODEP); Office of Science Education (OSE); Child Welfare Information Gateway; StopBullying.gov; U.S. Department of Education (ED); U.S. Environmental Protection Agency (EPA); U.S. Senate Committee on Health, Education, Labor, and Pensions; and WhiteHouse.gov.

In addition, this volume contains copyrighted documents from the following organization: The Nemours Foundation

It may also contain original material produced by Omnigraphics and reviewed by medical consultants.

About the Health Reference Series

The *Health Reference Series* is designed to provide basic medical information for patients, families, caregivers, and the general public. Each volume takes a particular topic and provides comprehensive coverage. This is especially important for people who may be dealing with a newly diagnosed disease or a chronic disorder in themselves or in a family member. People looking for preventive guidance, information about disease warning signs, medical statistics, and risk factors for health problems will also find answers to their questions in the *Health Reference Series*. The *Series*, however, is not intended to serve as a tool for diagnosing illness, in prescribing treatments, or as a substitute for the physician/patient relationship. All people concerned about medical symptoms or the possibility of disease are encouraged to seek professional care from an appropriate health care provider.

A Note about Spelling and Style

Health Reference Series editors use *Stedman's Medical Dictionary* as an authority for questions related to the spelling of medical terms and the *Chicago Manual of Style* for questions related to grammatical structures, punctuation, and other editorial concerns. Consistent adherence is not always possible, however, because the individual volumes within the *Series* include many documents from a wide variety of different producers, and the editor's primary goal is to present material from each source as accurately as is possible. This sometimes means that information in different chapters or sections may follow other guidelines and alternate spelling authorities.

Medical Review

Omnigraphics contracts with a team of qualified, senior medical professionals who serve as medical consultants for the *Health Reference Series*. As necessary, medical consultants review reprinted and originally written material for currency and accuracy. Citations including the phrase, "Reviewed (month, year)" indicate material reviewed by this team. Medical consultation services are provided to the *Health Reference Series* editors by:

Dr. Vijayalakshmi, MBBS, DGO, MD
Dr. Senthil Selvan, MBBS, DCH, MD
Dr. K. Sivanandham, MBBS, DCH, MS (Research), PhD

Our Advisory Board

We would like to thank the following board members for providing initial guidance on the development of this series:

- Dr. Lynda Baker, Associate Professor of Library and Information Science, Wayne State University, Detroit, MI

- Nancy Bulgarelli, William Beaumont Hospital Library, Royal Oak, MI

- Karen Imarisio, Bloomfield Township Public Library, Bloomfield Township, MI

- Karen Morgan, Mardigian Library, University of Michigan-Dearborn, Dearborn, MI

- Rosemary Orlando, St. Clair Shores Public Library, St. Clair Shores, MI

Health Reference Series *Update Policy*

The inaugural book in the *Health Reference Series* was the first edition of *Cancer Sourcebook* published in 1989. Since then, the *Series* has been enthusiastically received by librarians and in the medical community. In order to maintain the standard of providing high-quality health information for the layperson the editorial staff at Omnigraphics felt it was necessary to implement a policy of updating volumes when warranted.

Medical researchers have been making tremendous strides, and it is the purpose of the *Health Reference Series* to stay current with the most recent advances. Each decision to update a volume is made on an individual basis. Some of the considerations include how much new information is available and the feedback we receive from people who use the books. If there is a topic you would like to see added to the update list, or an area of medical concern you feel has not been adequately addressed, please write to:

Managing Editor
Health Reference Series
Omnigraphics
615 Griswold, Ste. 901
Detroit, MI 48226

Part One

Understanding and Identifying Learning Disabilities

Chapter 1

The Brain and Its Function

Chapter Contents

Section 1.1

Brain Basics: How the Brain Works

This section includes text excerpted from "Brain Basics: Know
Your Brain," National Institute of Neurological Disorders
and Stroke (NINDS), April 17, 2015.

The brain is the most complex part of the human body. This three-pound organ is the seat of intelligence, interpreter of the senses, initiator of body movement, and controller of behavior. Lying in its bony shell and washed by protective fluid, the brain is the source of all the qualities that define our humanity. The brain is the crown jewel of the human body.

For centuries, scientists and philosophers have been fascinated by the brain, but until recently they viewed the brain as nearly incomprehensible. Now, however, the brain is beginning to relinquish its secrets. Scientists have learned more about the brain in the last ten years than in all previous centuries because of the accelerating pace of research in neurological and behavioral science and the development of new research techniques. As a result, Congress named the 1990s the Decade of the Brain. At the forefront of research on the brain and other elements of the nervous system is the National Institute of Neurological Disorders and Stroke (NINDS), which conducts and supports scientific studies in the United States and around the world.

This section is a basic introduction to the human brain. It may help you understand how the healthy brain works, how to keep it healthy, and what happens when the brain is diseased or dysfunctional.

Architecture of the Brain

The brain is like a committee of experts. All the parts of the brain work together, but each part has its own special properties. The brain can be divided into three basic units: the **forebrain**, the **midbrain**, and the **hindbrain**.

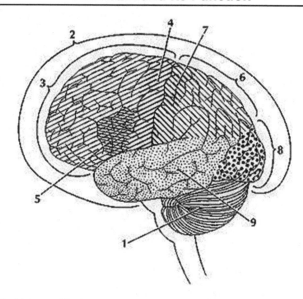

Figure 1.1. *Human Brain*

The hindbrain includes the upper part of the spinal cord, the brain stem, and a wrinkled ball of tissue called the **cerebellum (1)**. The hindbrain controls the body's vital functions such as respiration and heart rate. The cerebellum coordinates movement and is involved in learned rote movements. When you play the piano or hit a tennis ball you are activating the cerebellum. The uppermost part of the brainstem is the midbrain, which controls some reflex actions and is part of the circuit involved in the control of eye movements and other voluntary movements. The forebrain is the largest and most highly developed part of the human brain: it consists primarily of the **cerebrum (2)** and the structures hidden beneath it. When people see pictures of the brain it is usually the cerebrum that they notice. The cerebrum sits at the top most part of the brain and is the source of intellectual activities. It holds your memories, allows you to plan, enables you to imagine and think. It allows you to recognize friends, read books, and play games.

The cerebrum is split into two halves (hemispheres) by a deep fissure. Despite the split, the two cerebral hemispheres communicate with each other through a thick tract of nerve fibers that lies at the base of this fissure. Although the two hemispheres seem to be mirror images of each other, they are different. For instance, the ability to form words seems to lie primarily in the left hemisphere, while the right hemisphere seems to control many abstract reasoning skills.

For some as-yet-unknown reason, nearly all of the signals from the brain to the body and vice-versa crossover on their way to and from the brain. This means that the right cerebral hemisphere primarily controls the left side of the body and the left hemisphere primarily controls the right side. When one side of the brain is damaged, the opposite side of the body is affected. For example, a stroke in the right hemisphere of the brain can leave the left arm and leg paralyzed.

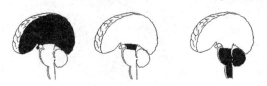

Figure 1.2. *Forebrain, Midbrain, and Hindbrain*

Geography of Thought

Each cerebral hemisphere can be divided into sections, or lobes, each of which specializes in different functions. To understand each lobe and its specialty we will take a tour of the cerebral hemispheres, starting with the two **frontal lobes (3)**, which lie directly behind the forehead. When you plan a schedule, imagine the future, or use reasoned arguments, these two lobes do much of the work. One of the ways the frontal lobes seem to do these things is by acting as short-term storage sites, allowing one idea to be kept in mind while other ideas are considered. In the rearmost portion of each frontal lobe is a **motor area (4)**, which helps control voluntary movement. A nearby place on the left frontal lobe called **Broca's area (5)** allows thoughts to be transformed into words.

When you enjoy a good meal—the taste, aroma, and texture of the food—two sections behind the frontal lobes called the **parietal lobes (6)** are at work. The forward parts of these lobes, just behind the motor areas, are the primary **sensory areas (7)**. These areas receive information about temperature, taste, touch, and movement from the rest of the body. Reading and arithmetic are also functions in the repertoire of each parietal lobe.

As you look at the words and pictures on this page, two areas at the back of the brain are at work. These lobes, called the **occipital lobes (8)**, process images from the eyes and link that information with images stored in memory. Damage to the occipital lobes can cause blindness.

The last lobes on our tour of the cerebral hemispheres are the **temporal lobes (9)**, which lie in front of the visual areas and nest under the parietal and frontal lobes. Whether you appreciate symphonies or rock music, your brain responds through the activity of these lobes. At the top of each temporal lobe is an area responsible for receiving information from the ears. The underside of each temporal lobe plays a crucial role in forming and retrieving memories, including those associated with music. Other parts of this lobe seem to integrate memories and sensations of taste, sound, sight, and touch.

Cerebral Cortex

Coating the surface of the cerebrum and the cerebellum is a vital layer of tissue the thickness of a stack of two or three dimes. It is called the cortex, from the Latin word for bark. Most of the actual information processing in the brain takes place in the cerebral cortex. When people talk about "gray matter" in the brain they are talking about this thin rind. The cortex is gray because nerves in this area lack the insulation that makes most other parts of the brain appear to be white. The folds in the brain add to its surface area and therefore increase the amount of gray matter and the quantity of information that can be processed.

Inner Brain

Deep within the brain, hidden from view, lie structures that are the gatekeepers between the spinal cord and the cerebral hemispheres. These structures not only determine our emotional state, they also modify our perceptions and responses depending on that state, and allow us to initiate movements that you make without thinking about them. Like the lobes in the cerebral hemispheres, the structures described below come in pairs: each is duplicated in the opposite half of the brain.

The **hypothalamus (10)**, about the size of a pearl, directs a multitude of important functions. It wakes you up in the morning, and gets the adrenaline flowing during a test or job interview. The hypothalamus is also an important emotional center, controlling the molecules that make you feel exhilarated, angry, or unhappy. Near the hypothalamus lies the **thalamus (11)**, a major clearinghouse for information going to and from the spinal cord and the cerebrum.

An arching tract of nerve cells leads from the hypothalamus and the thalamus to the **hippocampus (12)**. This tiny nub acts as a memory indexer—sending memories out to the appropriate part of the cerebral hemisphere for long-term storage and retrieving them when necessary. The basal ganglia (not shown) are clusters of nerve cells surrounding the thalamus. They are responsible for initiating and integrating movements. Parkinson disease, which results in tremors, rigidity, and a stiff, shuffling walk, is a disease of nerve cells that lead into the basal ganglia.

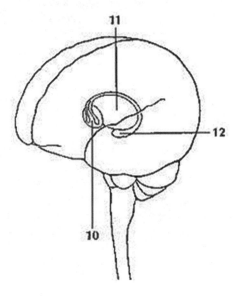

Figure 1.3. *Inner Brain*

Making Connections

The brain and the rest of the nervous system are composed of many different types of cells, but the primary functional unit is a cell called the neuron. All sensations, movements, thoughts, memories, and feelings are the result of signals that pass through neurons. Neurons consist of three parts. The **cell body (13)** contains the nucleus, where most of the molecules that the neuron needs to survive and function are manufactured. **Dendrites (14)** extend out from the cell body like the branches of a tree and receive messages from other nerve cells. Signals then pass from the dendrites through the cell body and may travel away from the cell body down an **axon (15)** to another neuron, a muscle cell, or cells in some other organ. The neuron is usually surrounded by many support cells. Some types of cells wrap around the axon to form an insulating **sheath (16)**. This sheath can include a fatty molecule called myelin, which provides insulation for the axon and helps nerve signals travel faster and farther. Axons may be very short, such as those that carry signals from one cell in the cortex to another cell less than a hair's width away. Or axons may be very long, such as those that carry messages from the brain all the way down the spinal cord.

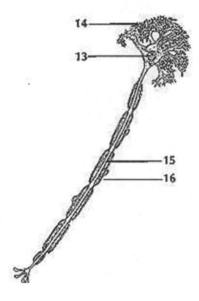

Figure 1.4. *Neuron*

Scientists have learned a great deal about neurons by studying the synapse—the place where a signal passes from the neuron to another cell. When the signal reaches the end of the axon it stimulates the release of **tiny sacs (17)**. These sacs release chemicals known as **neurotransmitters (18)** into the **synapse (19)**. The neurotransmitters cross the synapse and attach to **receptors (20)** on the neighboring cell. These receptors can change the properties of the receiving cell. If the receiving cell is also a neuron, the signal can continue the transmission to the next cell.

Some Key Neurotransmitters at Work

Acetylcholine is called an **excitatory neurotransmitter** because it generally makes cells more excitable. It governs muscle contractions and causes glands to secrete hormones. Alzheimer disease, which initially affects memory formation, is associated with a shortage of acetylcholine.

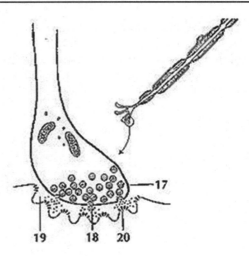

Figure 1.5. *Synapse*

GABA (gamma-aminobutyric acid) is called an inhibitory neurotransmitter because it tends to make cells less excitable. It helps control muscle activity and is an important part of the visual system. Drugs that increase GABA levels in the brain are used to treat epileptic seizures and tremors in patients with Huntington disease.

Serotonin is a neurotransmitter that constricts blood vessels and brings on sleep. It is also involved in temperature regulation. Dopamine is an inhibitory neurotransmitter involved in mood and the control of complex movements. The loss of dopamine activity in some portions of the brain leads to the muscular rigidity of Parkinson disease. Many medications used to treat behavioral disorders work by modifying the action of dopamine in the brain.

Section 1.2

How the Brain Develops

This section includes text excerpted from "Understanding the Effects
of Maltreatment on Brain Development," U.S. Department
of Health and Human Services (HHS), April 2015.

Understanding Brain Development

What we have learned about the process of brain development helps
us understand more about the roles both genetics and the environment
play in our development. It appears that genetics predispose us to
develop in certain ways, but our experiences, including our interactions
with other people, have a significant impact on how our predisposi-
tions are expressed. In fact, research now shows that many capacities
thought to be fixed at birth are actually dependent on a sequence of
experiences combined with heredity. Both factors are essential for
optimum development of the human brain.

Early Brain Development

The raw material of the brain is the nerve cell, called the *neuron.*
During fetal development, neurons are created and migrate to form
the various parts of the brain. As neurons migrate, they also differentiate, or specialize, to govern specific functions in the body in response
to chemical signals. This process of development occurs sequentially
from the "bottom up," that is, from areas of the brain controlling the
most primitive functions of the body (e.g., heart rate, breathing) to the
most sophisticated functions (e.g., complex thought).

The first areas of the brain to fully develop are the brainstem and
midbrain; they govern the bodily functions necessary for life, called
the autonomic functions. At birth, these lower portions of the nervous
system are very well developed, whereas the higher regions (the limbic
system and cerebral cortex) are still rather primitive. Higher function
brain regions involved in regulating emotions, language, and abstract
thought grow rapidly in the first three years of life.

Growing Child's Brain

Brain development, or learning, is actually the process of creating, strengthening, and discarding connections among the neurons; these connections are called *synapses*. Synapses organize the brain by forming pathways that connect the parts of the brain governing everything we do—from breathing and sleeping to thinking and feeling. This is the essence of postnatal brain development, because at birth, very few synapses have been formed. The synapses present at birth are primarily those that govern our bodily functions such as heart rate, breathing, eating, and sleeping.

The development of synapses occurs at an astounding rate during a child's early years in response to that child's experiences. At its peak, the cerebral cortex of a healthy toddler may create two million synapses per second. By the time children are two years old, their brains have approximately 100 trillion synapses, many more than they will ever need. Based on the child's experiences, some synapses are strengthened and remain intact, but many are gradually discarded. This process of synapse elimination—or pruning—is a normal part of development. By the time children reach adolescence, about half of their synapses have been discarded, leaving the number they will have for most of the rest of their lives.

Another important process that takes place in the developing brain is *myelination*. Myelin is the white fatty tissue that forms a sheath to insulate mature brain cells, thus ensuring clear transmission of neurotransmitters across synapses. Young children process information slowly because their brain cells lack the myelin necessary for fast, clear nerve impulse transmission. Like other neuronal growth processes, myelination begins in the primary motor and sensory areas (the brainstem and cortex) and gradually progresses to the higher-order regions that control thought, memories, and feelings. Also, like other neuronal growth processes, a child's experiences affect the rate and growth of myelination, which continues into young adulthood.

By three years of age, a baby's brain has reached almost 90 percent of its adult size. The growth in each region of the brain largely depends on receiving stimulation, which spurs activity in that region. This stimulation provides the foundation for learning.

Adolescent Brain Development

Studies using MRI techniques show that the brain continues to grow and develop into young adulthood (at least to the mid twenties). White matter, or brain tissue, volume has been shown to increase in adults as old as 32. Right before puberty, adolescent brains experience a growth spurt that occurs mainly in the frontal lobe, which is the area that governs planning, impulse control, and reasoning. During the teenage years, the brain goes through a process of pruning synapses—somewhat like the infant and toddler brain— and also sees an increase in white matter and changes to neurotransmitter systems. As the teenager grows into young adulthood, the brain develops more myelin to insulate the nerve fibers and speed neural processing, and this myelination occurs last in the frontal lobe. MRI comparisons between the brains of teenagers and the brains of young adults have shown that most of the brain areas were the same—that is, the teenage brain had reached maturity in the areas that govern such abilities as speech and sensory capabilities.

The major difference was the immaturity of the teenage brain in the frontal lobe and in the myelination of that area.

Normal puberty and adolescence lead to the maturation of a physical body, but the brain lags behind in development, especially in the areas that allow teenagers to reason and think logically. Most teenagers act impulsively at times, using a lower area of their brains— their "gut reaction"—because their frontal lobes are not yet mature. Impulsive behavior, poor decisions, and increased risk-taking are all part of the normal teenage experience. Another change that happens during adolescence is the growth and transformation of the limbic system, which is responsible for our emotions. Teenagers may rely on their more primitive limbic system in interpreting emotions and reacting since they lack the more mature cortex that can override the limbic response.

Plasticity—The Influence of Environment

Researchers use the term plasticity to describe the brain's ability to change in response to repeated stimulation. The extent of a brain's plasticity is dependent on the stage of development and the particular brain system or region affected. For instance, the lower parts of the brain, which control basic functions such as breathing and heart rate, are less flexible, or plastic, than the higher functioning cortex, which controls thoughts and feelings. While cortex plasticity decreases as a child gets older, some degree of plasticity remains. In fact, this brain plasticity is what allows us to keep learning into adulthood and throughout our lives.

The developing brain's ongoing adaptations are the result of both genetics and experience. Our brains prepare us to expect certain experiences by forming the pathways needed to respond to those experiences. For example, our brains are "wired" to respond to the sound of speech; when babies hear people speaking, the neural systems in their brains responsible for speech and language receive the necessary stimulation to organize and function. The more babies are exposed to people speaking, the stronger their related synapses become. If the appropriate exposure does not happen, the pathways developed in anticipation may be discarded. This is sometimes referred to as the concept of "use it or lose it." It is through these processes of creating, strengthening, and discarding synapses that our brains adapt to our unique environment.

The ability to adapt to our environment is a part of normal development. Children growing up in cold climates, on rural farms, or in large sibling groups learn how to function in those environments. Regardless of the general environment, though, all children need stimulation and nurturance for healthy development. If these are lacking (e.g., if a child's caretakers are indifferent, hostile, depressed, or cognitively impaired), the child's brain development may be impaired. Because the brain adapts to its environment, it will adapt to a negative environment just as readily as it will adapt to a positive one.

Sensitive Periods

Researchers believe that there are sensitive periods for development of certain capabilities. These refer to windows of time in the developmental process when certain parts of the brain may be most susceptible to particular experiences. Animal studies have shed light on sensitive periods, showing, for example, that animals that are artificially blinded during the sensitive period for developing vision may never develop the capability to see, even if the blinding mechanism is later removed.

It is more difficult to study human sensitive periods, but we know that, if certain synapses and neuronal pathways are not repeatedly activated, they may be discarded, and their capabilities may diminish. For example, infants have a genetic predisposition to form strong attachments to their primary caregivers, but they may not be able to achieve strong attachments, or trusting, durable bonds if they are in a severely neglectful situation with little one-on-one caregiver contact. Children from Romanian institutions who had been severely neglected had a much better attachment response if they were placed in foster care—and thus received more stable parenting—before they were 24 months old. This indicates that there is a sensitive period for attachment, but it is likely that there is a general sensitive period rather than a true cut-off point for recovery.

While sensitive periods exist for development and learning, we also know that the plasticity of the brain often allows children to recover from missing certain experiences. Both children and adults may be able to make up for missed experiences later in life, but it is likely to be more difficult. This is especially true if a young child was deprived of certain stimulation, which resulted in the pruning of synapses (neuronal connections) relevant to that stimulation and the loss of neuronal pathways. As children progress through each developmental stage, they will learn and master each step more easily if their brains have built an efficient network of pathways to support optimal functioning.

Memories

The organizing framework for children's development is based on the creation of memories. When repeated experiences strengthen a neuronal pathway, the pathway becomes encoded, and it eventually becomes a memory. Children learn to put one foot in front of the other to walk. They learn words to express themselves. And they learn that a smile usually brings a smile in return. At some point, they no longer have to think much about these processes—their brains manage these experiences with little effort because the memories that have been created allow for a smooth, efficient flow of information.

The creation of memories is part of our adaptation to our environment. Our brains attempt to understand the world around us and fashion our interactions with that world in a way that promotes our survival and, hopefully, our growth, but if the early environment is abusive or neglectful, our brains may create memories of these experiences that adversely color our view of the world throughout our life.

Babies are born with the capacity for *implicit memory*, which means that they can perceive their environment and recall it in certain unconscious ways. For instance, they recognize their mother's voice from an unconscious memory. These early implicit memories may have a significant impact on a child's subsequent attachment relationships.

In contrast, *explicit memory*, which develops around age two, refers to conscious memories and is tied to language development. Explicit memory allows children to talk about themselves in the past and future or in different places or circumstances through the process of conscious recollection.

Sometimes, children who have been abused or suffered other trauma may not retain or be able to access explicit memories of their experiences; however, they may retain implicit memories of the physical or emotional sensations, and these implicit memories may produce flashbacks, nightmares, or other uncontrollable reactions. This may be the case with very young children or infants who suffer abuse or neglect.

Section 1.3

Executive Function

"Executive Function," © 2016 Omnigraphics. Reviewed June 2016.

Overview

Executive function refers to a key set of mental skills that helps the brain organize information and direct behavior. Most aspects of executive function are controlled by the prefrontal cortex, an area of the brain that lies directly behind the forehead. This part of the brain matures during puberty, which generally leads to an improved ability to perform higher-level tasks requiring organization and planning. The main steps involved in executive function are:

- analyze what needs to be done;
- plan how to approach it;
- organize the steps to be accomplished;
- develop timelines for performing each step;
- adjust the approach, steps, or timelines as needed; and
- complete the task within the time allowed.

The brains of people with strong executive function skills can execute this process very quickly. But people with weaknesses in executive function tend to exhibit a pattern of chronic difficulty in organizing information and performing complex tasks. They may experience problems in getting started on a project, establishing priorities, making plans, following directions, remembering details, making decisions, using information in a logical way, paying attention, staying on task, switching focus, and managing time. Executive function disorder (EFD) also makes it more difficult for people to control impulses and regulate their behavior in response to different situations.

Causes and Symptoms

Although the cause of EFD is unknown, research suggests that genes may play an important role in its development. The different ways in which children and young people use executive skills are heavily influenced by heredity. In addition, studies have shown that executive function issues often coexist with learning disabilities and attention problems, such as dyslexia and attention deficit hyperactivity disorder (ADHD). Other brain differences may affect the development of EFD as well, including neurological conditions, mood disorders, autism, fetal alcohol syndrome, and damage to the prefrontal cortex from concussions, strokes, or brain tumors.

EFD can produce a wide range of symptoms that vary by individual. Even in one individual, the symptoms may change over time. Some of the common challenges that may indicate problems with executive function include:

- deciding how to begin a task;
- figuring out how much time a task will require;
- paying attention to directions;
- concentrating on the task at hand and avoiding distractions;
- refocusing on the task after being interrupted;
- switching from one task to another, or from small details to the big picture;
- remembering multiple steps;
- incorporating outside feedback;
- changing the plan if needed; and
- completing tasks in a timely manner.

Weaknesses in executive function skills may also manifest themselves in behavior issues, particularly in problems controlling impulses and emotions or regulating responses to different stimuli or situations. Many people with EFD have trouble with impulse control, or the ability to stop and think before speaking or acting. EFD can also affect emotional control, or the ability to manage emotions and avoid overreacting to small problems. People with EFD also tend to struggle with flexibility, or the ability to change course and come up with a new solution if one approach fails. Finally, self-monitoring can be a challenge for people with EFD. They may not be able to evaluate the effectiveness of their own strategies or use previous experience to improve future performance.

Diagnosis and Treatment

EFD is not listed as a separate condition in the American Psychiatric Association's *Diagnostic and Statistical Manual of Mental Disorders (DSM)*, which provides criteria for mental health professionals to use in making formal diagnoses. Instead, EFD usually occurs in conjunction with another health condition. Weakness in executive function is one of the criteria used to diagnose attention deficit hyperactivity disorder (ADHD), autism, and learning disabilities. In addition, people who are diagnosed with both learning disabilities and ADHD face an increased risk of severe executive dysfunction.

Although EFD is closely associated with other disorders, executive function can be evaluated—and skill deficits identified—by trained mental health professionals. The recommended process for diagnosing EFD includes the following steps:

- Keep a record of symptoms and behaviors.

- Get a complete medical examination to rule out physical causes, such as hearing impairments or seizure disorders.

- See a specialist for a full evaluation of executive function, which may include reviewing school records, filling out questionnaires or screening forms, taking an intelligence test, and conducting observations of behavior at home, at school, or at the clinician's office.

- Review the results and develop an intervention plan with strategies for dealing with the issues identified.

Once executive function issues have been identified, various educational strategies and behavioral approaches can help people with EFD overcome or adapt to their weaknesses. Although experts recommend early intervention during childhood, treatment can be effective at any age since the brain continues to develop. Several types of professionals may be involved in developing and administering treatment for EFD, including psychologists, speech therapists, and occupational therapists. Cognitive behavioral therapy is a proven method that can help people with EFD develop tools to monitor their thoughts and behavior.

Children with EFD may be eligible for special education services through school systems, including academic supports and accommodations. Many schools employ response to intervention (RTI) to identify students who perform below grade level and provide them with extra help, whether within small groups or through more intensive one-on-one instruction. Classroom teachers may also use informal support strategies, such as assigning students with EFD a seat in the front row to make it easier for them to pay attention.

There are also a number of strategies parents can try at home to help children with EFD, such as:

- making checklists to provide a visual reminder of the steps involved in completing a task, and to identify those that have already been accomplished;

- providing estimates of the time that should be budgeted for activities;

- using calendars and planners, whether on paper or on electronic devices, to keep track of schedules and aid in time management; and

- explaining feedback, which may help inflexible thinkers understand the value of taking different approaches to tasks.

Parents of children with EFD may also find it helpful to seek ideas, advice, and support from other parents who are dealing with the same issues. Many organizations and online communities offer such assistance. Experts also encourage parents of children with EFD to maintain a positive attitude. Since executive functioning skills continue to develop into adulthood, many children form effective strategies for dealing with EFD that enable them to reach their full potential.

References

1. Morin, Amanda. "Understanding Executive Functioning Issues," Understood.org, 2016.

2. ———. "Four Ways Kids Use Organization Skills to Learn," Understood.org, 2016.

Chapter 2

Early Learning and Speech and Language Development Milestones

Chapter Contents

Section 2.1

Early Learning

This section includes text excerpted from "Early Learning: Topic Information," *Eunice Kennedy Shriver* National Institute of Child Health (NICHD), August 27, 2015.

What Is Early Learning?

Children begin learning in the womb. From the moment they're born, interaction with the world around them helps them build crucial skills. For example:

- By three months of age, babies can recognize people they know.

- By 8 to 12 months, babies can recognize themselves in the mirror.

- From 18 months to preschool age, children can learn nine new words each day.

Children learn all kinds of basic skills and concepts from the people and world around them:

- In the first few years of life, children start to become independent, learning how to act and how to control their emotions and behaviors.

- They learn language; math skills such as shapes, numbers, and counting; pre-reading skills like how to hold a book and follow along as someone reads to them; and, with them, skills for lifelong learning.

- They also start forming relationships of trust and develop ways to handle and resolve problems.

Making sure children have good learning experiences during their early years—whether at home, in childcare, or in preschool—will support their lifelong learning, health, and well-being.

Why Is Early Learning Important?

Early learning paves the way for learning at school and throughout life. What children learn in their first few years of life—and how they learn it—can have long-lasting effects on their success and health as children, teens, and adults.

Studies show that supporting children's early learning can lead to:

- Higher test scores from preschool to age 21.
- Better grades in reading and math.
- A better chance of staying in school and going to college.
- Fewer teen pregnancies.
- Improved mental health.
- Lower risk of heart disease in adulthood.
- A longer lifespan.

What Are Some Factors That Affect Early Learning?

A child's home, family, and daily life have a strong effect on his or her ability to learn. Parents and guardians can control some things in their child's life and environment, but not everything.

Some factors that can affect early learning include:

- Parents' education.
- Family income.
- The number of parents in the home.
- Access to books and play materials.
- Stability of home life.
- Going to preschool.
- Quality of child care.
- Stress levels and exposure to stress (in the womb, as an infant, and as a child).
- The number of languages spoken at home.

Why Is It Important to Study Early Learning?

Early learning can improve children's health and well-being and have long-lasting benefits. Studying which factors affect early learning and education will help researchers:

- Design better ways to help at-risk children before they start school.

- Improve parent, caregiver, child care provider, and preschool teacher training.

- Use research findings to design better preschool and child care programs.

- Study innovative early intervention settings, such as pediatrician's offices and home visitor programs, and ways to make these programs convenient for parents and caretakers.

Recent examples include findings indicating that:

- Research shows that Head Start has positive effects on children's math, literacy, and vocabulary skills across the board. The program had an even greater impact—boosting early math skills most—among children whose parents spent little time reading to them or counting with them at home. Children whose homes provided a medium amount of such activities had the biggest gains in early literacy skills.

- Children who have trouble developing language skills may also have trouble controlling their impulses and behaviors.

- Bilingual speakers develop brain networks that help them filter out unnecessary information better than those who speak only one language. These brain networks might protect against Alzheimer disease and other age-related brain problems.

- Experience and genetic factors seem to influence whether a child will have "math anxiety"—very strong worries about math abilities that can be disabling.

How Can Parents and Caregivers Promote Early Learning?

A child's home, family, and daily life have a strong effect on his or her ability to learn. Parents and guardians can control some things in their child's life and environment, but not everything.

There are many things parents and caregivers can do to encourage their children's early learning.

You are your child's first teacher, and every day is filled with opportunities to help him or her learn. You can help by:

- Reading to your child, beginning when she or he is born.

- Pointing out and talking with your child about the names, colors, shapes, numbers, sizes, and quantities of objects in his or her environment.

- Listening and responding to your child as he or she learns to communicate.

- Practicing counting together.

Basic things like getting enough sleep and eating a healthy diet are also important for a child's brain development and ability to learn. Creating a stable home with routines and support encourages children to learn and explore. Loud background sounds in the home (televisions, stereos, video games) can be distracting and stressful to young children and should be turned off or the volume lowered when they are present.

Where Can I Find Information about Early Educational Programs for My Child?

Individual states offer different early education programs and resources. The website and contact information for the department of education in each state is accessible through this directory on the U.S. Department of Education (ED) website.

What Is "School Readiness"?

School readiness refers to having the skills, knowledge, abilities, and attitudes needed for success in school and for later learning and life.

School readiness includes:

- The child's ability to meet milestones appropriate for their stage of development, including motor skills, language development, and general knowledge; their curiosity and enthusiasm; and their ability to explore and try new things.

- The environment provided by the school, including high-quality instruction, leadership, appropriate teacher training, and support of relationships with parents and the community.

- Appropriate support from the child's family and community, such as daily learning opportunities and supporting the child's mental and physical health.

Section 2.2

Speech and Language Development Milestones

This section includes text excerpted from "Speech and Language Developmental Milestones," National Institute on Deafness and Other Communication Disorders (NIDCD), April 30, 2014.

How Do Speech and Language Develop?

The first three years of life, when the brain is developing and maturing, is the most intensive period for acquiring speech and language skills. These skills develop best in a world that is rich with sounds, sights, and consistent exposure to the speech and language of others.

There appear to be critical periods for speech and language development in infants and young children when the brain is best able to absorb language. If these critical periods are allowed to pass without exposure to language, it will be more difficult to learn.

What Are the Milestones for Speech and Language Development?

The first signs of communication occur when an infant learns that a cry will bring food, comfort, and companionship. Newborns also begin to recognize important sounds in their environment, such as the voice of their mother or primary caretaker. As they grow, babies begin to sort out the speech sounds that compose the words of their language. By six months of age, most babies recognize the basic sounds of their native language.

Children vary in their development of speech and language skills. However, they follow a natural progression or timetable for mastering the skills of language. A checklist of milestones for the normal development of speech and language skills in children from birth to five years of age is included on the following pages. These milestones help doctors and other health professionals determine if a child is on track or if he or she may need extra help. Sometimes a delay may be caused by hearing loss, while other times it may be due to a speech or language disorder.

What Is the Difference between a Speech Disorder and a Language Disorder?

Children who have trouble understanding what others say (receptive language) or difficulty sharing their thoughts (expressive language) may have a language disorder. Specific language impairment (SLI) is a language disorder that delays the mastery of language skills. Some children with SLI may not begin to talk until their third or fourth year.

Children who have trouble producing speech sounds correctly or who hesitate or stutter when talking may have a speech disorder. Apraxia of speech is a speech disorder that makes it difficult to put sounds and syllables together in the correct order to form words.

What Should I Do If My Child's Speech or Language Appears to Be Delayed?

Talk to your child's doctor if you have any concerns. Your doctor may refer you to a speech-language pathologist, who is a health professional trained to evaluate and treat people with speech or language disorders. The speech-language pathologist will talk to you about your child's communication and general development. He or she will also use special spoken tests to evaluate your child. A hearing test is often included in the evaluation because a hearing problem can affect speech and language development. Depending on the result of the evaluation, the speech-language pathologist may suggest activities you can do at home to stimulate your child's development. They might also recommend group or individual therapy or suggest further evaluation by an audiologist (a healthcare professional trained to identify and measure hearing loss), or a developmental psychologist (a healthcare professional with special expertise in the psychological development of infants and children).

What Research Is Being Conducted on Developmental Speech and Language Problems?

The National Institute on Deafness and Other Communication Disorders (NIDCD) sponsors a broad range of research to better understand the development of speech and language disorders, improve diagnostic capabilities, and fine-tune more effective treatments. An ongoing area of study is the search for better ways to diagnose and differentiate among the various types of speech delay. A large study following approximately 4,000 children is gathering data as the children grow to establish reliable signs and symptoms for specific speech disorders, which can then be used to develop accurate diagnostic tests. Additional genetic studies are looking for matches between different genetic variations and specific speech deficits.

Researchers sponsored by the NIDCD have discovered one genetic variant, in particular, that is linked to SLI, a disorder that delays children's use of words and slows their mastery of language skills throughout their school years. The finding is the first to tie the presence of a distinct genetic mutation to any kind of inherited language impairment. Further research is exploring the role this genetic variant may also play in dyslexia, autism, and speech-sound disorders.

A long-term study looking at how deafness impacts the brain is exploring how the brain "rewires" itself to accommodate deafness. So far, the research has shown that adults who are deaf react faster and more accurately than hearing adults when they observe objects in motion. This ongoing research continues to explore the concept of "brain plasticity"—the ways in which the brain is influenced by health conditions or life experiences—and how it can be used to develop learning strategies that encourage healthy language and speech development in early childhood.

A recent workshop convened by the NIDCD drew together a group of experts to explore issues related to a subgroup of children with autism spectrum disorders who do not have functional verbal language by the age of 5. Because these children are so different from one another, with no set of defining characteristics or patterns of cognitive strengths or weaknesses, development of standard assessment tests or effective treatments has been difficult. The workshop featured a series of presentations to familiarize participants with the challenges facing these children and helped them to identify a number of research gaps and opportunities that could be addressed in future research studies.

What Are Voice, Speech, and Language?

Voice, speech, and language are the tools we use to communicate with each other.

Voice is the sound we make as air from our lungs is pushed between vocal folds in our larynx, causing them to vibrate.

Speech is talking, which is one way to express language. It involves the precisely coordinated muscle actions of the tongue, lips, jaw, and vocal tract to produce the recognizable sounds that make up language.

Language is a set of shared rules that allow people to express their ideas in a meaningful way. Language may be expressed verbally or by writing, signing, or making other gestures, such as eye blinking or mouth movements.

Section 2.3

What Research Says about Language Acquisition

This section contains text excerpted from the following sources: Text under the heading "Children's Language Skills Are Stable from Toddlerhood to Adolescence" is excerpted from "Children's Language Skills Are Stable from Toddlerhood to Adolescence," *Eunice Kennedy Shriver* National Institute of Child Health and Human Development (NICHD), April 9, 2015; Text under the heading "Infants Exposed to Multiple Languages Show Enhanced Interpersonal Skills" is excerpted from "Infants Exposed to Multiple Languages Show Enhanced Interpersonal Skills," *Eunice Kennedy Shriver* National Institute of Child Health and Human Development (NICHD), March 24, 2016.

Children's Language Skills Are Stable from Toddlerhood to Adolescence

Children begin learning language in their first months after birth, and language skills continue to develop throughout life. Some children experience delays in learning language skills early on, while others develop their language skills more quickly.

Researchers in the *Eunice Kennedy Shriver* National Institute of Child Health and Human Development's (NICHD) Section on Child and Family Research within the Division of Intramural Research assessed whether children with high skills compared to their peers tended to remain relatively high skilled throughout childhood. The researchers used multiple methods, including sophisticated statistical techniques, to control for other variables that affect language skill and to assess the language skills of more than 300 children. Children's language skills were measured at ages 20 months, 4 years, 10 years, and 14 years.

The findings showed strong long-term stability in language skills from the end of infancy to adolescence. Language skills were more stable from ages 4 to 10 to 14 years than from ages 20 months to 4 years, suggesting language skill is likely to be more changeable at earlier ages.

Infants Exposed to Multiple Languages Show Enhanced Interpersonal Skills

Infants exposed to more than one language may be better able than their monolingual counterparts to see a situation from another point of view, according to a study funded in part by the National Institutes of Health. The study investigated whether a multilingual environment can influence developing communication skills before infants are able to speak.

The researchers conducted an interactive visual communication task with infants ages 14 to 17 months. An adult sat across a table from an infant. Between them were two identical props—one that both could see, and the other visible only to the infant. When the investigator asked for the prop, the infants from multilingual backgrounds were more likely to hand the investigator the prop that both could see, rather than the one that only the infant could see.

"These results showed a level of sophisticated thinking among the infants from multilingual backgrounds," said Layla Esposito, Ph.D., program officer at NIH's *Eunice Kennedy Shriver* National Institute of Child Health and Human Development (NICHD), which provided funding for the study. "Compared to the monolingual infants, multilingual infants realized that the adult could only see one prop, and they were aware enough to reach for the one that both could see."

The study appears online in Developmental Science. The researchers enrolled 32 infant boys and 32 infant girls divided equally between those exposed to English only and those exposed to more than one language (primarily Spanish and English).

While the infants could see both props, the investigator could only see one and extended a hand across the table with the palm facing up to engage the infant. When the investigator asked for the prop, infants with multilingual exposure consistently chose the one that the adult could see. The monolingual infants randomly chose between the two props, making no distinction.

"Apparently, babies who aren't speaking yet can pick up nonverbal cues from others," said Dr. Esposito. "Infants from multilingual backgrounds appear more adept at picking up these cues and better able to see a situation from another point of view."

Katherine Kinzler, Ph.D., an associate professor of psychology and human development at Cornell University and one of the authors of the study, said that more research is needed to determine the extent to which exposure to another language influences communication skills across the lifespan.

Chapter 3

Learning Disabilities Defined

What Are Learning Disabilities?

Learning disability (LD) is a general term that describes specific kinds of learning problems. A learning disability can cause a person to have trouble learning and using certain skills. The skills most often affected are: reading, writing, listening, speaking, reasoning, and doing math.

"Learning disabilities" is not the only term used to describe these difficulties. Others include:

- **dyslexia**—which refers to difficulties in reading

- **dysgraphia**—which refers to difficulties in writing

- **dyscalculia**—which refers to difficulties in math

All of these are considered learning disabilities.

Learning disabilities vary from person to person. One person with LD may not have the same kind of learning problems as another person with LD. A person has trouble with reading and writing. Another person with LD may have problems with understanding math. Still another person may have trouble in both of these areas, as well as with understanding what people are saying.

Researchers think that learning disabilities are caused by differences in how a person's brain works and how it processes information.

This chapter includes text excerpted from "Learning Disabilities (LD)," Center for Parent Information and Resources (CPIR), July 2015.

Children with learning disabilities are not "dumb" or "lazy." In fact, they usually have average or above average intelligence. Their brains just process information differently.

There is no "cure" for learning disabilities. They are life-long. However, children with LD can be high achievers and can be taught ways to get around the learning disability. With the right help, children with LD can and do learn successfully.

How Common Are Learning Disabilities?

Very common! As many as 1 out of every 5 people in the United States has a learning disability. Almost 1 million children (ages 6 through 21) have some form of a learning disability and receive special education in school. In fact, one-third of all children who receive special education have a learning disability.

What Are the Signs of a Learning Disability?

While there is no one "sign" that a person has a learning disability, there are certain clues. Most relate to elementary school tasks, because learning disabilities tend to be identified in elementary school. This is because school focuses on the very things that may be difficult for the child—reading, writing, math, listening, speaking, reasoning. A child probably won't show all of these signs, or even most of them. However, if a child shows a number of these problems, then parents and the teacher should consider the possibility that the child has a learning disability.

When a child has a learning disability, he or she:

- may have trouble learning the alphabet, rhyming words, or connecting letters to their sounds
- may make many mistakes when reading aloud, and repeat and pause often
- may not understand what he or she reads
- may have real trouble with spelling
- may have very messy handwriting or hold a pencil awkwardly
- may struggle to express ideas in writing
- may learn language late and have a limited vocabulary

- may have trouble remembering the sounds that letters make or hearing slight differences between words

- may have trouble understanding jokes, comic strips, and sarcasm

- may have trouble following directions

- may mispronounce words or use a wrong word that sounds similar

- may have trouble organizing what he or she wants to say or not be able to think of the word he or she needs for writing or conversation

- may not follow the social rules of conversation, such as taking turns, and may stand too close to the listener

- may confuse math symbols and misread numbers

- may not be able to retell a story in order (what happened first, second, third)

- may not know where to begin a task or how to go on from there

If a child has unexpected problems learning to read, write, listen, speak, or do math, then teachers and parents may want to investigate more. The same is true if the child is struggling to do any one of these skills. The child may need to be evaluated to see if he or she has a learning disability.

Chapter 4

Causes of Learning Disabilities

Chapter Contents

Section 4.1

What Are the Causes and Risk Factors of Learning Disabilities?

This section contains text excerpted from the following sources: Text
in this section begins with excerpts from "What Causes Learning
Disabilities?" *Eunice Kennedy Shriver* National Institute of Child
Health and Human Development (NICHD), February 28, 2014;
Text under the heading "Risk Factors" is excerpted from
"Developmental Disabilities," Centers for Disease Control
and Prevention (CDC), July 9, 2015.

Researchers do not know exactly what causes learning disabilities
(LD), but they appear to be related to differences in brain structure.
These differences are present from birth and often are inherited. To
improve understanding of learning disabilities, researchers at the
Eunice Kennedy Shriver National Institute of Child Health and Human
Development (NICHD) and elsewhere are studying areas of the brain
and how they function. Scientists have found that learning disabilities
are related to areas of the brain that deal with language and have used
imaging studies to show that the brain of a dyslexic person develops
and functions differently from a typical brain.

Sometimes, factors that affect a developing fetus, such as alcohol or
drug use, can lead to a learning disability. Other factors in an infant's
environment may play a role as well. These can include poor nutrition
and exposure to toxins such as lead in water or paint. In addition,
children who do not receive the support necessary to promote their
intellectual development early on may show signs of learning disabilities once they start school.

Sometimes a person may develop a learning disability later in life. Possible causes in such a case include dementia or a traumatic brain injury (TBI).

Risk Factors

Developmental disabilities begin anytime during the developmental
period and usually last throughout a person's lifetime. Most developmental disabilities begin before a baby is born, but some can happen
after birth because of injury, infection, or other factors.

Most developmental disabilities are thought to be caused by a complex mix of factors. These factors include genetics; parental health and behaviors (such as smoking and drinking) during pregnancy; complications during birth; infections the mother might have during pregnancy or the baby might have very early in life; and exposure of the mother or child to high levels of environmental toxins, such as lead. For some developmental disabilities, such as fetal alcohol syndrome, which is caused by drinking alcohol during pregnancy, we know the cause. But for most, we don't.

Following are some examples of what we know about specific developmental disabilities:

- At least 25% of hearing loss among babies is due to maternal infections during pregnancy, such as cytomegalovirus (CMV) infection; complications after birth; and head trauma.

- Some of the most common known causes of intellectual disability include fetal alcohol syndrome; genetic and chromosomal conditions, such as Down syndrome and fragile X syndrome; and certain infections during pregnancy, such as toxoplasmosis.

- Children who have a sibling are at a higher risk of also having an autism spectrum disorder.

- Low birthweight, premature birth, multiple birth, and infections during pregnancy are associated with an increased risk for many developmental disabilities.

- Untreated newborn jaundice (high levels of bilirubin in the blood during the first few days after birth) can cause a type of brain damage known as kernicterus. Children with kernicterus are more likely to have cerebral palsy, hearing and vision problems, and problems with their teeth. Early detection and treatment of newborn jaundice can prevent kernicterus.

Who Is Affected?

Developmental disabilities occur among all racial, ethnic, and socioeconomic groups. Recent estimates in the United States show that about one in six, or about 15%, of children aged 3 through 17 years have a one or more developmental disabilities, such as:

- Attention-deficit/hyperactivity disorder (ADHD)
- autism spectrum disorder

- cerebral palsy
- hearing loss
- intellectual disability
- learning disability
- vision impairment
- and other developmental delays

For over a decade, Centers for Disease Control and Prevention's (CDC) Autism and Developmental Disabilities Monitoring (ADDM) Network has been tracking the number and characteristics of children with autism spectrum disorder, cerebral palsy, and intellectual disability in several diverse communities throughout the United States.

Living with a Developmental Disability

Children and adults with disabilities need health care and health programs for the same reasons anyone else does—to stay well, active, and a part of the community.

Having a disability does not mean a person is not healthy or that he or she cannot be healthy. Being healthy means the same thing for all of us—getting and staying well so we can lead full, active lives. That includes having the tools and information to make healthy choices and knowing how to prevent illness.

Some health conditions, such as asthma, gastrointestinal symptoms, eczema and skin allergies, and migraine headaches, have been found to be more common among children with developmental disabilities. Thus, it is especially important for children with developmental disabilities to see a health care provider regularly.

Section 4.2

Environmental Contaminants and Learning Disabilities

This section includes text excerpted from "Neurodevelopmental Disorders," U.S. Environmental Protection Agency (EPA), October 31, 2015.

Neurodevelopmental Disorders

Neurodevelopmental disorders are disabilities associated primarily with the functioning of the neurological system and brain. Examples of neurodevelopmental disorders in children include attention-deficit/hyperactivity disorder (ADHD), autism, learning disabilities (LD), intellectual disability (also known as mental retardation), conduct disorders, cerebral palsy, and impairments in vision and hearing. Children with neurodevelopmental disorders can experience difficulties with language and speech, motor skills, behavior, memory, learning, or other neurological functions. While the symptoms and behaviors of neurodevelopmental disabilities often change or evolve as a child grows older, some disabilities are permanent. Diagnosis and treatment of these disorders can be difficult; treatment often involves a combination of professional therapy, pharmaceuticals, and home- and school-based programs.

Genetics can play an important role in many neurodevelopmental disorders, and some cases of certain conditions such as intellectual disability are associated with specific genes. However, most neurodevelopmental disorders have complex and multiple contributors rather than any one clear cause. These disorders likely result from a combination of genetic, biological, psychosocial, and environmental risk factors. A broad range of environmental risk factors may affect neurodevelopment, including (but not limited to) maternal use of alcohol, tobacco, or illicit drugs during pregnancy; lower socioeconomic status; preterm birth; low birthweight; the physical environment; and prenatal or childhood exposure to certain environmental contaminants.

Lead, methylmercury, and PCBs are widespread environmental contaminants associated with adverse effects on a child's developing brain and nervous system in multiple studies. The National Toxicology Program (NTP) has concluded that childhood lead exposure is associated with reduced cognitive function, including lower IQ (intelligence quotient) and reduced academic achievement. The NTP has also concluded that childhood lead exposure is associated with attention-related behavioral problems (including inattention, hyperactivity, and diagnosed attention-deficit/hyperactivity disorder) and increased incidence of problem behaviors (including delinquent, criminal, or antisocial behavior).

The U.S. Environmental Protection Agency (EPA) has determined that methylmercury is known to have neurotoxic and developmental effects in humans. Extreme cases of such effects were seen in people prenatally exposed during two high-dose mercury poisoning events in Japan and Iraq, who experienced severe adverse health effects such as cerebral palsy, mental retardation, deafness, and blindness. Prospective cohort studies have been conducted in island populations where frequent fish consumption leads to methylmercury exposure in pregnant women at levels much lower than in the poisoning incidents but much greater than those typically observed in the United States. Results from such studies in New Zealand and the Faroe Islands suggest that increased prenatal mercury exposure due to maternal fish consumption was associated with adverse effects on intelligence and decreased functioning in the areas of language, attention, and memory. These associations were not seen in initial results reported from a similar study in the Seychelles Islands. However, further studies in the Seychelles found associations between prenatal mercury exposure and some neurodevelopmental deficits after researchers had accounted for the developmental benefits of fish consumption. More recent studies conducted in the United States have found associations between neurodevelopmental effects and blood mercury levels within the range typical for U.S. women, after accounting for the beneficial effects of fish consumption during pregnancy.

Several studies of children who were prenatally exposed to elevated levels of polychlorinated biphenyls (PCBs) have suggested linkages between these contaminants and neurodevelopmental effects, including lowered intelligence and behavioral deficits such as inattention and impulsive behavior. Studies have also reported associations between PCB exposure and deficits in learning and memory. Most of these studies found that the effects are associated with exposure in the womb resulting from the mother having eaten food contaminated with PCBs, although some studies have reported relationships between adverse effects and PCB exposure during infancy and childhood. Although there is some inconsistency in the epidemiological literature, several reviews of the literature have found that the overall evidence supports a concern for effects of PCBs on children's neurological development. The Agency for Toxic Substances and Disease Registry has determined that "Substantial data suggest that PCBs play a role in neurobehavioral alterations observed in newborns and young children of women with PCB burdens near background levels." In addition, adverse effects on intelligence and behavior have been found in children of women who were highly exposed to mixtures of PCBs, chlorinated dibenzofurans, and other pollutants prior to conception.

A wide variety of other environmental chemicals have been identified as potential concerns for childhood neurological development, but have not been as well studied for these effects as lead, mercury, and PCBs. Concerns for these additional chemicals are based on both laboratory animal studies and human epidemiological research; in most cases, the epidemiological studies are relatively new and the literature is just beginning to develop. Among the chemicals being studied for potential effects on childhood neurological development are organophosphate pesticides, polybrominated diphenyl ether flame retardants (PBDEs), phthalates, bisphenol A (BPA), polycyclic aromatic hydrocarbons (PAHs), arsenic, and perchlorate. Exposure to all of these chemicals is widespread in the United States for both children and adults.

Organophosphate pesticides can interfere with the proper function of the nervous system when exposure is sufficiently high. Many children may have low capacity to detoxify organophosphate pesticides through age 7 years. In addition, recent studies have reported an association between prenatal organophosphate exposure and childhood ADHD in a U.S. community with relatively high exposures to organophosphate pesticides, as well as with exposures found within the general U.S. population. Other recent studies have described associations between prenatal organophosphate pesticide exposures and a variety of neurodevelopmental deficits in childhood, including reduced IQ (intelligence quotient), perceptual reasoning, and memory.

Studies of certain PBDEs have found adverse effects on behavior, learning, and memory in laboratory animals. A recent epidemiological study in New York City reported significant associations between children's prenatal exposure to PBDEs and reduced performance on IQ tests and other tests of neurological development in 6-year-old children. Another study in the Netherlands reported significant associations between children's prenatal exposure to PBDEs and reduced performance on some neurodevelopmental tests in 5- and 6-year-old children, while associations with improved performance were observed for other tests.

Two studies of a group of New York City children ages 4 to 9 years reported associations between prenatal exposure to certain phthalates and behavioral deficits, including effects on attention, conduct, and social behaviors. Some of the behavioral deficits observed in these studies are similar to those commonly displayed in children with ADHD and conduct disorder. Studies conducted in South Korea of children ages 8 to 11 years reported that children with higher levels of certain phthalate metabolites in their urine were more inattentive and hyperactive, displayed more symptoms of ADHD, and had lower IQ compared with those who had lower levels. The exposure levels in these studies are comparable to typical exposures in the U.S. population.

In 2008, the NTP concluded that there is "some concern" for effects of early-life (including prenatal) BPA exposure on brain development and behavior, based on findings of animal studies conducted at relatively low doses. An epidemiological study conducted in Ohio reported an association between prenatal exposure to BPA and effects on children's behavior (increased hyperactivity and aggression) at age 2 years. Another study of prenatal BPA exposure in New York City reported no association between prenatal BPA exposure and social behavior deficits in testing conducted at ages 7 to 9 years.

A series of recent studies conducted in New York City has reported that children of women who were exposed to increased levels of polycyclic aromatic hydrocarbons (PAHs, produced when gasoline and other materials are burned) during pregnancy are more likely to have experienced adverse effects on neurological development (for example, reduced IQ and behavioral problems).

Early-life exposure to arsenic has been associated with measures of reduced cognitive function, including lower scores on tests that measure neurobehavioral and intellectual development, in four studies conducted in Asia; however there are some inconsistencies in the findings of these studies. These findings are from countries where arsenic levels in drinking water are generally much higher than in the United States due to high levels of naturally occurring arsenic in groundwater. Perchlorate is a naturally occurring and man-made chemical that has been found in drinking Water and foods in the United States. Exposure to elevated levels of perchlorate inhibits iodide uptake into the thyroid gland, thus possibly disrupting the function of the thyroid and potentially leading to a reduction in the production of thyroid hormone.

Moderate deficits in maternal thyroid hormone levels during early pregnancy have been linked to reduced childhood IQ scores and other neurodevelopmental effects.

Interactions of environmental contaminants and other environmental factors may combine to increase the risk of neurodevelopmental disorders. For example, exposure to lead may have stronger effects on neurodevelopment among children with lower socioeconomic status. A child's brain and nervous system are vulnerable to adverse impacts from pollutants because they go through a long developmental process beginning shortly after conception and continuing through adolescence. This complex developmental process requires the precise coordination of cell growth and movement, and may be disrupted by even short-term exposures to environmental contaminants if they occur at critical stages of development. This disruption can lead to neurodevelopmental deficits that may have an effect on the child's achievements and behavior even when they do not result in a diagnosable disorder.

Attention-Deficit/Hyperactivity Disorder (ADHD)

Attention-deficit/hyperactivity disorder (ADHD) is a disruptive behavior disorder characterized by symptoms of inattention and/or hyperactivity-impulsivity, occurring in several settings and more frequently and severely than is typical for other individuals in the same stage of development. ADHD can make family and peer relationships difficult, diminish academic performance, and reduce vocational achievement.

As the medical profession has developed a greater understanding of ADHD through the years, the name of this condition has changed. The American Psychiatric Association adopted the name "attention deficit disorder" in the early 1980s and revised it to "attention-deficit/hyperactivity disorder" in 1987. Many children with ADHD have a mix inattention and hyperactivity/impulsivity behaviors, while some may display primarily hyperactive behavior traits, and others display primarily inattentive traits. It is possible for an individual's primary symptoms of ADHD to change over time. Children with ADHD frequently have other disorders, with parents reporting that about half of children with ADHD have a learning disability and about one in four have a conduct disorder.

Other disorders, including anxiety disorders, depression, and learning disabilities, can be expressed with signs and symptoms that resemble those of ADHD. A diagnosis of ADHD requires a certain amount of judgment on the part of a doctor, similar to diagnosis of other mental disorders. Despite the variability among children diagnosed with the disorder and the challenges involved in diagnosis, ADHD has good clinical validity, meaning that impaired children share similarities, exhibit symptoms, respond to treatment, and are recognized with general consistency across clinicians.

A great deal of research on ADHD has focused on aspects of brain functioning that are related to the behaviors associated with ADHD. Although this research is not definitive, it has found that children with ADHD generally have trouble with certain skills involved in problem-solving (referred to collectively as executive function). These skills include working memory (keeping information in mind while briefly doing something else), planning (organizing a sequence of activities to complete a task), response inhibition (suppressing immediate responses when they are inappropriate), and cognitive flexibility (changing an approach when a situation changes). Children with ADHD also generally have problems in maintaining sustained attention to a task (referred to as vigilance), and/or maintaining readiness to respond to new information (referred to as alertness).

While uncertainties remain, findings to date indicate that ADHD is caused by combinations of genetic and environmental factors. Much of the research on environmental factors has focused on the fetal environment. Maternal smoking during pregnancy has been associated with increased risk of ADHD in the child in numerous studies, however, this continues to be an active area of research as scientists consider whether other factors related to smoking (e.g., genetic factors, maternal mental health, stress, alcohol use, and low birth weight) may be responsible for associations attributed to smoking. Findings regarding ADHD and maternal consumption of alcohol during pregnancy are considered more limited and inconsistent. Preterm birth and low birth weight have also been found to increase the likelihood that a child will have ADHD. Psychosocial adversity (representing factors such as low socioeconomic status and in-home conflict) in childhood may also play a role in ADHD.

The potential role of environmental contaminants in contributing to ADHD, either alone or in conjunction with certain genetic susceptibilities or other environmental factors, is becoming better understood as a growing number of studies look explicitly at the relationship between ADHD and exposures to environmental contaminants.

Among environmental contaminants known or suspected to be developmental neurotoxicants, lead has the most extensive evidence of a potential contribution to ADHD. A number of recent epidemiological studies (all published since 2006, with data gathered beginning in 1999 or more recently) conducted in the United States and Asia have reported relationships between increased levels of lead in a child's blood and increased likelihood of ADHD. In most of these studies, blood lead levels were comparable to levels observed currently in the United States. The potential contribution of childhood lead exposure to the risk of ADHD may be amplified in children of women who smoked cigarettes during pregnancy.

In addition, several studies have reported relationships between blood lead levels and the aspects of brain functioning that are most affected in children with ADHD, including sustained attention, alertness, and problem-solving skills (executive functions, specifically cognitive flexibility, working memory, planning, and response inhibition). Similar results have been observed in laboratory animal studies. The NTP has concluded that childhood lead exposure is "associated with increased diagnosis of attention-related behavioral problems."

Although no studies evaluating a potential association between PCBs and ADHD itself have been published, a study in Massachusetts reported a relationship between levels of PCBs measured in cord blood and increased ADHD-like behaviors observed by teachers in children at ages 7 to 11 years. PCB levels in this study were generally lower than those measured in other epidemiological studies of PCBs and childhood neurological development. Other research findings also suggest that PCBs may play a role in contributing to ADHD. Several studies in U.S. and European populations, most having elevated exposure to PCBs through the diet, have found generally consistent associations with aspects of brain function that are most affected in children with ADHD, including alertness and problem-solving skills (executive functions, specifically response inhibition, working memory, cognitive flexibility, and planning). Studies in laboratory animals have similar findings regarding the mental functions affected by PCB exposure.

Studies of other environmental chemicals reporting associations with ADHD or related outcomes have been published in recent years, but findings tend to be much more limited than for lead and PCBs. Findings for phthalates and organophosphate pesticides were noted above. In addition, three studies have reported associations between ADHD or impulsivity and concentrations of certain perfluorinated chemicals measured in the blood of children. Studies of mercury have produced generally mixed findings of associations with ADHD or related symptoms and mental functions.

Learning Disability

Learning disability (or learning disorder) is a general term for a neurological disorder that affects the way in which a child's brain can receive, process, retain, and respond to information. A child with a learning disability may have trouble learning and using certain skills, including reading, writing, listening, speaking, reasoning, and doing math, although learning disabilities vary from child to child. Children with learning disabilities usually have average or above-average intelligence, but there are differences in the way their brains process information.

As with many other neurodevelopmental disorders, the causes of learning disabilities are not well understood. Often learning disabilities run in the family, suggesting that heredity may play a role in their development. Problems during pregnancy and birth, such as drug or alcohol use during pregnancy, low birth weight, lack of oxygen, or premature or prolonged labor, may also lead to learning disabilities.

As is the case with other neurodevelopmental outcomes, there are generally many more studies of lead exposure that are relevant to learning disabilities than for other environmental contaminants. Several studies have found associations between lead exposure and learning disabilities or reduced classroom performance that are independent of IQ.

Exposures to lead have been associated with impaired memory and difficulties or impairments in rule learning, following directions, planning, verbal abilities, speech processing, and classroom performance in children. Other findings that may indicate contributions from environmental contaminants to learning disabilities include a study that found associations of both maternal smoking during pregnancy and childhood exposure to environmental tobacco smoke with parent report of a child with a learning disability diagnosis; associations of prenatal mercury exposure with dysfunctions in children's language abilities and memory, and associations of prenatal PCB exposure with poorer concentration and memory deficits compared with unexposed children.

Autism Spectrum Disorders

Autism spectrum disorders (ASDs) are a group of developmental disabilities defined by significant social, communication, and behavioral impairments. The term "spectrum disorders" refers to the fact that although people with ASDs share some common symptoms, ASDs affect different people in different ways, with some experiencing very mild symptoms and others experiencing severe symptoms.

ASDs encompass autistic disorder and the generally less severe forms, Asperger syndrome and pervasive developmental disorder-not otherwise specified (PDD-NOS). Children with ASDs may lack interest in other people, have trouble showing or talking about feelings, and avoid or resist physical contact. A range of communication problems are seen in children with ASDs: some speak very well, while many children with an ASD do not speak at all. Another hallmark characteristic of ASDs is the demonstration of restrictive or repetitive interests or behaviors, such as lining up toys, flapping hands, rocking his or her body, or spinning in circles.

To date, no single risk factor sufficient to cause ASD has been identified; rather each case is likely to be caused by the combination of multiple genetic and environmental risk factors. Several ASD research findings and hypotheses may imply an important role for environmental contaminants. First, there has been a sharp upward trend in reported prevalence that cannot be fully explained by factors such as younger ages at diagnosis, migration patterns, changes in diagnostic criteria, inclusion of milder cases, or increased parental age. Also, the neurological signaling systems that are impaired in children with ASDs can be affected by certain environmental chemicals. For example, several pesticides are known to interfere with acetylcholine (Ach) and γ-aminobutyric acid (GABA) neurotransmission, chemical messenger systems that have been altered in certain subsets of autistic individuals. Some studies have reported associations between certain pharmaceuticals taken by pregnant women and increased incidence of autism, which may suggest that there are biological pathways by which other chemical exposures during pregnancy could increase the risk of autism.

Furthermore, some of the identified genetic risk factors for autism are de novo mutations, meaning that the genetic defect is not present in either of the parents' genes, yet can be found in the genes of the child when a new genetic mutation forms in a parent's germ cells (egg or sperm), potentially from exposure to contaminants Many environmental contaminants have been identified as agents capable of causing mutations in DNA, by leading to oxidative DNA damage and by inhibiting the body's normal ability to repair DNA damage. The role of parental age in increased autism risk might be explained by evidence that shows advanced parental age can contribute significantly to the frequency of de novo mutations in a parent's germ cells. Advanced parental age signifies a longer period of time when environmental exposures may act on germ cells and cause DNA damage and de novo mutations.

Finally, a recent study concluded that the role of genetic factors in ASDs has been overestimated, and that environmental factors play a greater role than genetic factors in contributing to autism. This study did not evaluate the role of any particular environmental factors, and in this context "environmental factors" are defined broadly to include any influence that is not genetic.

Studies, limited in number and often limited in research design, have examined the possible role that certain environmental contaminants may play in the development of ASDs. A number of these studies have focused on mercury exposures. Earlier studies reported higher levels of mercury in the blood, baby teeth, and urine of children with ASDs compared with control children; however, another more recent study reported no difference in the blood mercury levels of children with autism and typically developing children. Proximity to industrial and power plant sources of environmental mercury was reported to be associated with increased autism prevalence in a study conducted in Texas.

Thimerosal is a mercury-containing preservative that is used in some vaccines to prevent contamination and growth of harmful bacteria in vaccine vials. Since 2001, thimerosal has not been used in routinely administered childhood vaccines, with the exception of some influenza vaccines. The Institute of Medicine has rejected the hypothesis of a causal relationship between thimerosal-containing vaccines and autism.

Some studies have also considered air pollutants as possible contributors to autism. A study conducted in the San Francisco Bay Area reported an association between the amount of certain airborne pollutants at a child's place of birth (mercury, cadmium, nickel, trichloroethylene, and vinyl chloride) and the risk for autism, but a similar study in North Carolina and West Virginia did not find such a relationship. Another study in California reported that mothers who lived near a freeway at the time of delivery were more likely to have children diagnosed with autism, suggesting that exposure to traffic-related air pollutants may play a role in contributing to ASDs.

Finally, a study in Sweden reported an increased risk of ASDs in children born to families living in homes with polyvinyl chloride (PVC) flooring, which is a source of certain phthalates in indoor environments.

Intellectual Disability (Mental Retardation)

The most commonly used definitions of intellectual disability (also referred to as mental retardation) emphasize subaverage intellectual functioning before the age of 18, usually defined as an IQ less than 70 and impairments in life skills such as communication, self-care, home living, and social or interpersonal skills. Different severity categories, ranging from mild to severe retardation, are defined on the basis of IQ scores.

"Intellectual disability" is used as the preferred term for this condition in the disabilities sector, but the term "mental retardation" continues to be used in the contexts of law and public policy when designating eligibility for state and federal programs.

Researchers have identified some causes of intellectual disability, including genetic disorders, traumatic injuries, and prenatal events such as maternal infection or exposure to alcohol. However, the causes of intellectual disability are unknown in 30–50% of all cases. The causes are more frequently identified for cases of severe retardation (IQ less than 50), whereas the cause of mild retardation (IQ between 50 and 70) is unknown in more than 75% of cases. Exposures to environmental contaminants could be a contributing factor to the cases of mild retardation where the cause is unknown. Exposure to high levels of lead and mercury have been associated with intellectual disability.

Furthermore, lead, mercury, and PCBs all have been found to have adverse effects on intelligence and cognitive functioning in children, and recent studies have reported associations of a number of other environmental contaminants with childhood IQ deficits, including organophosphate pesticides, PBDEs, phthalates, and PAHs. Exposure to environmental contaminants that reduce IQ has the potential to increase the proportion of the population with IQ less than 70, thus increasing the incidence of intellectual disability in an exposed population.

Chapter 5

Signs and Symptoms of Learning Disabilities

What Are the Indicators of Learning Disabilities?

Many children have difficulty with reading, writing, or other learning-related tasks at some point, but this does not mean they have learning disabilities. A child with a learning disability often has several related signs, and these persist over time. The signs of learning disabilities vary from person to person. Common signs that a person may have learning disabilities include the following:

- Difficulty with reading and/or writing

- Problems with math skills

- Difficulty remembering

- Problems paying attention

- Trouble following directions

- Poor coordination

- Difficulty with concepts related to time

- Problems staying organized

This chapter includes text excerpted from "What Are the Indicators of Learning Disabilities?" *Eunice Kennedy Shriver* National Institute of Child Health and Human Development (NICHD),February 2, 2014.

A child with a learning disability also may exhibit one or more of the following:

- Impetuous behavior

- Inappropriate responses in school or social situations

- Difficulty staying on task (easily distracted)

- Difficulty finding the right way to say something

- Inconsistent school performance

- Immature way of speaking

- Difficulty listening well

- Problems dealing with new things in life

- Problems understanding words or concepts

These signs alone are not enough to determine that a person has a learning disability. A professional assessment is necessary to diagnose a learning disability.

Each learning disability has its own signs. Also, not every person with a particular disability will have all of the signs of that disability.

Children being taught in a second language that they are learning sometimes act in ways that are similar to the behaviors of someone with a learning disability. For this reason, learning disability assessment must take into account whether a student is bilingual or a second language learner.

Below are some common learning disabilities and the signs associated with them:

Dyslexia

People with dyslexia usually have trouble making the connections between letters and sounds and with spelling and recognizing words.

People with dyslexia often show other signs of the condition. These may include:

- Failure to fully understand what others are saying

- Difficulty organizing written and spoken language

- Delayed ability to speak

- Poor self-expression (for example, saying "thing" or "stuff" for words not recalled)

- Difficulty learning new vocabulary, either through reading or hearing

- Trouble learning foreign languages

- Slowness in learning songs and rhymes

- Slow reading as well as giving up on longer reading tasks

- Difficulty understanding questions and following directions

- Poor spelling

- Difficulty recalling numbers in sequence (for example, telephone numbers and addresses)

- Trouble distinguishing left from right

Dysgraphia

Dysgraphia is characterized by problems with writing. This disorder may cause a child to be tense and awkward when holding a pen or pencil, even to the extent of contorting his or her body. A child with very poor handwriting that he or she does not outgrow may have dysgraphia.

Other signs of this condition may include:

- A strong dislike of writing and/or drawing

- Problems with grammar

- Trouble writing down ideas

- A quick loss of energy and interest while writing

- Trouble writing down thoughts in a logical sequence

- Saying words out loud while writing

- Leaving words unfinished or omitting them when writing sentences

Dyscalculia

Signs of this disability include problems understanding basic arithmetic concepts, such as fractions, number lines, and positive and negative numbers.

Other symptoms may include:

- Difficulty with math-related word problems

- Trouble making change in cash transactions

- Messiness in putting math problems on paper

- Trouble recognizing logical information sequences (for example, steps in math problems)

- Trouble with understanding the time sequence of events

- Difficulty with verbally describing math processes

Dyspraxia

A person with dyspraxia has problems with motor tasks, such as hand-eye coordination, that can interfere with learning.
Some other symptoms of this condition include:

- Problems organizing oneself and one's things

- Breaking things

- Trouble with tasks that require hand-eye coordination, such as coloring within the lines, assembling puzzles, and cutting precisely

- Poor balance

- Sensitivity to loud and/or repetitive noises, such as the ticking of a clock

- Sensitivity to touch, including irritation over bothersome-feeling clothing

Chapter 6

Diagnosing Learning Disabilities

Chapter Contents

Section 6.1

How Are Learning Disabilities Diagnosed?

"How Are Learning Disabilities Diagnosed?"
© 2016 Omnigraphics. Reviewed June 2016.

Overview

Diagnosing learning disabilities (LDs) is difficult because LDs show up differently in different people and a learning disability in one area may be masked by accelerated ability in another. For instance, a child who has dyscalculia may not know how to add two numbers, but may write at a much higher grade level, leading teachers to think she is just being lazy about turning in her math homework.

Diagnosing Learning Disabilities in School-Aged Children and Adolescents

Learning disabilities often become evident when a child starts school. Teachers and other school professionals may identify students with suspected learning disabilities as they monitor the students' progress and their response to educational assistance. This is called the *response to intervention (RTI)* process. Parents may also bring their concerns about LDs in their children to the attention of school professionals.

If a student is suspected of having learning disabilities, further testing and evaluation will be needed.

The Individuals with Disabilities Education Act (IDEA) sets out clear rules and regulations on the process for evaluating children suspected of having LDs, so that students with LDs can take advantage of individualized educational plans (IEPs) when warranted. Under IDEA, an evaluation must be "full and individual" meaning it needs to be comprehensive in scope but tailored to the student as a distinct individual. Tests must be given in the language and at the level that the student understands best. Tests must investigate all the skills where the student has difficulty. The results must give relevant information to make informed decisions on the next steps in the student's educational plan.

In addition, the school staff must create an evaluation plan that informs the parents of all tests, observations, records they plan to use in the evaluation as well as providing the names of all evaluators.

The evaluation may include:

- **A physical examination** that looks for physical causes of LD such as vision, hearing, movement, or other health issues.

- **A psychological evaluation** to examine the student's emotional health and social skills, and determine how the student learns best.

- **Interviews** with the student, parents, and teachers to learn more about the student's academic history, behavior in and out of school, and other information that can help the evaluators with their diagnosis.

- **Behavioral assessment** is often accomplished using questionnaires filled out by teachers and parents about how the student interacts with the world in both normal and unusual situations.

- **Observation of the student** by teachers, the school psychologist, reading specialist, speech-language pathologist, and other educational professionals.

- **Standardized tests** that are selected by educational professionals based on the student's areas of strengths and weaknesses. These tests can test general ability or specific skills.

  - **Intelligence and achievement tests** are used to measure the student's intellectual potential, what he or she knows and can do, and areas of the student's strengths and weaknesses. There are a variety of standard intelligence and achievement tests geared to a person's age. The evaluators then use the results of these tests to focus on what further testing needs to done.

  - **Tests for reading, writing, and math** can include those that measure reading comprehension to determine the grade level at which a student should be taught; essential reading skills; oral reading (can the student read a passage aloud then answer questions on it?); pronunciation; general math skills.

  - **Tests for language, motor, and processing** skills look at issues that affect a student's learning skills. Results of this type of test may suggest problems with perception, memory, planning, motor skills, attention, and comprehension of both written and spoken communications.

- **Other information already on file** including report cards and state test scores.

Based on the results of the evaluation, the school's IEP administrator will work with the student's teachers and family to draw up a plan of study to accommodate the student's LDs and determine strategies for effective learning and living.

Diagnosing Learning Disabilities in Adults

An adult may suspect he or she has a learning disability if there are problems at work or school, such as trouble with reading, understanding charts, communicating effectively, or staying on task. There may be problems with everyday tasks including reading the newspaper, balancing the checkbook, or making decisions. Likewise, if an adult has struggled to learn or remember for a long time, he or she may decide it is time to find out why.

Adults should seek qualified professionals to conduct the assessment. These professionals are licensed to evaluate LD and include psychologists and psychiatrists.

The diagnostic process for identifying LDs in adults is similar to that of diagnosing a student. It includes interviews and observations, testing, an assessment of the results, and recommendations for living with the LD.

The assessment may include:

- **An interview** to gather information about the person's academic and career history, a review of any medical issues, and other information that can help the evaluator with the diagnosis.

- **A career interest inventory** to aid in determining what career areas are matches for the person's interests.

- **Standardized tests** that are selected by the professional based on the information given to them. As with students, these tests can test general ability or specific skills. Standardized tests are used to look at the person's intelligence, achievement, and ability to process information. Based on those results, further tests may be administered to identify specific LDs.

After the professional has gathered enough information, he or she will give the person the results of the assessment including the LD(s) identified and make recommendations for learning and living.

Because each person is different, the diagnosing of learning disabilities must be individually tailored to that person. Age and development play a part in determining whether a person has one or more LDs and which ones they are. In addition, LDs may not appear until later because the person has learned to cope with the LD or it has been masked by other strengths. Regardless of when an LD is first suspected, the final diagnosis must be made by a professional or group of professionals.

References

1. "Adult Learning Disability Assessment Process," Learning Disabilities Association of America, 2016.

2. "Adults with Learning Disabilities–An Overview," Learning Disabilities Association of America, 2016.

3. "How are Learning Disabilities Diagnosed?" National Institutes of Health, *Eunice Kennedy Shriver* National Institute of Child Health and Human Development, February 28, 2014.

4. Griffin, Rayma. "Who Can Diagnose Learning and Attention Issues in Adults?" Understood, 2016.

5. Morin, Amanda. "Understanding the Full Evaluation Process," Understood, July 11, 2014.

6. Patino, Erica. "Types of Behavior Assessments," Understood, May 30, 2014.

7. ———. "Types of Intelligence and Achievement Tests," Understood, June 5, 2014.

8. ———. "Types of Tests for Language, Motor and Processing Skills," Understood, June 5, 2014.

9. ———. "Types of Tests for Reading, Writing and Math," Understood, November 18, 2014.

Section 6.2

Evaluating Children for Learning Disabilities

Text in this section begins with excerpts from "Evaluating
Children for Disability," Center for Parent Information
and Resources (CPIR), May 2014.

Process of Evaluating Learning Disabilities

**Evaluation is an essential beginning step in the special edu-
cation process for a child with a disability**. Before a child can
receive special education and related services for the first time, a full
and individual initial evaluation of the child must be conducted to
see if the child has a disability and is eligible for special education.
**Informed parent consent must be obtained before this evalu-
ation may be conducted.**

The evaluation process is guided by requirements in our nation's
special education law, the Individuals with Disabilities Education Act
(IDEA).

Purposes of Evaluation

**The initial evaluation of a child is required by IDEA before
any special education and related services can be provided
to that child.** The purposes of conducting this evaluation are
straightforward:

- To see if the child is a "child with a disability," as defined by IDEA

- To gather information that will help determine the child's educational needs

- To guide decision making about appropriate educational programming for the child

IDEA's Definition of a "Child with a Disability"

IDEA lists different disability categories under which a child may
be found eligible for special education and related services.

These categories are:

- Autism
- Deafness
- Deaf-blindness
- Developmental delay
- Emotional disturbance
- Hearing impairment
- Intellectual disability
- Multiple disabilities
- Orthopedic impairment
- Other health impairment
- Specific learning disability
- Speech or language impairment
- Traumatic brain injury
- Visual impairment, including blindness

Having a disability, though, does not necessarily make a child eligible for special education. Consider this language from the IDEA regulations:

Child with a disability means a child evaluated in accordance with 300.304 through 300.311 as having [one of the disabilities listed above] and who, by reason thereof, needs special education and related services.

This provision includes the very important phrase "and who, by **reason thereof**" This means that, *because of the disability*, the child needs special education and related services. Many children have disabilities that do not bring with them the need for extra educational assistance or individualized educational programming. If a child has a disability but is not eligible under IDEA, he or she may be eligible for the protections afforded by other laws—such as Section 504 of the Rehabilitation Act of 1973, as amended. It's not uncommon for a child to have a 504 plan at school to address disability-related educational needs. Such a child will receive needed assistance but not under IDEA.

Identifying Children for Evaluation

Before a child's eligibility under IDEA can be determined, however, a full and individual evaluation of the child must be conducted. There are at least two ways in which a child may be identified to receive an evaluation under IDEA:

- **Parents may request that their child be evaluated.** Parents are often the first to notice that their child's learning, behavior, or development may be a cause for concern. If they're worried about their child's progress in school and think he or she might need extra help from special education services, they may call, email, or write to their child's teacher, the school's principal, or the Director of Special Education in the school district. If the school agrees that an evaluation is needed, it must evaluate the child at no cost to parents.

- **The school system may ask to evaluate the child.** Based on a teacher's recommendation, observations, or results from tests given to all children in a particular grade, a school may recommend that a child receive further screening or assessment to determine if he or she has a disability and needs special education and related services. The school system must ask parents for permission to evaluate the child, and parents must give their informed written permission before the evaluation may be conducted.

Giving Parents Notice

It is important to know that IDEA requires the school system to **notify parents in writing** that it would like to evaluate their child (or that it is refusing to evaluate the child). This is called giving **prior written notice**. It is not enough for the agency to tell parents that it would like to evaluate their child or that it refuses to evaluate their child. The school must also:

- explain why it wants to conduct the evaluation (or why it refuses)

- describe each evaluation procedure, assessment, record, or report used as a basis for proposing the evaluation (or refusing to conduct the evaluation)

- where parents can go to obtain help in understanding IDEA's provisions

- what other options the school considered and why those were rejected

- a description of any other factors that are relevant to the school's proposal (or refusal) to evaluate the child

The purpose behind this thorough explanation is to make sure that parents are fully informed, understand what is being proposed (or refused), understand what evaluation of their child will involve (or why the school system is refusing to conduct an evaluation of the child), and understand their right to refuse consent for evaluation, or to otherwise exercise their rights under IDEA's **procedural safeguards** if the school refuses to evaluate.

All written communication from the school must be in a form the general public can understand. It must be provided in parents' native language if they do not read English, or in the mode of communication they normally use (such as Braille or large print) unless it is clearly not feasible to do so. If parents' native language or other mode of communication is not a written language, the school must take steps to ensure:

- that the notice is translated orally (or by other means) to parents in their native language or other mode of communication

- that parents understand the content of the notice

- that there is written evidence that the above two requirements have been met

Parental Consent

Before the school may proceed with the evaluation, parents must give their informed written consent. This consent is for the evaluation only. It does not mean that the school has the parent's permission to provide special education services to the child. That requires a separate consent.

If parents refuse consent for an initial evaluation (or simply don't respond to the school's request), the school must carefully document all its attempts to obtain parent consent. It may also continue to pursue conducting the evaluation by using the law's **due process procedures** or its **mediation** procedures, unless doing so would be inconsistent with state law relating to parental consent.

However, if the child is homeschooled or has been placed in a private school by parents (meaning, the parents are paying for the cost of the private school), *the school may not override* parents' lack of consent for initial evaluation of the child. As the Department of Education notes:

once parents opt out of the public school system, States and school districts do not have the same interest in requiring parents to agree to the evaluation of their children. In such cases, it would be overly intrusive for the school district to insist on an evaluation over a parent's objection.

Timeframe for Initial Evaluation

Let's move on from the prerequisites for initial evaluation (parent notification and parent consent) to the actual process of initial evaluation and what the law requires. Let us assume that parents' informed consent has been given, and it's time to evaluate the child. **Must this evaluation be conducted within a certain period of time after parents give their consent?**

Yes. In its reauthorization of IDEA in 2004, Congress added a specific timeframe: The initial evaluation must be conducted **within 60 days** of receiving parental consent for the evaluation—or if the state establishes its own timeframe for conducting an initial evaluation, within *that* timeframe. (In other words: Any timeframe established by the state takes precedence over the 60-day timeline required by IDEA.)

The Scope of Evaluation

A child's initial evaluation must be full and individual, focused on that child and only that child. This is a longstanding provision of IDEA. An evaluation of a child under IDEA means much more than the child sitting in a room with the rest of his or her class taking an exam for that class, that school, that district, or that state. How the child performs on such exams will contribute useful information to an IDEA-related evaluation, but large-scale tests or group-administered instruments are not enough to diagnose a disability or determine what, if any, special education or related services the child might need, let alone plan an appropriate educational program for the child.

The evaluation must use a variety of assessment tools and strategies to gather relevant functional, developmental, and academic information about the child, including information provided by the parent. When conducting an initial evaluation, it's important to examine all areas of a child's functioning to determine not only if the child is a child with a disability, but also determine the child's educational needs. This full and individual evaluation includes evaluating the child's:

- health
- vision and hearing
- social and emotional status
- general intelligence
- academic performance
- communicative status
- motor abilities

As IDEA states, the school system must ensure that—the evaluation is sufficiently comprehensive to identify all of the child's special education and related services needs, whether or not commonly linked to the disability category in which the child has been classified.

Review Existing Data

Evaluation (and particularly reevaluation) typically begins with a review of existing evaluation data on the child, which may come from the child's classroom work, his or her performance on State or district assessments, information provided by the parents, and so on.

The purpose of this review is to decide if the existing data is sufficient to establish the child's eligibility and determine educational needs, or if additional information is needed. If the group determines there is sufficient information available to make the necessary determinations, the public agency must notify parents:

- of that determination and the reason for it
- that parents have the right to request assessment to determine the child's eligibility and educational needs

Unless the parents request an assessment, the public agency is not required to conduct one.

If it is decided that additional data is needed, the group then identifies what is needed to determine:

- whether your son or daughter has a particular category of disability (e.g., "other health impairment," "specific learning disability")

- your child's present levels of performance (that is, how he or she is currently doing in school) and his or her academic and developmental needs

- whether your child needs special education and related services

- if so, whether any additions or modifications are needed in the special education and related services to enable your child to meet the goals set out in the IEP to be developed and to participate, as appropriate, in the general curriculum

An example may help crystallize the comprehensive scope of evaluations: Consider a first-grader with suspected hearing and vision impairments who's been referred for an initial evaluation. In order to fully gather relevant functional, developmental, and academic information and identify all of the child's special education and related services needs, evaluation of this child will obviously need to focus on hearing and vision, as well as, cognitive, speech/language, motor, and social/behavioral skills, to determine:

- the degree of impairment in vision and hearing and the impact of these impairments on the child

- if there are additional impairments in other areas of functioning (including those not commonly linked to hearing and/or vision) that impact the child's aptitude, performance, and achievement

- what the child's educational needs are that must be addressed

With this example, any of the following individuals might be part of this child's evaluation team: audiologist, psychologist, speech-language pathologist, social worker, occupational or physical therapist, vision specialist, regular classroom teacher, educational diagnosticians, or others.

Assessment Tools and Strategies

The evaluation must use a variety of assessment tools and strategies. This has been one of the cornerstones of IDEA's evaluation requirements from its earliest days. Under IDEA, it is inappropriate and unacceptable to base any eligibility decision upon the results of only one procedure. Tests alone will not give a comprehensive picture of how a child performs or what he or she knows or does not know. Only by collecting data through a *variety of approaches* (e.g., observations, interviews, tests, curriculum-based assessment, and so on) and from a *variety of sources* (parents, teachers, specialists, child) can an adequate picture be obtained of the child's strengths and weaknesses.

IDEA also requires schools to use technically sound instruments and processes in evaluation. Technically sound instruments generally refers to assessments that have been shown through research to be valid and reliable. Technically sound processes requires that assessments and other evaluation materials be:

• administered by trained and knowledgeable personnel

• administered in accordance with any instructions provided by the producer of the assessments

• used for the purposes for which the assessments or measures are valid and reliable

In conjunction with using a variety of sound tools and processes, assessments must include those that are tailored to assess specific areas of educational need (for example, reading or math) and not merely those that are designed to provide a single general intelligence quotient, or IQ.

Taken together, all of this information can be used to determine whether the child has a disability under IDEA, the specific nature of the child's special needs, whether the child needs special education and related services and, if so, to design an appropriate program.

Consider Language, Communication Mode, and Culture

Another important component in evaluation is to ensure that assessment tools are not discriminatory on a racial or cultural basis. Evaluation must also be conducted in the child's typical, accustomed mode of communication (unless it is clearly not feasible to do so) and in a form that will yield accurate information about what the child knows and can do academically, developmentally, and functionally. For many, English is not the native language; others use sign to communicate, or assistive or alternative augmentative communication devices. To assess such a child using a means of communication or response not highly familiar to the child raises the probability that the evaluation results will yield minimal, if any, information about what the child knows and can do.

Specifically, consideration of language, culture, and communication mode means the following:

- If your child has limited English proficiency, materials and procedures used to assess your child must be selected and administered to ensure that they measure the extent to which your child has a disability and needs special education, rather than measuring your child's English language skills.

This provision in the law is meant to protect children of different racial, cultural, or language backgrounds from misdiagnosis. For example, children's cultural backgrounds may affect their behavior or test responses in ways that teachers or other personnel do not understand. Similarly, if a child speaks a language other than English or has limited English proficiency, he or she may not understand directions or words on tests and may be unable to answer correctly. As a result, a child may mistakenly appear to be a slow learner or to have a hearing or communication problem.

- If an assessment is not conducted under standard conditions–meaning that some condition of the test has been changed (such as the qualifications of the person giving the test or the method of giving the test)–a description of the extent to which it varied from standard conditions must be included in the evaluation report

- If your child has impaired sensory, manual, or speaking skills, the law requires that tests are selected and administered so as best to ensure that test results accurately reflect his or her aptitude or achievement level (or whatever other factors the test claims to measure), and not merely reflect your child's impaired sensory, manual, or speaking skills (unless the test being used is intended to measure those skills)

What about Evaluation for Specific Learning Disabilities?

IDEA's regulations specify additional procedures required to be used for determining the existence of a specific learning disability. It's important to note, though, that IDEA 2004 made dramatic changes in how children who are suspected of having a learning disability are to be evaluated.

- States must not require the use of a severe discrepancy between intellectual ability and achievement

- States must permit the use of a process based on the child's response to scientific, research-based intervention

- States may permit the use of other alternative research-based procedures for determining whether a child has a specific learning disability

- The team that makes the eligibility determination must include a regular education teacher and at least one person qualified to conduct individual diagnostic examinations of children, such as a school psychologist, speech-language pathologist, or remedial reading teacher

Determining Eligibility

Parents were not always included in the group that determined their child's eligibility and, in fact, were often excluded. Since the IDEA Amendments of 1997, **parents are to be part of the group that determines their child's eligibility** and are also to be provided a copy of the evaluation report, as well as documentation of the determination of the child's eligibility.

Some school systems will hold a meeting where they consider only the eligibility of the child for special education and related services. At this meeting, your child's assessment results should be explained. The specialists who assessed your child will explain what they did, why they used the tests they did, your child's results on those tests or other evaluation procedures, and what your child's scores mean when compared to other children of the same age and grade.

It is important to know that the group may not determine that a child is eligible if the determinant factor for making that judgment is the child's lack of instruction in reading or math or the child's limited English proficiency. The child must otherwise meet the law's definition of a "child with a disability"–meaning that he or she has one of the disabilities listed in the law and, because of that disability, needs special education and related services.

If the evaluation results indicate that your child meets the definition of one or more of the disabilities listed under IDEA and needs special education and related services, the results will form the basis for developing your child's IEP.

What Happens If You Don't Agree with the Evaluation Results?

If you, as parents of a child with a disability, disagree with the results of your child's evaluation as obtained by the public agency, you have the right to obtain what is known as an **Independent Educational Evaluation**, or IEE. An IEE means an evaluation conducted by a qualified examiner who is not employed by the public agency responsible for the education of your child. If you ask for an IEE, the public agency must provide you with, among other things, information about where an IEE may be obtained.

Who pays for the independent evaluation? The answer is that some IEEs are at public expense and others are paid for by the parents. For example, if you are the parent of a child with a disability and you disagree with the public agency's evaluation, you may request an IEE at public expense. "At public expense" means that the public agency either pays for the full cost of the evaluation or ensures that the evaluation is otherwise provided at no cost to you as parents. The public agency may grant your request and pay for the IEE, or it may initiate a hearing to show that its own evaluation was appropriate. The public agency may ask why you object to the public evaluation. However, the agency may not require you to explain, and it may not unreasonably delay either providing the IEE at public expense or initiating a due process hearing to defend the public evaluation.

If the public agency initiates a hearing and the final decision of the hearing officer is that the agency's evaluation was appropriate, then you still have the right to an IEE but not at public expense. As part of a due process hearing, a hearing officer may also request an IEE; if so, that IEE must be at public expense. Whenever an IEE is publicly funded, that IEE must meet the same criteria that the public agency uses when it initiates an evaluation. The public agency must tell you what these criteria are—such as location of the evaluation and the qualifications of the examiner—and they must be the same criteria the public agency uses when it initiates an evaluation, to the extent they are consistent with your right to an IEE. However, the public agency may not impose other conditions or timelines related to your obtaining an IEE at public expense.

Of course, you have the right to have your child independently evaluated at any time at your own expense. (Note: When the same tests are repeated within a short time period, the validity of the results can be seriously weakened.) The results of this evaluation must be considered by the public agency, if it meets agency criteria, in any decision made with respect to providing your child with FAPE. The results may also be presented as evidence at a hearing regarding your child.

What Happens down the Road?

After the initial evaluation, evaluations must be conducted at least every three years (generally called a triennial evaluation) after your child has been placed in special education. Reevaluations can also occur more frequently if conditions warrant, or if you or your child's teacher request a reevaluation. Informed parental consent is also necessary for reevaluations.

As with initial evaluations, reevaluations begin with the review of existing evaluation data, including evaluations and information provided by you, the child's parents. Your consent is not required for the review of existing data on your child. As with initial evaluation, this review is to identify what additional data, if any, are needed to determine whether your child continues to be a "child with a disability" and continues to need special education and related services. If the group determines that additional data are needed, then the public agency must administer tests and other evaluation materials as needed to produce the data. Prior to collecting this additional information, the agency must obtain your informed written consent.

Or, if the group determines that no additional data are needed to determine whether your child continues to be a "child with a disability," the public agency must notify you:

- of this determination and the reasons for it

- of your right, as parents, to request an assessment to determine whether, for the purposes of services under IDEA, your child continues to be a "child with a disability"

A *final note with respect to reevaluations*: Before determining that your child is no longer a "child with a disability" and, thus, no longer eligible for special education services under IDEA, the public agency must evaluate your child in accordance with all of the provisions described above. This evaluation, however, is not required before terminating your child's eligibility due to graduation with a regular high school diploma or due to exceeding the age eligibility for FAPE under State law.

Chapter 7

Prevalence of Learning Disabilities

National Health Interview Survey

The National Health Interview Survey (NHIS) provides nationally representative data on the prevalence of ADHD, learning disabilities, autism, and intellectual disability (mental retardation) in the United States each year. NHIS is a large-scale household interview survey of a representative sample of the civilian noninstitutionalized U.S. population, conducted by the National Center for Health Statistics (NCHS). The interviews are conducted in person at the participants' homes. From 1997–2005, interviews were conducted for approximately 12,000–14,000 children annually. From 2006–2008, interviews were conducted for approximately 9,000–10,000 children per year. From 2011–2013, interviews were conducted for approximately 11,000–13,000 children per year. The data are obtained by asking a parent or other knowledgeable household adult questions regarding the child's health status. NHIS asks "Has a doctor or health professional ever told you that your child had Attention Deficit/Hyperactivity Disorder (ADHD) or Attention Deficit Disorder (ADD)? Autism? Mental Retardation?" Another question on the NHIS survey asks "Has a representative from a school or a health professional ever told you that your child had a learning disability?"

This chapter includes text excerpted from "Neurodevelopmental Disorders," U.S. Environmental Protection Agency (EPA), October 2015.

Indicators

The four indicators that follow provide the best nationally representative data available on the prevalence of neurodevelopmental disorders among U.S. children over time. The indicators present the number of children ages 5 to 17 years reported to have ever been diagnosed with

ADHD (Indicator H6), learning disabilities (Indicator H7), autism (Indicator H8), and intellectual disability (Indicator H9). These four conditions are examples of neurodevelopmental disorders that may be influenced by exposures to environmental contaminants. Intellectual disability and learning disabilities are disorders in which a child's cognitive or intellectual development is affected, and ADHD is a disorder in which a child's behavioral development is affected. Autism spectrum disorders are disorders in which a child's behavior, communication, and social skills are affected. Indicators H6 to H9 have been updated since the publication of the America's Children and the Environment, Third Edition (January 2013) to include data through 2013.

Indicator H6: Percentage of children ages 5 to 17 years reported to have attention deficit hyperactivity disorder, by sex, 1997–2013

Indicator H7: Percentage of children ages 5 to 17 years reported to have a learning disability, by sex, 1997–2013

Indicator H8: Percentage of children ages 5 to 17 years reported to have autism, 1997–2013

Indicator H9: Percentage of children ages 5 to 17 years reported to have intellectual disability (mental retardation), 1997–2013

Data Presented in the Indicators

The following indicators display the prevalence of Attention Deficit Hyperactivity Disorder (ADHD), learning disabilities, autism, and intellectual disability among U.S. children, for the years 1997–2013. Diagnosing neurodevelopmental disorders in young children can be difficult: many affected children may not receive a diagnosis until they enter preschool or kindergarten. For this reason, the indicators here show children ages 5 to 17 years. Where data are sufficiently reliable, the indicators provide separate prevalence estimates for boys and girls.

Although the National Health Insurance Scheme (NHIS) provides national-level data on the prevalence of neurodevelopmental disorders over a span of many years, NHIS data could underestimate the prevalence of neurodevelopmental disorders. Reasons for underestimation may include late identification of affected children and the exclusion of institutionalized children from the NHIS survey population. A diagnosis of a neurodevelopmental disorder depends not only on the presence of particular symptoms and behaviors in a child, but on concerns being raised by a parent or teacher about the child's behavior, as well as the child's access to a doctor and the accuracy of the doctor's diagnosis. Further, the NHIS relies on parents reporting that their child has been diagnosed with a neurodevelopmental disorder, and the accuracy of parental responses could be affected by cultural and other factors.

Long-term trends in these conditions are difficult to detect with certainty due to a lack of data to track prevalence over many years, as well as changes in awareness and diagnostic criteria, which could explain at least part of the observed increasing trends. The NHIS questions also do not assess whether a child currently has a disorder; instead, they provide data on whether a child has ever been diagnosed with a disorder, regardless of their current status.

Survey responses for learning disabilities may be more uncertain than for the other three disorders presented. Whereas survey respondents are asked whether the child has been diagnosed with ADHD, autism, or intellectual disability (mental retardation) by a health professional, for learning disabilities an affirmative response may also include a school representative. It is possible that some parents may respond "yes" to the question regarding learning disabilities based on informal comments made at school, rather than a formal evaluation to determine whether the child has any specific learning disability; similarly, they may give a "yes" answer for children with diagnosed disorders that are not learning disabilities. For example, parents of children with intellectual disability might also respond "yes" to the learning disability question, thinking that any learning problems may apply, even though intellectual disability and learning disabilities are distinct conditions.

Because autism is the only autism spectrum disorder (ASD) referred to in the survey, it is not clear how parents of children with other ASDs, i.e., Asperger syndrome and PDD-NOS (Pervasive Developmental Disorder-Not Otherwise Specified), may have responded. The estimates shown by Indicator H8 could represent underestimates of ASD prevalence if parents of children with Asperger syndrome and PDD-NOS did not answer yes to the NHIS questions about autism.

In addition to the data shown in the indicator graphs, supplemental tables provide information regarding the prevalence of neurodevelopmental disorders for different age groups and prevalence by race/ethnicity, sex, and family income. These comparisons use the most current four years of data available. The data from four years are combined to increase the statistical reliability of the estimates for each race/ethnicity, sex, and family income group. The tables include prevalence estimates for the following race/ethnicity groups: White non-Hispanic, Black non-Hispanic, Asian non-Hispanic, Hispanic, and "All Other Races." The "All Others Races" category includes all other races not specified, together with those individuals who report more than one race. The limits of the sample design and sample size often prevent statistically reliable estimates for smaller race/ethnicity groups. The data are also tabulated for three income groups: all incomes, income below the poverty level, and greater than or equal to the poverty level.

Other Estimates of ADHD and Autism Prevalence

In addition to NHIS, other NCHS studies provide data on prevalence of ADHD and ASDs among children. The National Survey of Children's Health (NSCH), conducted in 2003 by NCHS, found that 7.8% of children ages 4 to 17 years had ever been diagnosed with ADHD. The same survey, when conducted again in 2007, found that 9.5% of children ages 4 to 17 years had ever been diagnosed with ADHD. Both estimates are somewhat higher than the ADHD prevalence estimates from the NHIS for those years. The 2007 NSCH also estimates that 7.2% of children ages 4 to 17 years currently have ADHD. The 2007 NSCH also provides information at the state level: North Carolina had the highest rate, with 15.6% of children ages 4 to 17 years having ever been diagnosed with ADHD; the rate was lowest in Nevada, at 5.6%.

In 2002 and 2006, the Centers for Disease Control and Prevention (CDC) performed thorough data gathering in selected areas to examine the prevalence of ASDs in eight-year-old children. The ASD prevalence estimate for 2002 was 0.66%, or 1 in 152 eight-year-old children, and the estimate for 2006 was 0.9%, or 1 in 110 eight-year-old children. The 2007 NSCH also provides an estimate of 1.1% of children ages 3 to 17 years reported to have ASDs, or about 1 in 90.

- From 1997 to 2013, the proportion of children ages 5 to 17 years reported to have ever been diagnosed with attention-deficit/ hyperactivity disorder (ADHD) increased from 6.3% in 1993 to 10.7% in 2012 and 9.9% in 2013.

- The increasing trend was statistically significant for children overall, and for both boys and girls considered separately.

- For the years 2010–2013, the percentage of boys reported to have ADHD (13.7%) was higher than the rate for girls (6.0%). This difference was statistically significant.

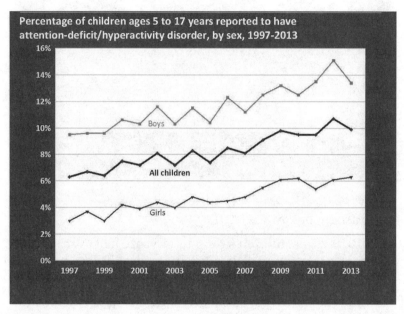

Figure 7.1. *Percentage of children ages 5 to 17 years reported to have attention-deficit/hyperactivity disorder, by sex, 1997-2013*

- In 2010–2013, 11.9% of White non-Hispanic children, 11.8% of children of "All Other Races," 10.1% of Black non-Hispanic children, 6.2% of Hispanic children, and 2.1% of Asian non- Hispanic children were reported to have ADHD.

  - These differences were statistically significant, with two exceptions: there was no statistically significant difference between children of "All Other Races" and White non- Hispanic children, or between children of "All Other Races" and Black non-Hispanic children.

- In 2010–2013, 13.1% of children from families living below the poverty level were reported to have ADHD compared with 9.1% of children from families living at or above the poverty level. This difference was statistically significant.

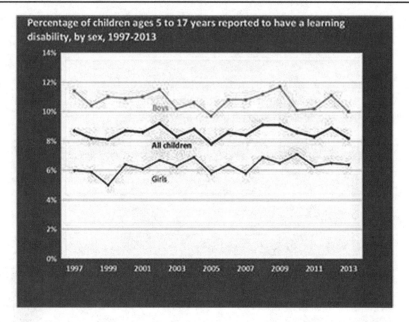

Figure 7.2. *Percentage of children ages 5 to 17 years reported to have learning disability, by sex, 1997-2013*

- In 2013, 8.2% of children ages 5 to 17 years had ever been diagnosed with a learning disability. There was little change in this percentage between 1997 and 2013.

- For the years 2010–2013, the percentage of boys reported to have a learning disability (10.4%) was higher than for girls (6.6%). This difference was statistically significant.

- The reported prevalence of learning disability varies by race and ethnicity. The highest percentages of learning disability are reported for American Indian or Alaska Native non-Hispanic children (12.7%), Black non-Hispanic children (9.8%), children of "All Other Races" (9.6%), and White non-Hispanic children (8.9%). By comparison, 7.6% of Hispanic children are reported to have a learning disability, and Asian non-Hispanic children have the lowest prevalence of learning disability, at 3.0%.

  - The prevalence of learning disability reported for Hispanic children and for Asian non-Hispanic children were lower than for the remaining race/ethnicity groups, and these differences were statistically significant. The difference in prevalence between Hispanic and Asian non-Hispanic children was also statistically significant.

80

- For the years 2010–2013, the percentage of children reported to have a learning disability was higher for children living below the poverty level (12.8%) compared with those living at or above the poverty level (7.4%), a statistically significant difference.

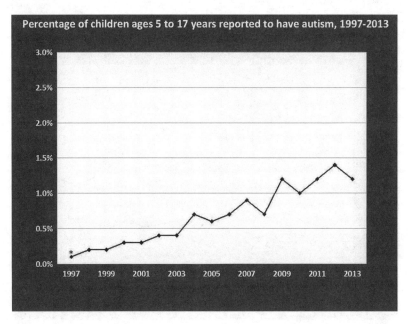

Figure 7.3. *Percentage of children ages 5 to 17 years reported to have autism, by sex, 1997-2013*

- The percentage of children ages 5 to 17 years reported to have ever been diagnosed with autism rose from 0.1% in 1997 to 1.2% in 2013. This increasing trend was statistically significant.

- For the years 2010–2013, the rate of reported autism was more than four times higher in boys than in girls, 1.9% and 0.4%, respectively. This difference was statistically significant.

- The reported prevalence of autism varies by race/ethnicity. The highest prevalence of autism is for children of "All Other Races" (1.7%) and White non-Hispanic children (1.4%). Autism prevalence was lower among Asian non-Hispanic children (1.1%), Black non-Hispanic children (0.8%), and Hispanic children (0.9%).

  - The prevalence of autism for both White non-Hispanic children and children of "All Other Races" was statistically significantly different from the prevalence for both Black non-Hispanic children and Hispanic children.

- For the years 2010–2013, the prevalence of autism was similar for children living below the poverty level and those living at or above the poverty level.

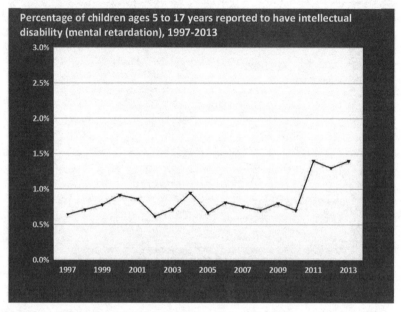

Figure 7.4. *Percentage of children ages 5 to 17 years reported to have intellectual disability (mental retardation), by sex, 1997-2013*

- In 2013, 1.4% of children ages 5 to 17 years were reported to have ever been diagnosed with intellectual disability (mental retardation). This percentage fluctuated between 0.6% and 0.9% from 1997 to 2010, and was between 1.3% and 1.4% from 2011 to 2013.

- In 2010–2013, the percentage of boys reported to have intellectual disability (1.6%) was higher than for girls (0.8 %). This difference was statistically significant.

- In 2010–2013, there was little difference by race/ethnicity in the reported prevalence of intellectual disability.

- In 2010–2013, 17% of children from families with incomes below the poverty level were reported to have intellectual disability, compared with 1.1% of children from families at or above the poverty level, a statistically significant difference.

Part Two

Types of Learning Disabilities

Chapter 8

Auditory Processing Disorder

Overview

Auditory processing disorder (APD), also known as central auditory processing disorder (CAPD), is a hearing problem that affects about 5% of school-aged children.

Kids with this condition can't process what they hear in the same way other kids do because their ears and brain don't fully coordinate. Something interferes with the way the brain recognizes and interprets sounds, especially speech.

With the right therapy, kids with APD can be successful in school and life. Early diagnosis is important, because when the condition isn't caught and treated early, a child can have speech and language delays or problems learning in school.

Trouble Understanding Speech

Kids with APD are thought to hear normally because they can usually hear sounds that are delivered one at a time in a very quiet environment (such as a sound-treated room). The problem is that they usually don't recognize slight differences between sounds in words, even when the sounds are loud and clear enough to be heard.

These kinds of problems usually happen when there is background noise, which is often the case in social situations. So kids with APD can have trouble understanding what is being said to them when they're in noisy places like a playground, sports events, the school cafeteria, and parties.

Symptoms

Symptoms of APD can range from mild to severe and can take many different forms. If you think your child might have a problem processing sounds, ask yourself these questions:

- Is your child easily distracted or unusually bothered by loud or sudden noises?
- Are noisy environments upsetting to your child?
- Does your child's behavior and performance improve in quieter settings?
- Does your child have difficulty following directions, whether simple or complicated?
- Does your child have reading, spelling, writing, or other speech-language difficulties?
- Are verbal (word) math problems difficult for your child?
- Is your child disorganized and forgetful?
- Are conversations hard for your child to follow?

APD is often misunderstood because many of the behaviors noted above also can accompany other problems, like learning disabilities, attention deficit hyperactivity disorder (ADHD), and even depression.

Causes

Often, the cause of a child's APD isn't known. Evidence suggests that head trauma, lead poisoning, and chronic ear infections could play a role. Sometimes, there can be multiple causes.

Diagnosis

If you think your child is having trouble hearing or understanding when people talk, have an audiologist (hearing specialist) exam your child. Only audiologists can diagnose auditory processing disorder.

Audiologists look for five main problem areas in kids with APD:

1. **Auditory figure-ground problems:** This is when a child can't pay attention if there's noise in the background. Noisy, loosely structured classrooms could be very frustrating.

2. **Auditory memory problems:** This is when a child has difficulty remembering information such as directions, lists, or study materials. It can be immediate ("I can't remember it now") and/or delayed ("I can't remember it when I need it for later").

3. **Auditory discrimination problems:** This is when a child has difficulty hearing the difference between words or sounds that are similar (COAT/BOAT or CH/SH). This can affect following directions and reading, spelling, and writing skills, among others.

4. **Auditory attention problems:** This is when a child can't stay focused on listening long enough to complete a task or requirement (such as listening to a lecture in school). Kids with CAPD often have trouble maintaining attention, although health, motivation, and attitude also can play a role.

5. **Auditory cohesion problems:** This is when higher-level listening tasks are difficult. Auditory cohesion skills—drawing inferences from conversations, understanding riddles, or comprehending verbal math problems—require heightened auditory processing and language levels. They develop best when all the other skills (levels 1 through 4 above) are intact.

Since most of the tests done to check for APD require a child to be at least seven or eight years old, many kids aren't diagnosed until then or later.

Helping Your Child

A child's auditory system isn't fully developed until age 15. So, many kids diagnosed with APD can develop better skills over time as their auditory system matures. While there is no known cure, speech-language therapy and assistive listening devices can help kids make sense of sounds and develop good communication skills.

A frequency modulation (FM) system is a type of assistive listening device that reduces background noise and makes a speaker's voice louder so a child can understand it. The speaker wears a tiny microphone and a transmitter, which sends an electrical signal to a wireless receiver that the child wears either on the ear or elsewhere on the body. It's portable and can be helpful in classroom settings.

A crucial part of making the FM system effective is ongoing therapy with a speech-language pathologist, who will help the child develop speaking and hearing skills. The speech-language pathologist or audiologist also may recommend tutoring programs.

Several computer-assisted programs are geared toward children with APD. They mainly help the brain do a better job of processing sounds in a noisy environment. Some schools offer these programs, so if your child has APD, be sure to ask school officials about what may be available.

At Home

Strategies applied at home and school can ease some of the problem behaviors associated with APD.

Kids with APD often have trouble following directions, so these suggestions may help:

- Reduce background noise whenever possible at home and at school

- Have your child look at you when you're speaking

- Use simple, expressive sentences

- Speak at a slightly slower rate and at a mildly increased volume

- Ask your child to repeat the directions back to you and to keep repeating them aloud (to you or to himself or herself) until the directions are completed

- For directions that are to be completed later, writing notes, wearing a watch, or maintaining a household routine can help. So can general organization and scheduling

- It can be frustrating for kids with APD when they're in a noisy setting and they need to listen. Teach your child to notice noisy environments and move to quieter places when listening is necessary

Other tips that might help:

- Provide your child with a quiet study place (not the kitchen table)

- Maintain a peaceful, organized lifestyle

- Encourage good eating and sleeping habits

- Assign regular and realistic chores, including keeping a neat room and desk

- Build your child's self-esteem

At School

It's important for the people caring for your child to know about APD. Be sure to tell teachers and other school officials about the APD and how it may affect learning. Kids with APD aren't typically put in special education programs, but you may find that your child is eligible for a 504 plan through the school district that would outline any special needs for the classroom.

Some things that may help:

- changing seating plans so your child can sit in the front of the classroom or with his or her back to the window

- study aids, like a tape recorder or notes that can be viewed online

- computer-assisted programs designed for kids with APD

Keep in regular contact with school officials about your child's progress. One of the most important things that both parents and teachers can do is to acknowledge that APD is real. Its symptoms and behaviors are not something that a child can control. What the child can control is recognizing the problems associated with APD and using the strategies recommended both at home and school.

A positive, realistic attitude and healthy self-esteem in a child with APD can work wonders. And kids with APD can go on to be just as successful as other classmates. Coping strategies and techniques learned in speech therapy can help them go far.

Chapter 9

Dyscalculia

What Is Dyscalculia?

People with dyscalculia have difficulty understanding numbers and learning math skills. Dyscalculia encompasses a wide range of learning disabilities related to math. Students with dyscalculia may:

- have difficulty learning to count or have a poor memory for numbers

- have trouble writing numbers, finding correct place values, and lining up equations

- have trouble remembering math facts

- be unable to follow a sequence of steps

- have difficulty understanding numbers, math symbols, and word problems

- find it hard to visualize patterns

- have difficulty measuring things

- have an exceptionally slow and difficult time solving math problems

- avoid games that require strategies involving math

This chapter includes excerpts from "Dyscalculia Special Needs Factsheet Print," © 1995–2016. The Nemours Foundation/KidsHealth®. Reprinted with permission.

- become extremely frustrated or anxious with schoolwork related to math

How Is Dyscalculia Identified?

Students with dyscalculia may:

- have difficulty learning to count or have a poor memory for numbers
- have trouble writing numbers, finding correct place values, and lining up equations
- have trouble remembering math facts
- be unable to follow a sequence of steps
- have difficulty understanding numbers, math symbols, and word problems
- find it hard to visualize patterns
- have difficulty measuring things
- have an exceptionally slow and difficult time solving math problems
- avoid games that require strategies involving math
- become extremely frustrated or anxious with schoolwork related to math

What Teachers Can Do?

If you suspect a student has dyscalculia, recommend seeking an educational evaluation to a parent or guardian, an administrator, or a school counselor.

Teachers can help students struggling with dyscalculia to become aware of their strengths and weaknesses. Helping students understand their learning styles and using alternative approaches can enable them to achieve confidence and success in math.

Additional math support in school and tutors outside the classroom can help students with dyscalculia focus on specific learning difficulties. Reinforcing math facts and practicing new skills can help make understanding math concepts easier.

Other strategies for inside and outside the classroom include:

- giving extra time to work on math-related assignments

- using graph paper for students who have difficulty organizing problems on paper

- planning and organizing students' approach to math problems

- using estimating as a way to approach solving math problems

- using objects and visuals to help solve problems

- starting with concrete examples before moving to harder, more abstract concepts

- explaining math concepts and terms clearly and encouraging students to ask questions

- providing a quiet place to work with few distractions

Chapter 10

Dysgraphia

What Is Dysgraphia?

Dysgraphia is a neurological disorder characterized by writing disabilities. Specifically, the disorder causes a person's writing to be distorted or incorrect. In children, the disorder generally emerges when they are first introduced to writing. They make inappropriately sized and spaced letters, or write wrong or misspelled words, despite thorough instruction. Children with the disorder may have other learning disabilities; however, they usually have no social or other academic problems. Cases of dysgraphia in adults generally occur after some trauma. The cause of the disorder is unknown, but in adults, it is usually associated with damage to the parietal lobe of the brain.

Is There Any Treatment?

Treatment for dysgraphia varies and may include treatment for motor disorders to help control writing movements. Other treatments may address impaired memory or other neurological problems. Some physicians recommend that individuals with dysgraphia use computers to avoid the problems of handwriting.

This chapter contains text excerpted from the following sources: Text beginning with the heading "What is Dysgraphia?" is excerpted from "NINDS Dysgraphia Information Page," National Institute of Neurological Disorders and Stroke (NINDS), September 16, 2011. Reviewed June 2016; Text under the heading "What Teachers Should Know?" is excerpted from "Dysgraphia Special Needs Factsheet," © 1995–2016. The Nemours Foundation/KidsHealth®. Reprinted with permission.

What Is the Prognosis?

Some individuals with dysgraphia improve their writing ability, but for others, the disorder persists.

What Research Is Being Done?

The National Institute of Neurological Disorders and Stroke (NINDS) and other institutes of the National Institutes of Health (NIH) support dysgraphia research through grants to major medical institutions across the country. Much of this research focuses on finding better ways to treat, and ultimately, prevent dysgraphia.

What Teachers Should Know?

Regardless of their reading ability, people with dysgraphia have difficulty writing, and may have problems with spelling, writing legibly, or putting their thoughts on paper.

Kids and teens with dysgraphia may have:

- poor fine-motor skills
- visual-spacial difficulties
- language-processing deficits

Students with dysgraphia may:

- frequently misspell words or incorrectly place words on a page
- have an exceptionally slow and difficult time writing
- have an awkward pencil grip
- have messy or illegible handwriting
- have trouble taking notes or tests or completing their schoolwork
- avoid writing and become extremely frustrated with schoolwork

What Teachers Can Do?

If you think a student might have dysgraphia, recommend seeking an educational evaluation to a parent or guardian, an administrator, or a school counselor.

Writing is one of the most important keys to academic success. Give students with dysgraphia plenty of extra time to practice their writing skills. Teach them how to organize their thoughts and encourage them to edit and proofread their work.

If students continue to struggle with handwriting, try:

- using graph paper, wide-ruled paper, or paper with raised lines
- allowing students with dysgraphia to choose the writing utensils they are most comfortable with
- making sure the pencil is properly positioned, using a tripod grasp, which means the pencil should rest near the base of the thumb and be held in place with the thumb, index, and middle fingers (certain kinds of pencil grips can be helpful, too)
- modifying the writing utensil grip as needed
- recommending occupational therapy to help with writing skills

Additional accommodations may be necessary, including:

- giving more time to complete tests and written assignments
- allowing for oral and visual assessments of knowledge
- using assistive technology, such as word processing and note-taking software

Chapter 11

Dyslexia

Chapter Contents

Section 11.1

Dyslexia Basics

This section includes text excerpted from "Reading and Reading Disorders: Overview," *Eunice Kennedy Shriver* National Institute Child Health and Human Development (NICHD), February 28, 2014.

Dyslexia Overview

Reading is a skill that is important for communication, education, and most fields of work. Reading disorders interfere with people's ability to read and affect how they learn to read. The *Eunice Kennedy Shriver* National Institute Child Health and Human Development (NICHD) conducts and supports a variety of research aimed at understanding the process of reading and identifying the best ways to help people who struggle with reading. The institute also aims to understand the mechanisms of reading disorders and the best interventions for improving reading skills among people with these disorders.

Common Names

- Reading disabilities
- Reading disorders

Medical or Scientific Names

- Reading disabilities
- Reading disorders
- Developmental reading disorders
- Dyslexia
- Developmental dyslexia

What Is Reading?

Reading is the multicomponent process by which a person gets information from written letters and words. A person can read using sight or touch, such as when a vision-impaired person reads braille.

How Does Reading Work?

Reading is a complex, multipart process.

Phonemic Awareness

Spoken words are made up of smaller pieces of sound—called phonemes.

The English language has about 40 phonemes. When someone says a word, the sound comes out as one continuous stream (Figure 11.1). The brain must be able to separate the sound pieces. For example, the word "bag" has three phonemes—/b/, /æ/, and /g/. Understanding that words are made up of individual sounds is a key part of learning to read. This understanding is called **phonemic awareness.**

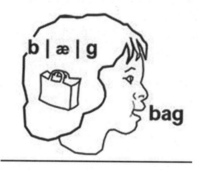

Figure 11.1. *Phonemes and Speech*

Phonemes make up spoken words, and words only make sense when these phonemes are combined in a particular order. Phonemic awareness can be taught and learned using activities such as rhyming games.

Another way to teach and learn this awareness is to work with single phonemes in spoken words, such as identifying the first sound in cat as /k/. Part of this learning is also realizing that a change to a single sound or phoneme can change the meaning of the word. For example, changing the /g/ in bag to a /t/ gives us the word bat, which has a different meaning from bag.

Alphabetic Principle and Phonics

Another part of learning to read (in alphabetic languages such as English) is understanding that letters of the alphabet, either by themselves or with other letters, stand for sounds or phonemes. This knowledge is called the alphabetic principle (Figure 11.2).

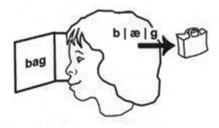

Figure 11.2. *The Alphabetic Principle*

When students learn how to apply their knowledge of the sounds in words (phonemic awareness), together with their skills at recognizing letters, and can use the letter-sound pairings to sound out printed words, it is called phonics.

To better understand phonics, think about how you read a made-up word like "blit" or "fratchet." Even though you don't know the made-up word or what it means, you can read it by figuring out what sounds the letters make, and then you can sound it out and pronounce it.

Phonemic awareness and phonics skills help readers sound out new words.

Vocabulary

Knowing that a word has meaning is an important part of learning to read. The words we know are called our **vocabulary**.

Learning vocabulary starts very early in life, such as when toddlers look at what you are talking about, or say their first words to get what they need or want. As toddlers grow, they learn more and more words. By the time they start to sound out words as part of learning to read, most children can recognize most of the words they are sounding out, recognizing that they have heard those words before and what the words mean. This is why having a good vocabulary is so important to reading.

Fluency

As a reader continues to develop phonics skills, a specific reading skill called fluency also improves. Fluency goes beyond just pronouncing or knowing words—it actually includes many parts, such as:

- Being able to read quickly

- Recognizing words and their meanings

- Saying words and sentences with feeling, and stressing the right word or phrase so that a sentence sounds natural and conveys the correct meaning

Comprehension

Understanding the information that words and sentences communicate is another important part of reading. This is called comprehension. Comprehension is actually the main goal of learning to read. There are many ways to improve comprehension:

- Building vocabulary can help a reader recognize more words and better understand the overall meaning of the text

- Understanding the structure of text-or how it is organized— helps readers know what to expect and where so that they can better comprehend what they are reading. Teachers show students different ways to understand the structure of the text in order to improve the students' comprehension

- Teachers can give students strategies or guidelines for understanding different types of texts, such as a newspaper, a fiction book, a textbook, or a menu

- Such strategies teach students to ask and answer questions about what they are reading, summarize paragraphs and stories they read, and draw conclusions about the information

Teaching students to think and write about what they are reading is an important way for them to use their skills to understand science, history, social studies, math, and many other subjects they will study throughout their education.

What Are Reading Disorders?

Reading disorders occur when a person has trouble with any part of the reading process. Reading and language-based learning disabilities are commonly called dyslexia. These disorders are present from a young age and usually result from specific differences in the way the brain processes language.

There are many different symptoms and types of reading disorders, and not everyone with a reading disorder has every symptom. People with reading disorders may have problems recognizing words that they already know and may also be poor spellers.

Other symptoms may include the following:

- Trouble with handwriting
- Difficulty reading quickly
- Problems reading with correct expression
- Problems understanding the written word

Reading disorders are not a type of intellectual and development disorder, and they are not a sign of lower intelligence or unwillingness to learn.

People with reading disorders may have other learning disabilities, too, including problems with writing or numbers.

Types of Reading Disorders

Dyslexia is a brain-based type of learning disability that specifically impairs a person's ability to read. Individuals with dyslexia typically read at levels significantly lower than expected despite having normal intelligence. Although the disorder varies from person to person, common characteristics among people with dyslexia are difficulty with phonological processing (the manipulation of sounds), spelling, and/or rapid visual-verbal responding. Dyslexia can be inherited in some families, and recent studies have identified a number of genes that may predispose an individual to developing dyslexia. Examples of specific types of reading disorders include:

- **Word decoding**. People who have difficulty sounding out written words; matching the letters to sounds to be able to read a word
- **Lack of fluency**. People who lack fluency have difficulty reading quickly, accurately, and with proper expression (if reading aloud)
- **Poor reading comprehension**. People with poor reading comprehension have trouble understanding what they read

A related problem is **alexia**, or an acquired inability to read. Unlike most reading disabilities, which are present from when a child starts to learn to read, people with alexia were once able to read but lost the ability after a stroke or an injury to the area of the brain involved with reading.

What Are the Symptoms of Reading Disorders?

Different people with reading disabilities have different combinations of symptoms and different areas of difficulty with reading.

The International Dyslexia Association lists the symptoms of dyslexia in people of different age groups. This list includes many different symptoms of reading disorders, such as problems with word decoding (sounding out words), comprehension, pronunciation, and fluency.

Symptoms can include:

- Problems sounding out words
- Difficulty recognizing known words
- Poor spelling
- Slow reading
- Problems reading out loud with correct expression
- Problems understanding what was just read

How Many People Are Affected by/at Risk for Reading Disorders?

According to the International Dyslexia Association (IDA), 5% to 6% of students in the United States receive special educational services for a disability in reading and language processing.

The IDA estimates, however, that up to 20% of the population as a whole has some of the symptoms of reading disorders.

How Are Reading Disorders Diagnosed?

Diagnosing reading disorders usually involves a series of tests of a person's memory, spelling abilities, visual perception, and reading skills. Family history, a child's history of response to instruction, IQ tests, and other assessments might also be involved.

The U.S. Department of Education (ED) offers services and assistance to support people with dyslexia and specific learning disabilities through its Office of Special Education Programs (OSEP).

The OSEP also supports the Parents Technical Assistance Center Network, which can help parents learn about their children's reading or other disabilities, assist them with connecting with and talking to professionals about their children's disabilities, and help them understand the laws and policies related to education for a child with a disability such as dyslexia.

What Causes Reading Disorders?

Research shows that reading disability is a specific, brain-based difficulty in learning to recognize and decipher printed words. But there is no single known cause of these difficulties.

Environmental factors—children's experiences in the classroom, for example, or whether they were read to every day as preschoolers—can play a significant role in most types of reading difficulty.

In addition, research suggests that difficulty with reading may be linked to a person's genetic makeup and, therefore, passed on from one generation to the next. For example, some cases of reading disability are associated with one or more alterations in genes that play a role in prenatal brain development.

What Are Common Treatments for Reading Disorders?

Early, intensive instruction in language and different aspects of reading by specialized teachers is the best way to improve reading skills. The most appropriate treatment strategy depends on the needs of the individual.

Reading disorders cannot be cured, but people with these disorders can overcome specific problems, learn to read, and improve fluency and comprehension with proper instruction, especially if they receive help and instruction early.

Because there is no single treatment for reading disorders, there is also no single resource that provides comprehensive information about treatment for reading disorders. However, a few good places to start are:

- U.S. Department of Education (ED), Institute of Education Sciences: What Works Clearinghouse

- U.S. Department of Education (ED), Office of Special Education and Rehabilitative Services

- International Dyslexia Association: Information on Interventions and Instructions

Where Can I Get Help for My Child's Reading Disorder?

Many organizations for people with reading and other learning disorders provide a wealth of resources to help these people and their parents get help.

A few places to start are:

- U.S. Department of Education (ED), Office of Special Education Programs (OSEP). OSEP offers services and assistance to support people with dyslexia and specific learning disabilities

- Parent Technical Assistance Center Network, also supported by OSEP. The Network can help parents learn about their children's reading or other disabilities, assist parents with connecting with and talking to professionals about their children's disabilities, and help parents understand the laws and policies related to education for a child with a disability, such as dyslexia

- National Dissemination Center for Children with Disabilities (NICHCY), offers information related to education for all kinds of disabilities, including reading disorders

- Special Education resources, maintained by the Learning Disabilities Association of America. These resources help parents understand the process of getting special education for their child and help them make sure the child is getting all the help he or she needs

- Help with Your Child, also maintained by the Learning Disabilities Association of America, provides a list of resources for parents of children with learning disabilities. These resources include descriptions of the professionals that may be able to help a child with reading disorders, tips for parents on helping their child at home, and resources for working effectively with teachers. It also offers information on special education

- The National Center for Learning Disabilities can help provide resources for getting your child evaluated at school and questions to ask an evaluator. It also provides information on dealing with daily living and parenting a child with a learning disability

Section 11.2

Dyslexia and the Brain: What Current Research Tells Us

This section includes text excerpted from "NICHD-Supported Research Sheds Light on a Family of Genes Involved in Dyslexia, Respiratory Health, and Organ Position," *Eunice Kennedy Shriver* National Institute Child Health and Human Development (NICHD), May 19, 2014.

Study of the CCDC40 Gene and Primary Ciliary Dyskinesia

In 2011, several researchers supported by the *Eunice Kennedy Shriver* National Institute Child Health and Human Development (NICHD), Developmental Biology and Structural Variation Branch (DBSVB) who were studying a gene called ccdc40 in zebrafish and mice learned that the gene is involved in development of cilia and also affects organ positioning during fetal development. The collaborators consulted Heymut Omran, M.D., then at the University of Freiburg and now at the University of Muenster (Germany), who was following a group of patients with the rare condition primary ciliary dyskinesia (PCD).

Cilia are microscopic, hair-like structures in the airways that normally act to sweep bacteria out of the respiratory system. In PCD, the cilia are improperly formed and do not move properly. As a result, people with PCD are prone to getting serious infections of the ear, lung, and sinus.

Omran reported that the cilia in the animals with mutated versions of the ccdc40 gene looked just like the abnormal cilia of his patients with PCD. Genetic testing of the patients revealed that two-thirds of them also had mutations in the CCDC40 gene. Many of them also had congenital heart defects and atypical positioning of the heart (with the heart on the right instead of the left side of the body), suggesting a possible genetic link between the cilia-induced respiratory disorder PCD and the heart problems seen in patients with this disorder.

That work was published in the journal Nature Genetics in 2011. According to Dr. Lorette Javois, director of the DBSVB's Program on Organogenesis (organ development), "This was a prime example of how our Branch's basic scientists work with clinicians to move the medical field forward by first learning what a dysfunctional gene does in an animal model and then in studying the gene in humans. This knowledge may contribute to new treatment strategies for PCD."

Study of the DYX1C1 Gene and Dyslexia

The Reading, Writing, and Related Learning Disabilities Program within the NICHD's Child Development and Behavior Branch (CDBB) focuses on altogether different conditions than PCD. Among the CDDB's research interests is the reading disorder dyslexia, which may be linked with abnormal migration of brain cells during fetal development. Individuals with dyslexia process language differently from most people. They may have trouble with handwriting, difficulty reading words accurately and with correct expression, and challenges with understanding the written word.

With NICHD support, a group of scientists was studying DYX1C1, a gene that seems be involved in dyslexia and in migration of brain cells during fetal development. They were "knocking out" (inactivating) the Dyx1c1 gene in zebrafish and mice, expecting to find abnormal brain cell migration patterns similar to those that have been found in human brains affected by dyslexia. While studying the animals, the scientists were surprised to observe instead that the animals' cilia did not function properly.

Based on the connection between mutations in CCDC40 and PCD, the scientists went on to investigate whether the DYX1C1 gene is also associated with PCD in humans.

Dr. Omran and Joseph J. LoTurco, Ph.D., of the University of Connecticut, in Storrs, led a team of more than 85 researchers in 7 countries to learn more about the function of the DYX1C1 gene. Resources for this effort were provided by the NICHD as well as other parts of the NIH, including the National Heart, Lung, and Blood Institute; the National Institute for Mental Health; and the National Center for Advancing Translational Sciences. They learned that mutations in the DYX1C1 gene do disrupt the normal structure of cilia.

Genetic analyses confirmed that all 12 of Dr. Omran's PCD patients had altered forms of the DYX1C1 gene, although none of them had dyslexia. This finding suggests that having an altered form of the gene does not cause dyslexia directly, even though it may affect risk for the condition.

"It's remarkable how a single gene can play such a wide variety of roles, with an impact on many different kinds of functions," Dr. LoTurco said, referring to the role of DYX1C1 in the formation of cilia in animals and in neuronal migration in humans. In late 2013, the research team published its findings about the DYX1C1 gene in the journal Nature Genetics.

NICHD Fosters a Spectrum of Research Leading to Unique Observations

This research might lead to new methods for detecting PCD or dyslexia so that appropriate interventions can start early. Although these study findings do not have direct implications for understanding dyslexia, Dr. LoTurco said, the results do provide researchers with additional leads for investigating genetic patterns that may be linked to the reading disorder.

The NICHD provided support that helped bridge animal research carried out by basic scientists with clinical research focusing on human health.

"With its broad portfolio of research projects, the NICHD supports scientists working in diverse fields and using different research models—from animals to humans—to enable discoveries such as this one," explained Brett Miller, Ph.D., director of the Reading, Writing, and Related Learning Disabilities Program within the CDBB.

He also underscored the importance of continuing research on DYX1C1 and CCDC40: "DBSVB and CDDB are two very different branches, but we're both supporting research that's converging on this family of genes and showing their importance in normal development."

Section 11.3

The READ Act Legislation on Dyslexia

This section includes text excerpted from "Bipartisan READ Act Provides Millions with Dyslexia a Brighter Future," Committee on Science, Space, and Technology, October 26, 2015.

Bipartisan READ Act Provides Millions with Dyslexia a Brighter Future

The House of Representatives unanimously approved the *Research Excellence and Advancements for Dyslexia Act (the READ Act)*, a bipartisan bill introduced by Science, Space, and Technology Committee Chairman Lamar Smith (R-Texas) on October 26, 2015 in Washington, D.C. Dyslexia affects an estimated 8.5 million school children and one in six Americans in some form. *The READ Act* supports important research to further our understanding of dyslexia, including better methods for early detection and teacher training. The bill passed out of Committee on October 8 with unanimous support.

Chairman Smith: "Despite the prevalence of dyslexia, many Americans remain undiagnosed, untreated and silently struggle at school or work. Too many children undiagnosed with dyslexia have difficulties in the classroom and sometimes drop out of school and face uncertain futures. Today we can shine a light on dyslexia and help millions of Americans have a brighter and more prosperous future. We need to enable those with dyslexia to achieve their maximum potential. *The READ Act* will help accomplish this."

The READ Act requires the president's annual budget request to Congress to include a line item for the Research in Disabilities Education program of the National Science Foundation (NSF). It also requires the NSF to devote at least $5 million annually to dyslexia research, which would focus on best practices in the following areas:

- Early identification of children and students with dyslexia

- Professional development about dyslexia for teachers and administrators

- Curricula development and evidence-based educational tools for children with dyslexia

The READ Act authorizes multi-directorate, merit-reviewed, and competitively awarded dyslexia research projects using funds appropriated for the NSF Research and Related Activities account and the Education and Human Resources Directorate.

Chairman Smith introduced *the READ Act* with Rep. Julia Brownley (D-Calif.), who are co-chairs of the bipartisan Congressional Dyslexia Caucus. The Caucus is comprised of over 100 Members of Congress and is dedicated to increasing public awareness about dyslexia and ensuring all students have equal educational opportunities.

Chapter 12

Gifted but Learning Disabled

Identification of Gifted/Learning Disabled (GLD)

The identification of gifted/learning disabled (GLD) students is not a straightforward process. A student with two exceptionalities is often described as twice exceptional and these students have been noted throughout our history. Many of these GLD people have made significant contributions to our society. For instance, Goldstein *(A diamond in the rough)* reminds us that,

Despite Einstein's brilliance in visual and spatial reasoning and problem-solving, researcher Bernard M. Patten wrote, as a schoolboy he had behavioral problems, was a rotten speller, and had trouble expressing himself. His report cards were dismal.

It is these traits that are often linked to the twice exceptional or GLD person. The gifted/learning disabled have been identified as a unique group of individuals with unique educational needs for three decades; however, identification and programming strategies have remained elusive for this particular group of students. To achieve, these students require remediation in their areas of need or disability while at the same time they require opportunities to enhance their strengths in their areas of giftedness.

Gifted/learning disabled students are also students at risk. Baum has previously explained that school comes easily for these students

This section includes text excerpted from "The Challenge of Identifying Gifted/ Learning Disabled Students," Education Resources Information Center (ERIC), U.S. Department of Education (ED), March 2013.

yet they are often unprepared for the challenges their disabilities create when they are presented with higher-level tasks as they progress in school. This ability/disability can produce, among many possible emotions and behaviors, frustration, anger, depression, carelessness, off-task behavior, and classroom disruption. These students may also suffer from low self-esteem and Waldron, Saphir, and Rosenblum point out that these students can feel they are a disappointment to their teachers and parents and tend to focus on what they cannot do, rather on what they can do.

Definitions

Learning Disabled

Learning disabled refer to a number of disorders which may affect the acquisition, organization, retention, understanding or use of verbal or nonverbal information. These disorders affect learning in individuals who otherwise demonstrate at least average abilities essential for thinking and/or reasoning. As such, learning disabilities are distinct from global intellectual deficiency. Learning disabilities result from impairments in one or more processes related to perceiving, thinking, remembering or learning. . . . . These disorders are not due primarily to hearing and/or vision problems, socio-economic factors, cultural or linguistic differences, lack of motivation or ineffective teaching.

In addition,

A learning disorder [be] evident in both academic and social situations . . . [and] involves one or more of the processes necessary for the proper use of spoken language or the symbols of communication, and is characterized by a condition that

a) is not primarily the result of:
   – impairment of vision;
   – impairment of hearing;
   – physical disability;
   – developmental disability;
   – primary emotional disturbance;
   – cultural difference; and
b) results in a significant discrepancy between academic achievement and assessed intellectual ability, with deficits in one or more of the following:
   – receptive language (listening, reading);
   – language processing (thinking, conceptualizing, integrating);
   – expressive language (talking, spelling, writing);
   – mathematical computations.

c) may be associated with one or more conditions diagnosed as:
 – a perceptual handicap;
 – a brain injury;
 – minimal brain dysfunction;
 – dyslexia;
 – developmental aphasia.

Gifted

Giftedness as exceptional potential and/or performance across a wide range of abilities in one or more of the following areas:

- general intellectual
- specific academic
- creative thinking
- social
- musical
- artistic
- kinesthetic

Exactly how to measure this is not indicated however the need to focus on the exceptional potential and/or performance in general intellectual and specific academic abilities is clear.

A gifted student have, an unusually advanced degree of general intellectual ability that requires differentiated learning experiences of a depth and breadth beyond those normally provided in the regular school program to satisfy the level of educational potential indicated.

Gifted / Learning Disabled

Combining the definitions for gifted and learning disabled results in the following definition for gifted/disabled that will be used for the remainder of this discussion. A gifted/learning disabled (GLD) student is a student of superior intellectual ability who demonstrates a significant discrepancy between their level of performance in a particular academic area and their expected level of performance based on their intellectual ability. In addition to superior intellectual ability and a performance/potential discrepancy, a processing deficit is also evident.

Although GLD students have been identified as a unique group since the 1970's, they remain under identified in the population of

115

disabled students. Because criteria used to establish giftedness varies between school jurisdictions, it is difficult to make identification comparisons. It is also difficult to establish common identification criteria. In sum, the characteristics of the gifted/learning disabled can impinge negatively on the identification process.

Three types of Gifted / Learning Disabled (GLD)

Because of their academic potential, the gifted/learning disabled student's achievement may not be as low as other students with learning disabilities. For this reason, they may be referred for special education less often than their non-gifted counterparts. Brody and Mills speculate that these students may fail to receive the specialized services they require because they fail to meet the criteria for either gifted or learning disabled programs. Gifted students are often able to compensate for their disabilities and are not achieving below grade level. They may not receive referrals unless there are behavioral issues. On the other hand, students who have learning disabilities may not be identified as gifted because they do not consistently display high achievement. Looking at the reasons behind the lack of referrals, researchers have identified three different types of GLD students:

1. gifted with mild learning disabilities

2. gifted with severe learning disabilities

3. masked abilities and disabilities

Type I–Mild Learning Disability

The first type of GLD students are those who are gifted with mild learning disabilities. These students tend to do well throughout elementary school and often participate in gifted programs at that level. They do not run into difficulty until they must do higher level work in the area of their disability and may go through periods of underachievement. Because they have previously done well, they are often not identified as learning disabled, but may be looked upon as lazy, lacking motivation, or as having poor self-esteem. Baum does caution that these may be valid causes of underachievement and must be considered as well.

Type II–Severe Learning Disability

The second type of student has severe learning disabilities, but is also gifted. These students are often identified as learning disabled, but rarely identified as gifted. They are noted for what they cannot do, rather for what they can do and attention becomes focused on their problems. Unless they are correctly identified and provided with appropriate programming, it is difficult for these students to reach their full potential.

Type III–Masked Abilities and Disabilities

The final type of student is generally not identified as gifted or learning disabled. Their gifts mask their disabilities and their disabilities mask their gifts. As a result of this masking they appear average and are not often referred for evaluation. Without a formal assessment, the discrepancy between their ability and their achievement is not noticed. These students may perform at grade level, but do not reach their full potential. This third group presents an interesting challenge, as their disability may lower their IQ (intelligence quotient) score so significantly that even with testing they may not be identified as gifted.

Compensation

Further complicating the identification of gifted/learning disabled students is the idea of compensation. Gifted students are excellent problem solvers. The more abstract reasoning they have, the better able they are to use reasoning in place of modality strength to solve problems. Compensation can be unconscious or conscious. One part of the brain may take over when another part is damaged. In some cases, students may be taught specific compensation techniques. While compensation can help the student adapt, it can also make an accurate diagnosis of a learning disability more difficult.

Recommended Methods of Identification

A Multi-Faceted Approach

Determining the best method to identify gifted/learning disabled students is not an easy task due to their dual issues. Nielson, in reviewing the Twice-Exceptional Child Projects (a research project funded by the U.S. government), found that gifted/learning disabled student's scores on the WISC-R resembled their gifted peers, while their reading and written language ability more closely resembled that of learning disabled students. Brody and Mills suggest that since gifted/learning disabled students represent a variety of giftedness in combination with various forms of learning disabilities, one pattern or set of scores that identifies all gifted/learning disabled students is not very likely. There is however a set of characteristics that seems to apply across all gifted/learning disabled students that should be the focus when identifying these students:

1. evidence of an outstanding talent or ability

2. evidence of a discrepancy between expected and actual achievement

3. evidence of a processing deficit

Chapter 13

Nonverbal Learning Disability (NLD)

Overview

Nonverbal learning disability (NLD) is a brain-based learning disability where individuals have difficulty with abstract thinking, spatial relationships, and identifying and interpreting concepts and patterns. Nonverbal learning disability occurs in 0.1 to 1 percent of the general population. It is also called non-verbal learning disorder (NVLD) or a right-hemisphere learning disorder.

People use the spoken word in various ways. Sometimes they say exactly what they mean. Sometimes they expect the listener to pick up another meaning from their facial expression or tone of voice. Sometimes they expect the listener to fill in information from past experience or some other source of information. For example "I love rainy days" when said directly is the truth. But, if the same phrase is said with a frown or eye roll and a growly tone, the speaker is being sarcastic, and is really telling the listener that she hates rainy days. Finally, if the speaker says, "You know how I feel about rainy days," the listener is expected to fill in some previously learned information. A person with a nonverbal learning disability cannot interpret the facial expressions and tone of voice of the sarcasm and thus takes the untrue statement as true. Nor can the listener draw on a pattern of previously learned information, and thus truly does not know how the speaker feels.

Signs of NLD

Children with NLD tend to be very smart. They talk freely, develop large vocabularies in comparison to other children their age, memorize facts, and read early. Intelligence tests show high verbal IQ (intelligence quotient) but low performance IQ due to visual-spatial difficulties.

There are five main areas of weakness in people with NLD. People with NLD may not exhibit weakness in all five areas, nor may they exhibit them all at once. The weaknesses tend to become more obvious as children progress in school and are required to rely more on identifying patterns and less on memorized facts.

The five main areas of weakness have been identified as:

1. **Visual/Spatial Awareness.** Children with NLD may have problems estimating distance, size, and/or shape of objects. They may be clumsy, spill drinks, bump into people or objects, or not be able to catch a ball. They may also have a poor sense of direction, such as being able to distinguish left from right.

2. **Motor Skills.** Children with NLD may have trouble mastering basic motor skills both large (such as dressing themselves, running, or riding a bike) or small (such as writing or using scissors).

3. **Abstract Thinking.** Children with NLD may have difficulty seeing or understanding the big picture. They can read a story and relate the details, but cannot answer questions about how the details fit together.

4. **Conceptual Skills.** Children with NLD may have trouble grasping the larger concept of a situation. For example, determining how pieces of a puzzle fit together to make a whole or identifying the steps needed to solve a problem. This contributes to problems especially with math.

5. **Social Skills.** Children with NLD may have trouble making friends or socializing in a group. They may interrupt or behave inappropriately in social situations. They use previously learned skills to cope with new social situations, whether appropriate or not.

In addition, because NLD occurs in the right side of the brain, children with NLD may have a distorted sense of touch or feel and poor coordination on the left side of the body.

These areas of weakness are often masked in pre-school and the early elementary grades when students are learning basic (rote) skills like reading and arithmetic. By the fourth or fifth grade, when students are required to process what they read or remember patterns from previous examples, the weaknesses start to become evident. At the same time, these very smart children may start exhibiting behavioral problems brought on by frustration in not "getting it" or feelings of being a social reject.

Diagnosis of NLD

The diagnosis of NLD is controversial. NLD is not listed in the American Psychiatric Association's Diagnostic and Statistical Manual of Mental Disorders, 5th ed., the manual used by doctors and therapists to diagnose learning disabilities. Nor is NLD recognized as a disability covered by the Individuals with Disabilities Education Act (IDEA). Nonetheless, if a child is exhibiting signs of NLD, there are steps parents should take to identify the problem.

- **A medical exam.** A thorough physical examination and a discussion of the child's learning problems will help the doctor rule out any physical causes for the learning problems.

- **A mental health professional.** Most likely the family doctor will refer the child to a neurologist or other specialist. The specialist will talk to the parents and child about what is happening, and may administer a variety of tests in the areas of speech and language, motor skills, and visual-spatial relationships. The results coupled with information from the parents and child will help the specialist analyze the strengths and weaknesses associated with NLD and make a diagnosis.

As with many learning disorders, the symptoms of NLD vary from child to child, thus a comprehensive assessment is needed to determine the individual child's needs. With the input and support of learning professionals and therapists as well as the family, steps can be taken to help the student with NLD.

Help for NLD

It is important to work with the child's school specialists to develop accommodations for the child's NLD. Formal accommodations may be developed through an Individualized Education Program (IEP) or 504 plan. If the child does not qualify for either plan, informal accommodations may be made in the classroom. Classroom accommodations may include modifying homework assignments and tests for time and content, presenting lectures with PowerPoint slides so the student can see as well as hear the material being covered, and/or working with a reading specialist to read a passage aloud then extract key terms and ideas.

Parents can help their child in various ways that will make things easier for both the student and the family. They can:

- Establish structure and routine

- Give clear instructions

- Keep a chart of the day's activities, both social and academic

- Make transitions easier by giving logical, step-by-step explanations of what is going to happen (We are going to IHOP restaurant for dinner. We need to leave in an hour.)

- Break down tasks into small steps in a logical sequence

- Play games with the child to have her identify emotions from facial expressions or voice tone

- Avoid sarcasm, or if it happens, use the experience to help the child identify the signs of sarcasm

- Set up one-on-one play dates with another child who shares an interest with yours. Play dates should be structured, monitored, and time bound

- Avoid situations that may overwhelm the child with too much sensory input—noise, smell, activity

There are other sources of help for parents and students. Social skills groups help the student in social situations. Parent behavioral training helps parents learn how to collaborate with teachers. Occupational and physical therapy may help the child improve movement and writing skills as well as build tolerance for outside experiences. Cognitive therapy can help the child deal with anxiety, depression, and other mental health issues.

Although NLD presents many challenges for both the student and the family, there is help available and with patience and effort, there will be improvement.

References

1. Epstein, Varda. "Nonverbal Learning Disorder: Is This What Your Child Has?" Kars4Kids, July 1, 2015.

2. Miller, Caroline. "What Is Nonverbal Learning Disorder?" Child Mind Institute, 2016.

3. Patino, Erica. "Understanding Nonverbal Learning Disabilities," Understood, May 21, 2014.

4. "Quick Facts On Nonverbal Learning Disorder," Child Mind Institute, 2016.

5. Thompson, Sue. "Nonverbal Learning Disorders," LDonline, 1996.

Chapter 14

Speech, Language, and Communication Disorders

Chapter Contents

Section 14.1

Delayed Speech or Language Development

This section includes excerpts from "Delayed Speech or Language
Development," © 1995–2016. The Nemours Foundation/
KidsHealth®. Reprinted with permission.

Your son is two years old and still isn't talking. He says a few
words, but compared with his peers you think he's way behind. You
remember that his sister could put whole sentences together at the
same age. Hoping he will catch up, you postpone seeking professional
advice. Some kids are early walkers and some are early talkers, you
tell yourself. Nothing to worry about.

This scenario is common among parents of kids who are slow to
speak. Unless they observe other areas of "slowness" during early
development, parents may hesitate to seek advice. Some may excuse
the lack of talking by reassuring themselves that "he'll outgrow it" or
"she's just more interested in physical things."

Knowing what's "normal" and what's not in speech and language
development can help you figure out if you should be concerned or if
your child is right on schedule.

Normal Speech and Language Development

It's important to discuss early speech and language development,
as well as other developmental concerns, with your doctor at every
routine well-child visit. It can be difficult to tell whether a child is just
immature in his or her ability to communicate or has a problem that
requires professional attention.

These developmental norms may provide clues:

Before 12 Months

It's important for kids this age to be watched for signs that they're
using their voices to relate to their environment. Cooing and babbling
are early stages of speech development. As babies get older (often
around 9 months), they begin to string sounds together, incorporate

the different tones of speech, and say words like "mama" and "dada" (without really understanding what those words mean).

Before 12 months of age, babies also should be attentive to sound and begin to recognize names of common objects (bottle, binky, etc.). Babies who watch intently but don't react to sound may be showing signs of hearing loss.

By 12 to 15 Months

Kids this age should have a wide range of speech sounds in their babbling (like p, b, m, d, or n), begin to imitate and approximate sounds and words modeled by family members, and typically say one or more words (not including "mama" and "dada") spontaneously. Nouns usually come first, like "baby" and "ball." Your child also should be able to understand and follow simple one-step directions ("Please give me the toy," etc.).

From 18 to 24 Months

Though there is a lot of variability, most toddlers are saying about 20 words by 18 months and 50 or more words by the time they turn 2. By age 2, kids are starting to combine two words to make simple sentences, such as "baby crying" or "Daddy big." A 2-year-old should be able to identify common objects (in person and in pictures), points to eyes, ears, or nose when asked, and follow two-step commands ("Please pick up the toy and give it to me," for example).

From 2 to 3 Years

Parents often see huge gains in their child's speech. Your toddler's vocabulary should increase (to too many words to count) and he or she should routinely combine three or more words into sentences.

Comprehension also should increase—by 3 years of age, a child should begin to understand what it means to "put it on the table" or "put it under the bed." Your child also should begin to identify colors and comprehend descriptive concepts (big versus little, for example).

The Difference between Speech and Language

Speech and language are often confused, but there is a distinction between the two:

- Speech is the verbal expression of language and includes articulation, which is the way sounds and words are formed

- Language is much broader and refers to the entire system of expressing and receiving information in a way that's meaningful. It's understanding and being understood through communication — verbal, nonverbal, and written

Although problems in speech and language differ, they often overlap. A child with a language problem may be able to pronounce words well but be unable to put more than two words together. Another child's speech may be difficult to understand, but he or she may use words and phrases to express ideas. And another child may speak well but have difficulty following directions.

Warning Signs of a Possible Problem

If you're concerned about your child's speech and language development, there are some things to watch for. An infant who isn't responding to sound or who isn't vocalizing is of particular concern.

Between 12 and 24 months, reasons for concern include a child who:

- isn't using gestures, such as pointing or waving bye-bye, by 12 months
- prefers gestures over vocalizations to communicate at 18 months
- has trouble imitating sounds by 18 months
- has difficulty understanding simple verbal requests

Seek an evaluation if a child over 2 years old:

- can only imitate speech or actions and doesn't produce words or phrases spontaneously
- says only certain sounds or words repeatedly and can't use oral language to communicate more than his or her immediate needs
- can't follow simple directions
- has an unusual tone of voice (such as raspy or nasal sounding)
- is more difficult to understand than expected for his or her age. Parents and regular caregivers should understand about half of a child's speech at 2 years and about three quarters at 3 years. By 4 years old, a child should be mostly understood, even by people who don't know the child

Causes of Delayed Speech or Language

Many things can cause delays in speech and language development. Speech delays in an otherwise normally developing child can sometimes be caused by oral impairments, like problems with the tongue or palate (the roof of the mouth). A short frenulum (the fold beneath the tongue) can limit tongue movement for speech production.

Many kids with speech delays have oral-motor problems, meaning there's inefficient communication in the areas of the brain responsible for speech production. The child encounters difficulty using and coordinating the lips, tongue, and jaw to produce speech sounds. Speech may be the only problem or may be accompanied by other oral-motor problems such as feeding difficulties. A speech delay may also be a part of (instead of indicate) a more "global" (or general) developmental delay.

Hearing problems are also commonly related to delayed speech, which is why a child's hearing should be tested by an audiologist whenever there's a speech concern. A child who has trouble hearing may have trouble articulating as well as understanding, imitating, and using language.

Ear infections, especially chronic infections, can affect hearing ability. Simple ear infections that have been adequately treated, though, should have no effect on speech. And, as long as there is normal hearing in at least one ear, speech and language will develop normally.

What Speech-Language Pathologists Do?

If you or your doctor suspect that your child has a problem, early evaluation by a speech-language pathologist is crucial. Of course, if there turns out to be no problem after all, an evaluation can ease your fears.

Although you can seek out a speech-language pathologist on your own, your primary care doctor can refer you to one.

In conducting an evaluation, a speech-language pathologist will look at a child's speech and language skills within the context of total development. Besides observing your child, the speech-language pathologist will conduct standardized tests and scales, and look for milestones in speech and language development.

The speech-language pathologist will also assess:

- what your child understands (called receptive language)
- what your child can say (called expressive language)

- if your child is attempting to communicate in other ways, such as pointing, head shaking, gesturing, etc.

- sound development and clarity of speech

- your child's oral-motor status (how a child's mouth, tongue, palate, etc., work together for speech as well as eating and swallowing)

If the speech-language pathologist finds that your child needs speech therapy, your involvement will be very important. You can observe therapy sessions and learn to participate in the process. The speech therapist will show you how you can work with your child at home to improve speech and language skills.

Evaluation by a speech-language pathologist may find that your expectations are simply too high. Educational materials that outline developmental stages and milestones may help you look at your child more realistically.

What Parents Can Do?

Like so many other things, speech development is a mixture of nature and nurture. Genetic makeup will, in part, determine intelligence and speech and language development. However, a lot of it depends on environment. Is a child adequately stimulated at home or at childcare? Are there opportunities for communication exchange and participation? What kind of feedback does the child get?

When speech, language, hearing, or developmental problems do exist, early intervention can provide the help a child needs. And when you have a better understanding of why your child isn't talking, you can learn ways to encourage speech development.

Here are a few general tips to use at home:

- **Spend a lot of time communicating with your child**, even during infancy—talk, sing, and encourage imitation of sounds and gestures.

- **Read to your child**, starting as early as 6 months. You don't have to finish a whole book, but look for age-appropriate soft or board books or picture books that encourage kids to look while you name the pictures. Try starting with a classic book (such as Pat the *Bunny*, in which your child imitates the patting motion) or books with textures that kids can touch. Later, let your child point to recognizable pictures and try to name them. Then move on to nursery rhymes, which have rhythmic appeal. Progress to predictable books (such as *Brown Bear, Brown Bear*) that let kids anticipate what happens. Your little one may even start to memorize favorite stories.

• **Use everyday situations** to reinforce your child's speech and language. In other words, talk your way through the day. For example, name foods at the grocery store, explain what you're doing as you cook a meal or clean a room, point out objects around the house, and as you drive, point out sounds you hear. Ask questions and acknowledge your child's responses (even when they're hard to understand). Keep things simple, but never use "baby talk."

Whatever your child's age, recognizing and treating problems early on is the best approach to help with speech and language delays. With proper therapy and time, your child will likely be better able to communicate with you and the rest of the world.

Section 14.2

Apraxia of Speech

This section includes text excerpted from "NINDS Dysgraphia
Information Page," National Institute on Deafness
and Other Communication Disorders (NIDCD),
June 7, 2010. Reviewed June 2016.

What Is Apraxia of Speech?

Apraxia of speech, also known as verbal apraxia or dyspraxia, is a speech disorder in which a person has trouble saying what he or she wants to say correctly and consistently. It is not due to weakness or paralysis of the speech muscles (the muscles of the face, tongue, and lips). The severity of apraxia of speech can range from mild to severe.

What Are the Types and Causes of Apraxia?

There are two main types of speech apraxia: acquired apraxia of speech and developmental apraxia of speech. Acquired apraxia of speech can affect a person at any age, although it most typically occurs in adults. It is caused by damage to the parts of the brain that are involved in speaking, and involves the loss or impairment of existing speech abilities. The disorder may result from a stroke, head injury, tumor, or other illness affecting the brain. Acquired apraxia of speech may occur together with muscle weakness affecting speech production (dysarthria) or language difficulties caused by damage to the nervous system (aphasia).

Developmental apraxia of speech (DAS) occurs in children and is present from birth. It appears to affect more boys than girls. This speech disorder goes by several other names, including developmental verbal apraxia, developmental verbal dyspraxia, articulatory apraxia, and childhood apraxia of speech. DAS is different from what is known as a developmental delay of speech, in which a child follows the "typical" path of speech development but does so more slowly than normal.

The cause or causes of DAS are not yet known. Some scientists believe that DAS is a disorder related to a child's overall language development. Others believe it is a neurological disorder that affects the brain's ability to send the proper signals to move the muscles involved in speech. However, brain imaging and other studies have not found evidence of specific brain lesions or differences in brain structure in children with DAS. Children with DAS often have family members who have a history of communication disorders or learning disabilities. This observation and recent research findings suggest that genetic factors may play a role in the disorder.

What Are the Symptoms?

People with either form of apraxia of speech may have a number of different speech characteristics, or symptoms. One of the most notable symptoms is difficulty putting sounds and syllables together in the correct order to form words. Longer or more complex words are usually harder to say than shorter or simpler words. People with apraxia of speech also tend to make inconsistent mistakes when speaking. For example, they may say a difficult word correctly but then have trouble repeating it, or they may be able to say a particular sound one day and have trouble with the same sound the next day. People with apraxia of speech often appear to be groping for the right sound or word, and may try saying a word several times before they say it correctly. Another common characteristic of apraxia of speech is the incorrect use of "prosody"—that is, the varying rhythms, stresses, and inflections of speech that are used to help express meaning.

Children with developmental apraxia of speech generally can understand language much better than they are able to use language to express themselves. Some children with the disorder may also have other problems. These can include other speech problems, such as dysarthria; language problems such as poor vocabulary, incorrect grammar, and difficulty in clearly organizing spoken information; problems with reading, writing, spelling, or math; coordination or "motor-skill" problems; and chewing and swallowing difficulties.

The severity of both acquired and developmental apraxia of speech varies from person to person. Apraxia can be so mild that a person has trouble with very few speech sounds or only has occasional problems pronouncing words with many syllables. In the most severe cases, a person may not be able to communicate effectively with speech, and may need the help of alternative or additional communication methods.

How Is It Diagnosed?

Professionals known as speech-language pathologists play a key role in diagnosing and treating apraxia of speech. There is no single factor or test that can be used to diagnose apraxia. In addition, speech-language experts do not agree about which specific symptoms are part of developmental apraxia. The person making the diagnosis generally looks for the presence of some, or many, of a group of symptoms, including those described above. Ruling out other contributing factors, such as muscle weakness or language-comprehension problems, can also help with the diagnosis.

To diagnose developmental apraxia of speech, parents and professionals may need to observe a child's speech over a period of time. In formal testing for both acquired and developmental apraxia, the speech-language pathologist may ask the person to perform speech tasks such as repeating a particular word several times or repeating a list of words of increasing length (for example, love, loving, lovingly). For acquired apraxia of speech, a speech-language pathologist may also examine a person's ability to converse, read, write, and perform non-speech movements. Brain-imaging tests such as magnetic resonance imaging (MRI) may also be used to help distinguish acquired apraxia of speech from other communication disorders in people who have experienced brain damage.

How Is It Treated?

In some cases, people with acquired apraxia of speech recover some or all of their speech abilities on their own. This is called spontaneous recovery. Children with developmental apraxia of speech will not outgrow the problem on their own. Speech-language therapy is often helpful for these children and for people with acquired apraxia who do not spontaneously recover all of their speech abilities.

Speech-language pathologists use different approaches to treat apraxia of speech, and no single approach has been proven to be the most effective. Therapy is tailored to the individual and is designed to treat other speech or language problems that may occur together with apraxia. Each person responds differently to therapy, and some people will make more progress than others. People with apraxia of speech usually need frequent and intensive one-on-one therapy. Support and encouragement from family members and friends are also important.

In severe cases, people with acquired or developmental apraxia of speech may need to use other ways to express themselves. These might include formal or informal sign language, a language notebook with pictures or written words that the person can show to other people, or an electronic communication device such as a portable computer that writes and produces speech.

What Research Is Being Done?

Researchers are searching for the causes of developmental apraxia of speech, including the possible role of abnormalities in the brain or other parts of the nervous system. They are also looking for genetic factors that may play a role in DAS. Other research on DAS is aimed at identifying more specific criteria and new techniques that can be used to diagnose the disorder and distinguish it from other communication disorders. Research on acquired apraxia of speech includes studies to pinpoint the specific areas of the brain that are involved in the disorder. In addition, researchers are studying the effectiveness of various treatment approaches for acquired and developmental apraxia of speech.

Chapter 15

Visual Processing Disorders

Overview

Visual processing disorders are weaknesses in the brain functions that process visual input. Although the eyes are the organs that actually receive visual images in the form of light, the brain must process these images and make sense of them. People with visual processing issues may have good eyesight, but their brains do not accurately receive or interpret the visual signals from their eyes. These weaknesses can create challenges in many areas of life, from recognizing letters and symbols, to distinguishing objects in space, to remembering things that have been seen.

Although visual processing issues are common in children with learning disabilities—and especially those with dyslexia—they are not considered learning disabilities by themselves. Nevertheless, they can have an impact on many areas of learning, such as reading, writing, vocabulary, verbal expression, memory, and attention. In addition to affecting learning, visual processing issues can impact socialization and self-esteem. Although medical research has not uncovered the cause of visual processing issues, the evidence suggests that preterm birth, low birth weight, and traumatic brain injury may increase the likelihood of visual processing issues.

Symptoms

Visual processing issues can be difficult to recognize, but there are some relatively common symptoms in children, including:

- being clumsy, or bumping into things;
- experiencing difficulty writing or coloring within the lines;
- reversing or misreading letters, words, and numbers;
- difficulty remembering sequences or numbers or spelling of words;
- trouble paying attention to visual tasks or being distracted by visual information;
- showing a lack of interest in movies, television, or video presentations;
- having trouble with reading comprehension or remembering information when reading silently—especially when combined with strong verbal skills and oral comprehension;
- having trouble copying notes or recognizing changes in classroom displays, signs, or notices;
- skipping words or lines while reading;
- having weak math skills, confusing mathematical signs and symbols, or omitting steps in equations;
- frequently rubbing the eyes or complaining about eye strain.

Diagnosis

Diagnosing a visual processing disorder involves several steps. The first step is to take notes and keep records of the problems experienced by the child. The next step involves taking the child to a pediatrician or pediatric optometrist to conduct a basic vision test and look for health issues involving the eyes. If there are no significant problems with the child's eye health, the next step is to obtain a reference to a neuropsychologist.

Neuropsychologists are trained to diagnose visual processing issues and can perform tests to determine the extent to which these weaknesses may be affecting the child's development. Researchers have identified eight different types of visual processing disorders, each of which affects different skills and creates its own challenges. The types of visual processing issues include:

- Visual discrimination

People with this type of issue have trouble comparing similar items—such as letters, shapes, patterns, or objects—and telling the difference between them. They may mix up letters like *d* and *b*, or *h* and *n*.

- Visual sequencing

People with this type of visual processing issue have difficulty distinguishing the order of letters, numbers, words, symbols, or images. They may misread letters or have trouble keeping their place on the page while reading.

- Visual figure-ground discrimination

This type of issue is characterized by difficulty seeing a shape or image against a background. People with this issue may not be able to locate a certain piece of information on a page or screen.

- Visual memory

People with this type of issue have difficulty remembering what they have seen or read, whether recently (short term) or some time ago (long term). They may struggle with reading comprehension, spelling familiar words, typing, using a calculator, or recalling a phone number.

- Visual spatial relationships

People with this type of issue have trouble seeing where objects are positioned in space, whether in relation to themselves or to other objects. They may experience challenges in understanding distances, reading maps, judging time, or picturing the relationship of objects described in writing or in a spoken narrative.

- Visual closure

People with this type of issue have trouble recognizing familiar objects when only parts are visible. They may not be able to identify a face if the mouth is missing, for instance, or to recognize a familiar word if a letter is missing.

- Letter and symbol reversal

People with this issue tend to reverse letters or numbers when reading or writing. They may also struggle with letter formation.

• Visual-motor processing

People with this issue have difficulty coordinating bodily movements using feedback from the eyes. They may appear uncoordinated or clumsy and bump into things. They may also struggle to write within lines or copy from a blackboard.

Treatment

Although there is no cure for visual processing disorders, there are many different strategies that can help people improve their skills and adapt to the challenges they face. Teachers and paraprofessionals at school may offer valuable assistance for children who are diagnosed with visual processing issues. Some of these children may qualify for special education services and receive an Individualized Education Program (IEP), which outlines the specific supports the school must provide. Schools also may provide informal supports to meet the children's needs, such as allowing them to use books with large print or have tests read aloud.

Parents and caregivers can also help children with visual processing disorders improve their skills. Experts recommend writing out schedules and instructions in large print, with each step numbered clearly, and color coding important points. It is also important to provide plenty of opportunities for children to practice visual processing skills through fun activities. Playing with jigsaw puzzles and games, reading "seek and find" books like *Where's Waldo?*, creating maps and travel logs, playing catch or rolling a ball back and forth, and estimating distances using a tape measure are all examples of activities that hone visual processing skills.

References

1. Arky, Beth. "Understanding Visual Processing Issues," Understood, 2016.

2. "Visual Processing Disorders—In Detail," LD Online, 2015.

3. "Visual Processing Issues: What You're Seeing," Understood, 2016.

Part Three

Other Disorders That Make
Learning Difficult

Chapter 16

Aphasia

What is Aphasia?

Aphasia is a neurological disorder caused by damage to the portions of the brain that are responsible for language. Primary signs of the disorder include difficulty in expressing oneself when speaking, trouble understanding speech, and difficulty with reading and writing. Aphasia is not a disease, but a symptom of brain damage. Most commonly seen in adults who have suffered a stroke, aphasia can also result from a brain tumor, infection, head injury, or dementia that damages the brain. It is estimated that about one million people in the United States today suffer from aphasia. The type and severity of language dysfunction depends on the precise location and extent of the damaged brain tissue.

What Are the Categories of Aphasia?

Generally, aphasia can be divided into four broad categories:

1. **Expressive aphasia** involves difficulty in conveying thoughts through speech or writing. The patient knows what he wants to say, but cannot find the words he needs.

This chapter includes text excerpted from "NINDS Aphasia Information Page," National Institute of Neurological Disorders and Stroke (NINDS), September 11, 2015.

2. **Receptive aphasia** involves difficulty understanding spoken or written language. The patient hears the voice or sees the print but cannot make sense of the words.

3. Patients with **anomic or amnesia aphasia**, the least severe form of aphasia, have difficulty in using the correct names for particular objects, people, places, or events.

4. **Global aphasia** results from severe and extensive damage to the language areas of the brain. Patients lose almost all language function, both comprehension and expression. They cannot speak or understand speech, nor can they read or write.

Is There Any Treatment?

In some instances, an individual will completely recover from aphasia without treatment. In most cases, however, language therapy should begin as soon as possible and be tailored to the individual needs of the patient. Rehabilitation with a speech pathologist involves extensive exercises in which patients read, write, follow directions, and repeat what they hear. Computer-aided therapy may supplement standard language therapy.

What Is the Prognosis?

The outcome of aphasia is difficult to predict given the wide range of variability of the condition. Generally, people who are younger or have less extensive brain damage fare better. The location of the injury is also important and is another clue to prognosis. In general, patients tend to recover skills in language comprehension more completely than those skills involving expression.

What Research Is Being Done?

The National Institute of Neurological Disorders and Stroke and the National Institute on Deafness and Other Communication Disorders conduct and support a broad range of scientific investigations to increase our understanding of aphasia, find better treatments, and discover improved methods to restore lost function to people who have aphasia.

Chapter 17

Attention Deficit Hyperactivity Disorder (ADHD)

Chapter Contents

Section 17.1

About Attention Deficit Hyperactivity Disorder

This section includes text excerpted from "Attention Deficit
Hyperactivity Disorder," National Institute of Mental
Health (NIMH), March 2016.

Definition

Attention deficit hyperactivity disorder (ADHD) is a brain disorder marked by an ongoing pattern of inattention and/or hyperactivity-impulsivity that interferes with functioning or development.

- **Inattention** means a person wanders off task, lacks persistence, has difficulty sustaining focus, and is disorganized; and these problems are not due to defiance or lack of comprehension.

- **Hyperactivity** means a person seems to move about constantly, including situations in which it is not appropriate when it is not appropriate, excessively fidgets, taps, or talks. In adults, it may be extreme restlessness or wearing others out with their activity.

- **Impulsivity** means a person makes hasty actions that occur in the moment without first thinking about them and that may have high potential for harm; or a desire for immediate rewards or inability to delay gratification. An impulsive person may be socially intrusive and excessively interrupt others or make important decisions without considering the long-term consequences.

Signs and Symptoms

Inattention and hyperactivity/impulsivity are the key behaviors of ADHD. Some people with ADHD only have problems with one of the behaviors, while others have both inattention and hyperactivity-impulsivity. Most children have the combined type of ADHD.

In preschool, the most common ADHD symptom is hyperactivity.

It is normal to have some inattention, unfocused motor activity and impulsivity, but for people with ADHD, these behaviors:

- are more severe.
- occur more often.
- interfere with or reduce the quality of how they functions socially, at school, or in a job.

Inattention

People with symptoms of inattention may often:

- Overlook or miss details, make careless mistakes in schoolwork, at work, or during other activities.
- Have problems sustaining attention in tasks or play, including conversations, lectures, or lengthy reading.
- Not seem to listen when spoken to directly.
- Not follow through on instructions and fail to finish schoolwork, chores, or duties in the workplace or start tasks but quickly lose focus and get easily sidetracked.
- Have problems organizing tasks and activities, such as what to do in sequence, keeping materials and belongings in order, having messy work and poor time management, and failing to meet deadlines.
- Avoid or dislike tasks that require sustained mental effort, such as schoolwork or homework, or for teens and older adults, preparing reports, completing forms or reviewing lengthy papers.
- Lose things necessary for tasks or activities, such as school supplies, pencils, books, tools, wallets, keys, paperwork, eyeglasses, and cell phones.
- Be easily distracted by unrelated thoughts or stimuli.
- Be forgetful in daily activities, such as chores, errands, returning calls, and keeping appointments.

Hyperactivity-Impulsivity

People with symptoms of hyperactivity-impulsivity may often:

- Fidget and squirm in their seats.
- Leave their seats in situations when staying seated is expected, such as in the classroom or in the office.

- Run or dash around or climb in situations where it is inappropriate or, in teens and adults, often feel restless.

- Be unable to play or engage in hobbies quietly.

- Be constantly in motion or "on the go," or act as if "driven by a motor."

- Talk nonstop.

- Blurt out an answer before a question has been completed, finish other people's sentences, or speak without waiting for a turn in conversation.

- Have trouble waiting his or her turn.

- Interrupt or intrude on others, for example in conversations, games, or activities.

Diagnosis of ADHD requires a comprehensive evaluation by a licensed clinician, such as a pediatrician, psychologist, or psychiatrist with expertise in ADHD. For a person to receive a diagnosis of ADHD, the symptoms of inattention and/or hyperactivity-impulsivity must be chronic or long-lasting, impair the person's functioning, and cause the person to fall behind normal development for his or her age. The doctor will also ensure that any ADHD symptoms are not due to another medical or psychiatric condition. Most children with ADHD receive a diagnosis during the elementary school years. For an adolescent or adult to receive a diagnosis of ADHD, the symptoms need to have been present prior to age 12.

ADHD symptoms can appear as early as between the ages of three and six and can continue through adolescence and adulthood. Symptoms of ADHD can be mistaken for emotional or disciplinary problems or missed entirely in quiet, well-behaved children, leading to a delay in diagnosis. Adults with undiagnosed ADHD may have a history of poor academic performance, problems at work, or difficult or failed relationships.

ADHD symptoms can change over time as a person ages. In young children with ADHD, hyperactivity-impulsivity is the most predominant symptom. As a child reaches elementary school, the symptom of inattention may become more prominent and cause the child to struggle academically. In adolescence, hyperactivity seems to lessen and may show more often as feelings of restlessness or fidgeting, but inattention and impulsivity may remain. Many adolescents with ADHD also struggle with relationships and antisocial behaviors. Inattention, restlessness, and impulsivity tend to persist into adulthood.

Risk Factors

Scientists are not sure what causes ADHD. Like many other illnesses, a number of factors can contribute to ADHD, such as:

- Genes.
- Cigarette smoking, alcohol use, or drug use during pregnancy.
- Exposure to environmental toxins during pregnancy.
- Exposure to environmental toxins, such as high levels of lead, at a young age.
- Low birth weight.
- Brain injuries.

ADHD is more common in males than females, and females with ADHD are more likely to have problems primarily with inattention. Other conditions, such as learning disabilities, anxiety disorder, conduct disorder, depression, and substance abuse, are common in people with ADHD.

Treatment and Therapies

While there is no cure for ADHD, currently available treatments can help reduce symptoms and improve functioning. Treatments include medication, psychotherapy, education or training, or a combination of treatments.

Medication

For many people, ADHD medications reduce hyperactivity and impulsivity and improve their ability to focus, work, and learn. Medication also may improve physical coordination. Sometimes several different medications or dosages must be tried before finding the right one that works for a particular person. Anyone taking medications must be monitored closely and carefully by their prescribing doctor.

Stimulants. The most common type of medication used for treating ADHD is called a "stimulant." Although it may seem unusual to treat ADHD with a medication that is considered a stimulant, it works because it increases the brain chemicals dopamine and norepinephrine, which play essential roles in thinking and attention.

Under medical supervision, stimulant medications are considered safe. However, there are risks and side effects, especially when misused or taken in excess of the prescribed dose. For example, stimulants can raise blood pressure and heart rate and increase anxiety. Therefore, a person with other health problems, including high blood pressure, seizures, heart disease, glaucoma, liver or kidney disease, or an anxiety disorder should tell their doctor before taking a stimulant.

Talk with a doctor if you see any of these side effects while taking stimulants:

- decreased appetite.

- sleep problems.

- tics (sudden, repetitive movements or sounds).

- personality changes.

- increased anxiety and irritability.

- stomachaches.

- headaches.

Non-stimulants. A few other ADHD medications are non-stimulants. These medications take longer to start working than stimulants, but can also improve focus, attention, and impulsivity in a person with ADHD. Doctors may prescribe a non-stimulant: when a person has bothersome side effects from stimulants; when a stimulant was not effective; or in combination with a stimulant to increase effectiveness.

Although not approved by the U.S. Food and Drug Administration (FDA) specifically for the treatment of ADHD, some antidepressants are sometimes used alone or in combination with a stimulant to treat ADHD. Antidepressants may help all of the symptoms of ADHD and can be prescribed if a patient has bothersome side effects from stimulants. Antidepressants can be helpful in combination with stimulants if a patient also has another condition, such as an anxiety disorder, depression, or another mood disorder.

Doctors and patients can work together to find the best medication, dose, or medication combination.

Psychotherapy

Adding psychotherapy to treat ADHD can help patients and their families to better cope with everyday problems.

Behavioral therapy is a type of psychotherapy that aims to help a person change his or her behavior. It might involve practical assistance, such as help organizing tasks or completing schoolwork, or working through emotionally difficult events. Behavioral therapy also teaches a person how to:

- monitor his or her own behavior.

- give oneself praise or rewards for acting in a desired way, such as controlling anger or thinking before acting.

Parents, teachers, and family members also can give positive or negative feedback for certain behaviors and help establish clear rules, chore lists, and other structured routines to help a person control his or her behavior. Therapists may also teach children social skills, such as how to wait their turn, share toys, ask for help, or respond to teasing. Learning to read facial expressions and the tone of voice in others, and how to respond appropriately can also be part of social skills training.

Cognitive behavioral therapy can also teach a person mindfulness techniques, or meditation. A person learns how to be aware and accepting of one's own thoughts and feelings to improve focus and concentration. The therapist also encourages the person with ADHD to adjust to the life changes that come with treatment, such as thinking before acting, or resisting the urge to take unnecessary risks.

Family and marital therapy can help family members and spouses find better ways to handle disruptive behaviors, to encourage behavior changes, and improve interactions with the patient.

Education and Training

Children and adults with ADHD need guidance and understanding from their parents, families, and teachers to reach their full potential and to succeed. For school-age children, frustration, blame, and anger may have built up within a family before a child is diagnosed. Parents and children may need special help to overcome negative feelings. Mental health professionals can educate parents about ADHD and how it affects a family. They also will help the child and his or her parents develop new skills, attitudes, and ways of relating to each other.

Parenting skills training (behavioral parent management training) teaches parents the skills they need to encourage and reward positive behaviors in their children. It helps parents learn how to use a system of rewards and consequences to change a child's behavior. Parents are taught to give immediate and positive feedback for behaviors they want to encourage, and ignore or redirect behaviors that they want to discourage. They may also learn to structure situations in ways that support desired behavior.

Stress management techniques can benefit parents of children with ADHD by increasing their ability to deal with frustration so that they can respond calmly to their child's behavior.

Support groups can help parents and families connect with others who have similar problems and concerns. Groups often meet regularly to share frustrations and successes, to exchange information about recommended specialists and strategies, and to talk with experts.

Tips to Help Kids and Adults with ADHD Stay Organized

For Kids

Parents and teachers can help kids with ADHD stay organized and follow directions with tools such as:

- Keeping a routine and a schedule. Keep the same routine every day, from wake-up time to bedtime. Include times for homework, outdoor play, and indoor activities. Keep the schedule on the refrigerator or on a bulletin board in the kitchen. Write changes on the schedule as far in advance as possible.

- Organizing everyday items. Have a place for everything, and keep everything in its place. This includes clothing, backpacks, and toys.

- Using homework and notebook organizers. Use organizers for school material and supplies. Stress to your child the importance of writing down assignments and bringing home the necessary books.

- Being clear and consistent. Children with ADHD need consistent rules they can understand and follow.

- Giving praise or rewards when rules are followed. Children with ADHD often receive and expect criticism. Look for good behavior, and praise it.

For Adults

A professional counselor or therapist can help an adult with ADHD learn how to organize his or her life with tools such as:

- Keeping routines.

- Making lists for different tasks and activities.

- Using a calendar for scheduling events.

- Using reminder notes.

- Assigning a special place for keys, bills, and paperwork.

- Breaking down large tasks into more manageable, smaller steps so that completing each part of the task provides a sense of accomplishment.

Join a Study

Clinical trials are research studies that look at new ways to prevent, detect, or treat diseases and conditions, including ADHD. During clinical trials, investigated treatments might be new drugs or new combinations of drugs, new surgical procedures or devices, or new ways to use existing treatments. In many trials, some participants are randomly assigned to the "control" group and receive an inactive "placebo" treatment or a standard intervention currently in use; sometimes the control subjects are later given a chance to try the experimental treatment. The object is to be able to compare the effect of the experimental treatment with standard or no treatment. The goal of clinical trials is to determine if a new test or treatment works and is safe. Although individual participants may benefit from being part of a clinical trial, participants should be aware that the primary purpose of a clinical trial is to gain new scientific knowledge so that others may be better helped in the future.

Section 17.2

ADHD and Other Conditions

This section includes text excerpted from "Attention-Deficit/
Hyperactivity Disorder (ADHD)," Centers for Disease Control
and Prevention (CDC), January 6, 2016.

Other Concerns and Conditions

Attention deficit hyperactivity disorder (ADHD) often occurs with other disorders. About half of children with ADHD referred to clinics have other disorders as well as ADHD.

The combination of ADHD with other disorders often presents extra challenges for children, parents, educators, and healthcare providers. Therefore, it is important for doctors to screen every child with ADHD for other disorders and problems. This page provides an overview of the more common conditions and concerns that can occur with ADHD. Talk with your doctor if you have concerns about your child's symptoms.

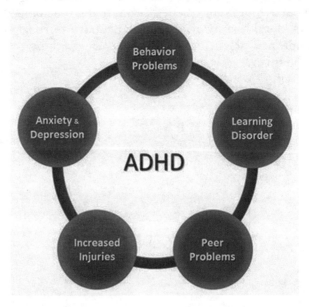

Figure 17.1. *Symptoms of ADHD*

Behavior or Conduct Problems

Children occasionally act angry or defiant around adults or respond aggressively when they are upset. When these behaviors persist over time, or are severe, they can become a behavior disorder. Children with ADHD are more likely to be diagnosed with a behavior disorder such as Oppositional Defiant Disorder (ODD) or Conduct Disorder (CD). About one in four children with ADHD have a diagnosed behavior disorder.

Oppositional Defiant Disorder

When children act out persistently so that it causes serious problems at home, in school, or with peers, they may be diagnosed with Oppositional Defiant Disorder (ODD). ODD is one of the most common disorders occurring with ADHD. ODD usually starts before eight years of age, but can also occur in adolescents. Children with ODD may be most likely to act oppositional or defiant around people they know well, such as family members or a regular care provider. Children with ODD show these behaviors more often than other children their age.

Examples of ODD behaviors include:

- Often losing their temper.

- Arguing with adults or refusing to comply with adults' rules or requests.

- Often getting angry, being resentful, or wanting to hurt someone who they feel has hurt them or caused problems for them.

- Deliberately annoying others; easily becoming annoyed with others.

- Often blaming other people for their own mistakes or misbehavior.

Conduct Disorder

Conduct Disorder (CD) is diagnosed when children show a behavioral pattern of aggression toward others, and serious violations of rules and social norms at home, in school, and with peers. These behaviors often lead to breaking the law and being jailed. Having ADHD makes a child more likely to be diagnosed with CD. Children with CD are more likely to get injured, and have difficulties getting along with peers.

Examples of CD behaviors include:

- Breaking serious rules, such as running away, staying out at night when told not to, or skipping school.
- Being aggressive in a way that causes harm, such as bullying, fighting, or being cruel to animals.
- Lying and stealing, or damaging other people's property on purpose.

Treatment for Disruptive Behavior Disorders

Starting treatment early is important. Treatment is most effective if it fits the needs of the child and family. The first step to treatment is to have a comprehensive evaluation by a mental health professional. Some of the signs of behavior problems, such as not following rules, are also signs of ADHD, so it is important to get a careful evaluation to see if a child has both conditions. For younger children, the treatment with the strongest evidence is behavioral parent training, where a therapist helps the parent learn effective ways to strengthen the parent-child relationship and respond to the child's behavior. For school-age children and teens, an often-used effective treatment is combination training and therapy that includes the child, the family, and the school. Sometimes medication is part of the treatment.

Learning Disorder

Many children with ADHD also have a learning disorder (LD). This is in addition to other symptoms of ADHD, such as difficulties paying attention, staying on task, or being organized, which also keep a child from doing well in school.

Having a learning disorder means that a child has a clear difficulty in one or more areas of learning, even when their intelligence is not affected. Learning disorders include:

- Dyslexia—difficulty with reading
- Dyscalculia—difficulty with math
- Dysgraphia—difficulty with writing

Data from the 2004-6 National Health Interview Survey suggests that almost half of children 6-17 years of age diagnosed with ADHD may also have LD. The combination of problems caused by ADHD and LD can make it particularly hard for a child to succeed in school.

Properly diagnosing each disorder is crucial, so that the child can get the right kind of help for each.

Treatment for Learning Disorders

Children with learning disorders often need extra help and instruction that is specialized for them. Having a learning disorder can qualify a child for special education services in school. Because children with ADHD often have difficulty in school, the first step is a careful evaluation to see if the problems are also caused by a learning disorder. Schools usually do their own testing to see if a child needs intervention. Parents, healthcare providers, and the school can work together to find the right referrals and treatment.

Anxiety and Depression

Anxiety

Many children have fears and worries. However, when a child experiences so many fears and worries that they interfere with school, home, or play activities, it is an anxiety disorder. Children with ADHD are more likely than those without to develop an anxiety disorder. Almost one in five children with ADHD have a diagnosed anxiety disorder.

Examples of anxiety disorders include:

- Separation anxiety—being very afraid when they are away from family

- Social anxiety—being very afraid of school and other places where they may meet people

- General anxiety—being very worried about the future and about bad things happening to them

Depression

Occasionally being sad or feeling hopeless is a part of every child's life. When children feel persistent sadness and hopelessness, it can cause problems. Children with ADHD are more likely than children without ADHD to develop childhood depression. Children may be more likely to feel hopeless and sad when they can't control their ADHD symptoms and the symptoms interfere with doing well at school or getting along with family and friends. About one in seven children with ADHD have a diagnosis of depression.

Examples of behaviors often seen when children are depressed include:

- Feeling sad or hopeless a lot of the time.
- Not wanting to do things that are fun.
- Having a hard time focusing.
- Feeling worthless or useless.

Children with ADHD already have a hard time focusing on things that are not very interesting to them. Depression can make it hard to focus on things that are normally fun. Changes in eating and sleeping habits can also be a sign of depression. For children with ADHD who take medication, changes in eating and sleeping can also be side-effects from the medication rather than signs of depression. Talk with your doctor if you have concerns.

Extreme depression can lead to thoughts of suicide. For youth ages 10-24 years, suicide is the leading form of death.

Treatment for Anxiety and Depression

The first step to treatment is to talk with a healthcare provider to get an evaluation. Some signs of depression, like having a hard time focusing, are also signs of ADHD, so it is important to get a careful evaluation to see if a child has both conditions. A mental health professional can develop a therapy plan that works best for the child and family. Early treatment is important, and can include child therapy, family therapy, or a combination of both. The school can also be included in therapy programs. For very young children, involving parents in treatment is very important. Cognitive behavioral therapy is one form of therapy that is used to treat anxiety or depression, particularly in older children. It helps the child change negative thoughts into more positive, effective ways of thinking. Consultation with a health provider can help determine if medication should also be part of the treatment.

Difficult Peer Relationships

ADHD can make peer relationships or friendships very difficult. Having friends is important to children's well-being and may be very important to their long-term development.

Although some children with ADHD have no trouble getting along with other children, others have difficulty in their relationships with their peers; for example, they might not have close friends, or might even be rejected by other children. Children who have difficulty making friends might also more likely have anxiety, behavioral and mood disorders, substance abuse, or delinquency as teenagers.

- Parents of children with ADHD report that their child has almost three times as many peer problems as a child without ADHD.

- Parents report that children with ADHD are almost ten times as likely to have difficulties that interfere with friendships.

How Does ADHD Interfere with Peer Relationships?

Exactly how ADHD contributes to social problems is not fully understood. Children who are inattentive sometimes seem shy or withdrawn to their peers. Children with symptoms of impulsivity/hyperactivity may be rejected by their peers because they are intrusive, may not wait their turn, or may act aggressively. In addition, children with ADHD are also more likely than those without ADHD to have other disorders that interfere with getting along with others.

Having ADHD Does Not Mean a Child Won't Have Friends

Not everyone with ADHD has difficulty getting along with others. For those children who do have difficulty, many things can be done to help them with relationships. The earlier a child's difficulties with peers are noticed, the more successful intervention may be. Although researchers don't have definitive answers on what works best for children with ADHD, some things parents might consider as they help their child build and strengthen peer relationships are:

- Pay attention to how children get along with peers. These relationships can be just as important as grades to school success.

- Regularly talk with people who play important roles in your child's life (such as teachers, school counselors, after-school activity leaders, healthcare providers, etc.). Keep updated on your child's social development in community and school settings.

- Involve your child in activities with other children. Talk with other parents, sports coaches and other involved adults about any progress or problems that may develop with your child.

- Peer programs can be helpful, particularly for older children and teenagers. Social skills training alone has not shown to be effective, but peer programs where children practice getting along with others can help. Schools and communities often have such programs available. You may want to talk to your healthcare provider and someone at your child's school about programs that might help.

Risk of Injuries

Children and adolescents with ADHD are likely to get hurt more often and more severely than peers without ADHD. Research indicates that children with ADHD are significantly more likely to

- Get injured while walking or riding a bicycle.

- Have head injuries.

- Injure more than one part of their body.

- Be hospitalized for unintentional poisoning.

- Be admitted to intensive care units or have an injury resulting in disability.

More research is needed to understand why children with ADHD get injured, but it is likely that being inattentive and impulsive puts children at risk. For example, a young child with ADHD may not look for oncoming traffic while riding a bicycle or crossing the street, or may do something dangerous without thinking of the possible consequences. Teenagers with ADHD who drive are more likely to have problems with driving, including breaking traffic rules, getting traffic tickets, and being in a crash than drivers without ADHD.

There are many ways to protect children from harm and keep them safe. Parents and other adults can take these steps to protect children with ADHD.

- Always have your child wear a helmet when riding a bike, skateboard, scooter, or skates. Remind children as often as necessary to watch for cars and to teach them how to be safe around traffic.

- Supervise children when they are involved in activities or in places where injuries are more likely, such as when climbing or when in or around a swimming pool.

- Keep potentially harmful household products, medications, and tools out of the reach of young children.

- Teens with ADHD are at extra risk when driving. They need to be extra careful to avoid distractions like driving with other teens in the car, talking on a cell phone, texting, eating, or playing with the radio. Like all teens, they need to avoid alcohol and drug use, and driving when drowsy.

• Parents should discuss rules of the road, why they are important to follow, and consequences for breaking them with their teens. Parents can create parent-teen driving agreements that put these rules in writing to set clear expectations and limits.

Chapter 18

Cerebral Palsy (CP)

Jennifer's Story

Jen was born 11 weeks early and weighed only 2½ pounds. The doctors were surprised to see what a strong, wiggly girl she was. But when Jen was just a few days old, she stopped breathing and was put on a ventilator. After 24 hours she was able to breathe on her own again. The doctors did a lot of tests to find out what had happened, but they couldn't find anything wrong. The rest of Jen's time in the hospital was quiet, and after two months she was able to go home. Everyone thought she would be just fine.

At home, Jen's mom noticed that Jen was really sloppy when she drank from her bottle. As the months went by, Jen's mom noticed other things she didn't remember seeing with Jen's older brother. At six months, Jen didn't hold her head up straight. She cried a lot and would go stiff with rage. When Jen went back for her six-month checkup, the doctor was concerned by what he saw and what Jen's mom told him. He suggested that Jen's mom take the little girl to a doctor who could look closely at Jen's development. Jen's mom took her to a *developmental specialist* who finally put a name to all the little things that hadn't seemed right with Jen–*cerebral palsy*.

What is Cerebral Palsy?

Cerebral palsy—also known as CP—is a condition caused by injury to the parts of the brain that control our ability to use our

---

This chapter includes text excerpted from "Cerebral Palsy," Early Childhood Learning & Knowledge Center (ECLKC), March 15, 2016.

muscles and bodies. Cerebral means having to do with the brain. Palsy means weakness or problems with using the muscles. Often the injury happens before birth, sometimes during delivery, or, like Jen, soon after being born.

CP can be mild, moderate, or severe. Mild CP may mean a child is clumsy. Moderate CP may mean the child walks with a limp. He or she may need a special leg brace or a cane. More severe CP can affect all parts of a child's physical abilities. A child with moderate or severe CP may have to use a wheelchair and other special equipment.

Sometimes children with CP can also have learning problems, problems with hearing or seeing (called sensory problems), or intellectual disabilities. Usually, the greater the injury to the brain, the more severe the CP. However, CP doesn't get worse over time, and most children with CP have a normal life span.

How Common is Cerebral Palsy?

Cerebral palsy occurs in approximately 2 per 1000 live births. This frequency rate hasn't changed in more than four decades, even with the significant advances in the medical care of newborns.

What Are the Signs of Cerebral Palsy?

There are four main types of CP:

1. *Spastic CP* is where there is too much muscle tone or tightness. Movements are stiff, especially in the legs, arms, and/or back. Children with this form of CP move their legs awkwardly, turning in or scissoring their legs as they try to walk. This form of CP occurs in 50-75% of all cases.

2. *Athetoid CP (also called dyskinetic CP)* can affect movements of the entire body. Typically, this form of CP involves slow, uncontrolled body movements and low muscle tone that makes it hard for the person to sit straight and walk. This form occurs in 10-20% of all cases.

3. *Ataxic CP* involves poor coordination, balance, and depth perception and occurs in approximately 5-10% of all cases.

4. *Mixed CP* is a combination of the symptoms listed above. A child with mixed CP has both high and low tone muscle. Some

muscles are too tight, and others are too loose, creating a mix of stiffness and involuntary movements.

More words used to describe the different types of CP include:

- *Diplegia* — This means only the legs are affected.

- *Hemiplegia* — This means one half of the body (such as the right arm and leg) is affected.

- *Quadriplegia* — This means both arms and legs are affected, sometimes including the facial muscles and torso.

Is There Help Available?

Yes, there's a lot of help available, beginning with the free evaluation of the child. The nation's special education law, the Individuals with Disabilities Education Act (IDEA), requires that all children suspected of having a disability be evaluated without cost to their parents to determine if they do have a disability and, because of the disability, need special services under IDEA. Those special services are:

Early intervention A system of services to support infants and toddlers with disabilities (before their 3rd birthday) and their families.

Special education and related services Services available through the public school system for school-aged children, including preschoolers (ages 3-21).

Under IDEA, children with CP are usually found eligible for services under the category of "Orthopedic Impairment." *IDEA's definition of orthopedic impairment reads as follows:*

...a severe orthopedic impairment that adversely affects a child's educational performance. The term includes impairments caused by a congenital anomaly, impairments caused by disease (e.g., poliomyelitis, bone tuberculosis), and impairments from other causes (e.g.,cerebral palsy, amputations, and fractures or burns that cause contractures).

To access early intervention services for a child up to his or her 3rd birthday, consult the Center for Parent Information and Resources (CIPR). You'll find a listing for early intervention under the first section, State Agencies. The agency listed there will be able to put you in contact with the early intervention program in your community.

To access special education services for a school-aged child, get in touch with your local public school system. Calling the elementary school in your neighborhood is an excellent place to start.

What about Treatment?

With early and ongoing treatment the effects of CP can be reduced. Many children learn how to get their bodies to work for them in other ways. For example, one infant whose CP keeps him from crawling may be able to get around by rolling from place to place.

Typically, children with CP may need different kinds of therapy, including:

- *Physical therapy (PT)*, which helps the child develop stronger muscles such as those in the legs and trunk. Through PT, the child works on skills such as walking, sitting, and keeping his or her balance.

- *Occupational therapy (OT)*, which helps the child develop fine motor skills such as dressing, feeding, writing, and other daily living tasks.

- *Speech-language pathology (S/L)*, which helps the child develop his or her communication skills. The child may work in particular on speaking, which may be difficult due to problems with muscle tone of the tongue and throat.

- All of these are available as related services in both early intervention programs (for very young children) and special education (for school-aged children).

Children with CP may also find a variety of special equipment helpful. For example, braces (also called AFOs) may be used to hold the foot in place when the child stands or walks. Custom splints can provide support to help a child use his or her hands. A variety of therapy equipment and adapted toys are available to help children play and have fun while they are working their bodies. Activities such as swimming or horseback riding can help strengthen weaker muscles and relax the tighter ones.

New medical treatments are being developed all the time. Sometimes surgery, Botox injections, or other medications can help lessen the effects of CP, but there is no cure for the condition. It's also important to understand that cerebral palsy is not contagious, not inherited, and not progressive. The symptoms will differ from person to person and change as children and their nervous systems mature.

What about School?

A child with CP can face many challenges in school and is likely to need individualized help. Fortunately, states are responsible for meeting the educational needs of children with disabilities.

As we've said, for children up to the 3rd birthday, services are provided through an early intervention system. Staff work with the child's family to develop what is known as an **Individualized Family Services Plan**, or IFSP. The IFSP will describe the child's unique needs as well as the services the child will receive to address those needs. The IFSP will also emphasize the unique needs of the family, so that parents and other family members will know how to help their young child with CP. Early intervention services may be provided on a sliding-fee basis, meaning that the costs to the family will depend upon their income.

For school-aged children, including preschoolers, special education and related services will be provided through the school system. School staff will work with the child's parents to develop an **Individualized Education Program**, or IEP. The IEP is similar to an IFSP in that it describes the child's unique needs and the services that have been designed to meet those needs. Special education and related services, which can include PT, OT, and speech-language pathology, are provided at no cost to parents.

In addition to therapy services and special equipment, children with CP may need what is known as assistive technology. Examples of assistive technology include:

- *Communication devices*, which can range from the simple to the sophisticated. Communication boards, for example, have pictures, symbols, letters, or words attached. The child communicates by pointing to or gazing at the pictures or symbols. Augmentative communication devices are more sophisticated and include voice synthesizers that enable the child to "talk" with others.

- *Computer technology*, which can range from electronic toys with special switches to sophisticated computer programs operated by simple switch pads or keyboard adaptations.

The ability of the brain to find new ways of working after an injury is remarkable. Even so, it can be difficult for parents to imagine what their child's future will be like. Good therapy and handling can help, but the most important "treatment" the child can receive is love and encouragement, with lots of typical childhood experiences, family, and friends. With the right mix of support, equipment, extra time, and accommodations, all children with CP can be successful learners and full participants in life.

Tips for Parents

- Learn about CP. The more you know, the more you can help yourself and your child. The resources and organizations listed at the end of this publication have a lot of information on CP to offer.

- Love and play with your child. Treat your son or daughter as you would a child without disabilities. Take your child places, read together, have fun.

- Learn from professionals and other parents how to meet your child's special needs, but try not to turn your lives into one round of therapy after another.

- Ask for help from family and friends. Caring for a child with CP is hard work. Teach others what to do and give them plenty of opportunities to practice while you take a break.

- Keep informed about new treatments and technologies that may help. New approaches are constantly being worked on and can make a huge difference to the quality of your child's life. However, be careful about unproven new "fads."

- Learn about assistive technology that can help your child. This may include a simple communication board to help your child express needs and desires, or may be as sophisticated as a computer with special software.

- Be patient, keep up your hope for improvement. Your child, like every child, has a whole lifetime to learn and grow.

- Work with professionals in early intervention or in your school to develop an IFSP or an IEP that reflects your child's needs and abilities. Be sure to include related services such as speech-language pathology, physical therapy, and occupational therapy if your child needs these. Don't forget about assistive technology either!

Tips for Teachers

- Learn more about CP. The resources and organizations listed organizations listed at the end of this publication have a lot of information about CP to offer.

- This may seem obvious, but sometimes the "look" of CP can give the mistaken impression that a child who has CP cannot learn as much as others. Focus on the individual child and learn first-hand what needs and capabilities he or she has.

- Tap into the strategies that teachers of students with learning disabilities use for their students. Become knowledgeable about different learning styles. Then you can use the approach best suited for a particular child, based upon that child's learning abilities as well as physical abilities.

- Be inventive. Ask yourself (and others), "How can I adapt this lesson for this child to maximize active, hands-on learning?"

- Learn to love assistive technology. Find experts within and outside your school to help you. Assistive technology can mean the difference between independence for your student or not.

- Always remember, parents are experts, too. Talk candidly with your student's parents. They can tell you a great deal about their daughter or son's special needs and abilities.

- Effective teamwork for the child with CP needs to bring together professionals with diverse backgrounds and expertise. The team must combine the knowledge of its members to plan, implement, and coordinate the child's services.

Chapter 19

Chromosomal Disorders

Chapter Contents

Section 19.1

Down Syndrome

This section includes text excerpted from "Birth Defects," Centers for
Disease Control and Prevention (CDC), March 3, 2016.

Facts about Down Syndrome

Down syndrome is a condition in which a person has an extra chromosome. Chromosomes are small "packages" of genes in the body.
Babies with Down syndrome have an extra copy of one of these chromosomes, chromosome 21.

Down Syndrome

Down syndrome is a condition in which a person has an extra chromosome. Chromosomes are small "packages" of genes in the body.
They determine how a baby's body forms during pregnancy and how
the baby's body functions as it grows in the womb and after birth.
Typically, a baby is born with 46 chromosomes. Babies with Down
syndrome have an extra copy of one of these chromosomes, chromosome 21. A medical term for having an extra copy of a chromosome is
'trisomy.' Down syndrome is also referred to as Trisomy 21. This extra
copy changes how the baby's body and brain develop, which can cause
both mental and physical challenges for the baby.

Even though people with Down syndrome might act and look similar, each person has different abilities. People with Down syndrome
usually have an IQ (intelligence quotient) in the mildly-to-moderately
low range and are slower to speak than other children.

Some common physical features of Down syndrome include:

- A flattened face, especially the bridge of the nose
- Almond-shaped eyes that slant up
- A short neck
- Small ears

- A tongue that tends to stick out of the mouth

- Tiny white spots on the iris (colored part) of the eye

- Small hands and feet

- A single line across the palm of the hand (palmar crease)

- Small pinky fingers that sometimes curve toward the thumb

- Poor muscle tone or loose joints

- Shorter in height as children and adults

Types of Down Syndrome

There are three types of Down syndrome. People often can't tell the difference between each type without looking at the chromosomes because the physical features and behaviors are similar.

- **Trisomy 21:** About 95% of people with Down syndrome have Trisomy 21. With this type of Down syndrome, each cell in the body has three separate copies of chromosome 21 instead of the usual 2 copies.

- **Translocation Down syndrome:** This type accounts for a small percentage of people with Down syndrome (about 3%). This occurs when an extra part or a whole extra chromosome 21 is present, but it is attached or "trans-located" to a different chromosome rather than being a separate chromosome 21.

- **Mosaic Down syndrome:** This type affects about 2% of the people with Down syndrome. Mosaic means mixture or combination. For children with mosaic Down syndrome, some of their cells have three copies of chromosome 21, but other cells have the typical two copies of chromosome 21. Children with mosaic Down syndrome may have the same features as other children with Down syndrome. However, they may have fewer features of the condition due to the presence of some (or many) cells with a typical number of chromosomes.

Other Problems

Many people with Down syndrome have the common facial features and no other major birth defects. However, some people with Down syndrome might have one or more major birth defects or other medical problems. Some of the more common health problems among children with Down syndrome are listed below.

- Hearing loss (up to 75% of people with Down syndrome may be affected)

- Obstructive sleep apnea, which is a condition where the person's breathing temporarily stops while asleep (between 50-75%)

- Ear infections (between 50-70%)

- Eye diseases (up to 60%), like cataracts and eye issues requiring glasses

- Heart defects present at birth (50%)

Other less common health problems among people with Down syndrome include:

- Intestinal blockage at birth requiring surgery

- Hip dislocation

- Thyroid disease

- Anemia (red blood cells can't carry enough oxygen to the body) and iron deficiency (anemia where the red blood cells don't have enough iron)

- Leukemia in infancy or early childhood

- Hirschsprung disease

Healthcare providers routinely monitor children with Down syndrome for these conditions. If they are diagnosed, treatment is offered.

Occurrence

Down syndrome remains the most common chromosomal condition diagnosed in the United States. Each year, about 6,000 babies born in the United States have Down syndrome. This means that Down syndrome occurs in about 1 out of every 700 babies.

Causes and Risk Factors

The extra chromosome 21 leads to the physical features and developmental challenges that can occur among people with Down syndrome. Researchers know that Down syndrome is caused by an extra chromosome, but no one knows for sure why Down syndrome occurs or how many different factors play a role.

One factor that increases the risk for having a baby with Down syndrome is the mother's age. Women who are 35 years or older when they become pregnant are more likely to have a pregnancy affected by Down syndrome than women who become pregnant at a younger age. However, the majority of babies with Down syndrome are born to mothers less than 35 years old, because there are many more births among younger women.

Diagnosis

There are two basic types of tests available to detect Down syndrome during pregnancy. Screening tests are one type and diagnostic tests are another type. A screening test can tell a woman and her health-care provider whether her pregnancy has a lower or higher chance of having Down syndrome. So screening tests help decide whether a diagnostic test might be needed. Screening tests do not provide an absolute diagnosis, but they are safer for the mother and the baby. Diagnostic tests can typically detect whether or not a baby will have Down syndrome, but they can be more risky for the mother and baby. Neither screening nor diagnostic tests can predict the full impact of Down syndrome on a baby; no one can predict this.

Screening Tests

Screening tests often include a combination of a blood test, which measures the amount of various substances in the mother's blood (e.g., MS-AFP, Triple Screen, Quad-screen), and an ultrasound, which creates a picture of the baby. During an ultrasound, one of the things the technician looks at is the fluid behind the baby's neck. Extra fluid in this region could indicate a genetic problem. These screening tests can help determine the baby's risk of Down syndrome. Rarely, screening tests can give an abnormal result even when there is nothing wrong with the baby. Sometimes, the test results are normal and yet they miss a problem that does exist.

A new test available since 2010 for certain chromosome problems, including Down syndrome, screens the mother's blood to detect small pieces of the developing baby's DNA (Deoxyribonucleic acid) that are circulating in the mother's blood. This test is recommended for women who are more likely to have a pregnancy affected by Down syndrome.

The test is typically completed during the first trimester (first three months of pregnancy) and it is becoming more widely available.

Diagnostic Tests

Diagnostic tests are usually performed after a positive screening test in order to confirm a Down syndrome diagnosis. Types of diagnostic tests include:

- Chorionic villus sampling (CVS)—examines material from the placenta

- Amniocentesis—examines the amniotic fluid (the fluid from the sac surrounding the baby)

- Percutaneous umbilical blood sampling (PUBS)—examines blood from the umbilical cord

These tests look for changes in the chromosomes that would indicate a Down syndrome diagnosis.

Treatments

Down syndrome is a lifelong condition. Services early in life will often help babies and children with Down syndrome to improve their physical and intellectual abilities. Most of these services focus on helping children with Down syndrome develop to their full potential. These services include speech, occupational, and physical therapy, and they are typically offered through early intervention programs in each state. Children with Down syndrome may also need extra help or attention in school, although many children are included in regular classes.

Section 19.2

47,XYY Syndrome

This section includes text excerpted from "47,XYY Syndrome,"
Genetics Home Reference (GHR), National Institutes
of Health (NIH), January 2009. Reviewed June 2016.

What Is 47,XYY Syndrome?

47,XYY syndrome is characterized by an extra copy of the Y chromosome in each of a male's cells. Although males with this condition may be taller than average, this chromosomal change typically causes no unusual physical features. Most males with 47,XYY syndrome have normal sexual development and are able to father children.

47,XYY syndrome is associated with an increased risk of learning disabilities and delayed development of speech and language skills. Delayed development of motor skills (such as sitting and walking), weak muscle tone (hypotonia), hand tremors or other involuntary movements (motor tics), and behavioral and emotional difficulties are also possible. These characteristics vary widely among affected boys and men.

A small percentage of males with 47,XYY syndrome are diagnosed with autistic spectrum disorders, which are developmental conditions that affect communication and social interaction.

How Common Is 47,XYY Syndrome?

This condition occurs in about 1 in 1,000 newborn boys. 5 to 10 boys with 47,XYY syndrome are born in the United States each day.

What Are the Genetic Changes Related to 47,XYY Syndrome?

People normally have 46 chromosomes in each cell. Two of the 46 chromosomes, known as X and Y, are called sex chromosomes because they help determine whether a person will develop male or female sex characteristics. Females typically have two X chromosomes (46,XX), and males have one X chromosome and one Y chromosome (46,XY).

175

47,XYY syndrome is caused by the presence of an extra copy of the Y chromosome in each of a male's cells. As a result of the extra Y chromosome, each cell has a total of 47 chromosomes instead of the usual 46. It is unclear why an extra copy of the Y chromosome is associated with tall stature, learning problems, and other features in some boys and men.

Some males with 47,XYY syndrome have an extra Y chromosome in only some of their cells. This phenomenon is called 46,XY/47,XYY mosaicism.

Can 47,XYY Syndrome Be Inherited?

Most cases of 47,XYY syndrome are not inherited. The chromosomal change usually occurs as a random event during the formation of sperm cells. An error in cell division called nondisjunction can result in sperm cells with an extra copy of the Y chromosome. If one of these atypical reproductive cells contributes to the genetic makeup of a child, the child will have an extra Y chromosome in each of the body's cells.

46,XY/47,XYY mosaicism is also not inherited. It occurs as a random event during cell division in early embryonic development. As a result, some of an affected person's cells have one X chromosome and one Y chromosome (46,XY), and other cells have one X chromosome and two Y chromosomes (47,XYY).

What Other Names Do People Use for 47,XYY Syndrome?

- Jacobs syndrome
- XYY Karyotype
- XYY syndrome
- YY syndrome

Section 19.3

Fragile X Syndrome (FXS)

This section includes text excerpted from "Fragile X
Syndrome (FXS)," Centers for Disease Control and
Prevention (CDC), April 15, 2015.

Facts about Fragile X Syndrome

Fragile X syndrome (FXS) is a genetic disorder. A genetic disorder
means that there are changes to the person's genes. FXS is caused by
changes in the fragile X mental retardation 1 (FMR1) gene. The FMR1
gene usually makes a protein called fragile X mental retardation protein (FMRP). FMRP is needed for normal brain development. People
who have FXS do not make this protein. People who have other fragile
X-associated disorders have changes in their FMR1 gene but usually
make some of the protein.

FXS affects both males and females. However, females often have
milder symptoms than males. The exact number of people who have
FXS is unknown, but it has been estimated that about 1 in 5,000 males
are born with the disorder.

Signs and Symptoms

Signs that a child might have FXS include:

- Developmental delays (not sitting, walking, or talking at the
  same time as other children the same age)

- Learning disabilities (trouble learning new skills)

- Social and behavior problems (such as not making eye contact,
  anxiety, trouble paying attention, hand flapping, acting, and
  speaking without thinking, and being very active)

Males who have FXS usually have some degree of intellectual disability that can range from mild to severe. Females with FXS can have
normal intelligence or some degree of intellectual disability. Autism spectrum disorders (ASDs) also occur more frequently in people with FXS.

Testing/Diagnosis

FXS can be diagnosed by testing a person's DNA (Deoxyribonucleic acid) from a blood test. A doctor or genetic counselor can order the test. Testing also can be done to find changes in the FMR1 gene that can lead to fragile X-associated disorders.

A diagnosis of FXS can be helpful to the family because it can provide a reason for a child's intellectual disabilities and behavior problems. This allows the family and other caregivers to learn more about the disorder and manage care so that the child can reach his or her full potential. However, the results of DNA tests can affect other family members and raise many issues. So, anyone who is thinking about FXS testing should consider having genetic counseling prior to getting tested.

Treatments

There is no cure for FXS. However, treatment services can help people learn important skills. Services can include therapy to learn to talk, walk, and interact with others. In addition, medicine can be used to help control some issues, such as behavior problems. To develop the best treatment plan, people with FXS, parents, and healthcare providers should work closely with one another, and with everyone involved in treatment and support—which may include teachers, childcare providers, coaches, therapists, and other family members. Taking advantage of all the resources available will help guide success.

Early Intervention Services

Early intervention services help children from birth to three years old (36 months) learn important skills. These services may improve a child's development. Even if the child has not been diagnosed with FXS, he or she may be eligible for services. These services are provided through an early intervention system in each state. Through this system, you can ask for an evaluation. In addition, treatment for particular symptoms, such as speech therapy for language delays, often does not need to wait for a formal diagnosis. While early intervention is extremely important, treatment services at any age can be helpful.

Finding Support

Having support and community resources can help increase confidence in managing FXS, enhance quality of life, and assist in meeting the needs of all family members. It might be helpful for parents of children with FXS to talk with one another. One parent might have learned how to address some of the same concerns another parent has. Often, parents of children with special needs can give advice about good resources for these children.

Remember that the choices of one family might not be best for another family, so it's important that parents understand all options and discuss them with their child's health care providers.

- Contact the National Fragile X Foundation at 1-800-688-8765 or ntlfx@fragilex.org to get information about treatments, educational strategies, therapies and intervention.

- Connect with a Community Support Network (CSN) at the National Fragile X Foundation. CSNs are organized and run by parent volunteers and provide support to families.

Section 19.4

Klinefelter Syndrome (KS)

This section includes text excerpted from "Klinefelter Syndrome (KS): Overview," Eunice Kennedy Shriver National Institute of Child Health and Human Development (NICHD), October 25, 2013.

Overview

Klinefelter syndrome (KS) describes a set of physical, language, and social development symptoms in males who have an extra X chromosome. Its main feature is infertility. Outward signs of KS can be subtle, so symptoms often are not recognized, and may not be treated in a timely manner. The *Eunice Kennedy Shriver* National Institute of Child Health and Human Development (NICHD) is one of many federal agencies and NIH Institutes working to understand KS, discover why it occurs, and identify and treat its symptoms.

Common Name

- Klinefelter syndrome

Medical or Scientific Names

- Klinefelter syndrome
- 47,XXY
- XXY syndrome or condition
- XXY trisomy
- 47,XXY/46,XY or mosaic syndrome (rare variation)
- Poly-X Klinefelter syndrome, including the following rare variations:
- 48,XXYY (or tetrasomy)
- 48,XXXY (or tetrasomy)
- 49,XXXXY (or pentasomy)

What is Klinefelter Syndrome?

The term "Klinefelter syndrome," or KS, describes a set of features that can occur in a male who is born with an extra X chromosome in his cells. It is named after Dr. Henry Klinefelter, who identified the condition in the 1940s.

Usually, every cell in a male's body, except sperm and red blood cells, contains 46 chromosomes. The 45th and 46th chromosomes—the X and Y chromosomes—are sometimes called "sex chromosomes" because they determine a person's sex. Normally, males have one X and one Y chromosome, making them XY. Males with KS have an extra X chromosome, making them XXY.

KS is sometimes called "47,XXY" (47 refers to total chromosomes) or the "XXY condition." Those with KS are sometimes called "XXY males."

Some males with KS may have both XY cells and XXY cells in their bodies. This is called "mosaic." Mosaic males may have fewer symptoms of KS depending on the number of XY cells they have in their bodies and where these cells are located. For example, males who have normal XY cells in their testes may be fertile.

In very rare cases, males might have two or more extra X chromosomes in their cells, for instance XXXY or XXXXY, or an extra Y, such as XXYY. This is called poly-X Klinefelter syndrome, and it causes more severe symptoms.

What Causes Klinefelter Syndrome (KS)?

The extra chromosome results from a random error that occurs when a sperm or egg is formed; this error causes an extra X cell to be included each time the cell divides to form new cells. In very rare cases, more than one extra X or an extra Y is included.

Language and Learning Problems in Klinefelter Syndrome

Most males with KS have normal intelligence quotients (IQs) and successfully complete education at all levels. (IQ is a frequently used intelligence measure, but does not include emotional, creative, or other types of intelligence.) Between 25% and 85% of all males with KS have some kind of learning or language-related problem, which makes it more likely that they will need some extra help in school. Without this help or intervention, KS males might fall behind their classmates as schoolwork becomes harder.

KS males may experience some of the following learning and language-related challenges:

- **A delay in learning to talk.** Infants with KS tend to make only a few different vocal sounds. As they grow older, they may have difficulty saying words clearly. It might be hard for them to distinguish differences between similar sounds.

- **Trouble using language to express their thoughts and needs.** Boys with KS might have problems putting their thoughts, ideas, and emotions into words. Some may find it hard to learn and remember some words, such as the names of common objects.

- **Trouble processing what they hear.** Although most boys with KS can understand what is being said to them, they might take longer to process multiple or complex sentences. In some cases, they might fidget or "tune out" because they take longer to process the information. It might also be difficult for KS males to concentrate in noisy settings. They might also be less able to understand a speaker's feelings from just speech alone.

- **Reading difficulties.** Many boys with KS have difficulty understanding what they read (called poor reading comprehension). They might also read more slowly than other boys.

By adulthood, most males with KS learn to speak and converse normally, although they may have a harder time doing work that involves extensive reading and writing.

Social and Behavioral Symptoms

Many of the social and behavioral symptoms in KS may result from the language and learning difficulties. For instance, boys with KS who have language difficulties might hold back socially and could use help building social relationships.

Boys with KS, compared to typically developing boys, tend to be:

- Quieter

- Less assertive or self-confident

- More anxious or restless

- Less physically active

- More helpful and eager to please

- More obedient or more ready to follow directions

In the teenage years, boys with KS may feel their differences more strongly. As a result, these teen boys are at higher risk of depression, substance abuse, and behavioral disorders. Some teens might withdraw, feel sad, or act out their frustration and anger.

As adults, most men with KS have lives similar to those of men without KS. They successfully complete high school, college, and other levels of education. They have successful and meaningful careers and professions. They have friends and families.

Contrary to research findings published several decades ago, males with KS are no more likely to have serious psychiatric disorders or to get into trouble with the law.

What Are the Treatments for Symptoms in Klinefelter Syndrome (KS)?

It's important to remember that because symptoms can be mild, many males with KS are never diagnosed ore treated.

The earlier in life that KS symptoms are recognized and treated, the more likely it is that the symptoms can be reduced or eliminated. It is especially helpful to begin treatment by early puberty. Puberty is a time of rapid physical and psychological change, and treatment can successfully limit symptoms. However, treatment can bring benefits at any age.

The type of treatment needed depends on the type of symptoms being treated.

Treating Language and Learning Symptoms

Some, but not all, children with KS have language development and learning delays. They might be slow to learn to talk, read, and write, and they might have difficulty processing what they hear. But various interventions, such as speech therapy and educational assistance, can help to reduce and even eliminate these difficulties. The earlier treatment begins, the better the outcomes.

Parents might need to bring these types of problems to the teacher's attention. Because these boys can be quiet and cooperative in the classroom, teachers may not notice the need for help.

Boys and men with KS can benefit by visiting therapists who are experts in areas such as coordination, social skills, and coping. XXY males might benefit from any or all of the following:

- **Physical therapists** design activities and exercises to build motor skills and strength and to improve muscle control, posture, and balance.

- **Occupational therapists** help build skills needed for daily functioning, such as social and play skills, interaction and conversation skills, and job or career skills that match interests and abilities.

- **Behavioral therapists** help with specific social skills, such as asking other kids to play and starting conversations. They can also teach productive ways of handling frustration, shyness, anger, and other emotions that can arise from feeling "different."

- **Mental health therapists or counselors** help males with KS find ways to cope with feelings of sadness, depression, self-doubt, and low self-esteem. They can also help with substance abuse problems. These professionals can also help families deal with the emotions of having a son with KS.

- **Family therapists** provide counseling to a man with KS, his spouse, partner, or family. They can help identify relationship problems and help patients develop communication skills and understand other people's needs.

Parents of XXY males have also mentioned that taking part in **physical activities at low-key levels**, such as karate, swimming, tennis, and golf, were helpful in improving motor skills, coordination, and confidence.

With regard to education, some boys with KS will qualify to receive state-sponsored special needs services to address their developmental and learning symptoms. But, because these symptoms may be mild, many XXY males will not be eligible for these services. Families can contact a local school district official or special education coordinator to learn more about whether XXY males can receive the following free services:

- **The Early Intervention Program for Infants and Toddlers with Disabilities** is required by two national laws, the Individuals with Disabilities and Education Improvement Act (IDEIA) and the Individuals with Disabilities Education Act (IDEA). Every state operates special programs for children from birth to age 3, helping them develop in areas such as behavior, development, communication, and social play.

- An **Individualized Education Plan (IEP)** for school is created and administered by a team of people, starting with parents and including teachers and school psychologists. The team works together to design an IEP with specific academic, communication, motor, learning, functional, and socialization goals, based on the child's educational needs and specific symptoms.

Treating Social and Behavioral Symptoms

Many of the professionals and methods for treating learning and language symptoms of the XXY condition are similar to or the same as the ones used to address social and behavioral symptoms.

For instance, boys with KS may need help with social skills and interacting in groups. Occupational or behavioral therapists might be able to assist with these skills. Some school districts and health centers might also offer these types of skill-building programs or classes.

In adolescence, symptoms such as lack of body hair could make XXY males uncomfortable in school or other social settings, and this discomfort can lead to depression, substance abuse, and behavioral problems or "acting out." They might also have questions about their masculinity or gender identity. In these instances, consulting a psychologist, counselor, or psychiatrist may be helpful.

Contrary to research results released decades ago, current research shows that XXY males are no more likely than other males to have serious psychiatric disorders or to get into trouble with the law.

How Do Health Care Providers Diagnose Klinefelter Syndrome (KS)?

The only way to confirm the presence of an extra chromosome is by a karyotype test. A health care provider will take a small blood or skin sample and send it to a laboratory, where a technician inspects the cells under a microscope to find the extra chromosome. A karyotype test shows the same results at any time in a person's life.

Tests for chromosome disorders, including KS, may be done before birth. To obtain tissue or liquid for this test, a pregnant woman undergoes chorionic villus sampling or amniocentesis. These types of prenatal testing carry a small risk for miscarriage and are not routinely conducted unless the woman has a family history of chromosomal disorders, has other medical problems, or is above 35 years of age.

Is there a cure for Klinefelter syndrome (KS)?

Currently, there is no way to remove chromosomes from cells to "cure" the XXY condition.

But many symptoms can be successfully treated, minimizing the impact the condition has on length and quality of life. Most adult XXY men have full independence and have friends, families, and normal social relationships. They live about as long as other men, on average.

Section 19.5

Prader-Willi Syndrome (PWS)

This section includes text excerpted from "Prader-Willi Syndrome (PWS): Overview," National Institute of Child Health and Human Development (NICHD), January 14, 2014.

Prader-Willi Syndrome (PWS) is the most common of the genetic disorders that cause life-threatening obesity in children. The syndrome affects many aspects of the person's life, including eating, behavior and mood, physical growth, and intellectual development. The *Eunice Kennedy Shriver* National Institute of Child Health and Human Development (NICHD) is one of many federal agencies and NIH Institutes working to understand PWS. The NICHD supports and conducts research on the factors that cause the syndrome and how best to diagnose and treat it.

Common Name

- Prader-Willi syndrome

Medical or Scientific Names

- Prader-Willi
- Prader-Labhart-Willi syndrome
- PWS
- Willi-Prader syndrome
- Prader-Willi-Fanconi syndrome
- PW

What is Prader-Willi Syndrome?

The term PWS refers to a genetic disorder that affects many parts of the body. Genetic testing can successfully diagnose 99% of infants with PWS.

The syndrome usually results from deletions or partial deletions on chromosome 15 that affect the regulation of gene expression, or how genes turn on and off. Andrea Prader and Heinrich Willi first described the syndrome in the 1950s.

One of the main symptoms of PWS is the inability to control eating. In fact, PWS is the leading genetic cause of life-threatening obesity. Other symptoms include low muscle tone and poor feeding as an infant, delays in intellectual development, and difficulty controlling emotions.

There is no cure for PWS, but people with the disorder can benefit from a variety of treatments to improve their symptoms. These treatments depend on the individual's needs, but they often include strict dietary supervision, physical therapy, behavioral therapy, and treatment with growth hormone, among others. As adults, people with PWS usually do best in special group homes for people with this disorder. Some can work in sheltered environments.

Intellectual Symptoms

Individuals with PWS have varying levels of intellectual disabilities. Learning disabilities are common, as are delays in starting to talk and in the development of language.

Behavioral and Psychiatric Problems in Prader-Willi Syndrome

Imbalances in hormone levels may contribute to behavioral and psychiatric problems. Behavioral problems may include temper tantrums, extreme stubbornness, obsessive-compulsive symptoms, picking the skin, and general trouble in controlling emotions. The individual will often repeat questions or statements. Sleep disturbances may include excessive daytime sleepiness and disruptions of sleep. Many individuals with PWS have a high pain threshold.

Stages of Prader-Willi Syndrome Symptoms

The appearance of PWS symptoms occurs in two recognized stages:

Stage 1 (Infancy to age 2 years)

- "Floppiness" and poor muscle tone
- Weak cries and a weak sucking reflex
- Inability to breastfeed, which may require feeding support, such as tube feeding
- Developmental delays
- Small genital organs

Stage 2 (Ages 2 to 8)

- Unable to feel satisfied with normal intake of food
- Inability to control eating, which can lead to overeating if not monitored
- Food-seeking behaviors
- Low metabolism
- Weight gain and obesity
- Daytime sleepiness and sleep problems

- Intellectual disabilities

- Small hands and feet

- Short stature

- Curvature of the spine (scoliosis)

- High pain threshold

- Behavioral problems, including the display of obsessive-compulsive symptoms, picking the skin, and difficulty controlling emotions

- Small genitals, often resulting in infertility in later life

What Causes Prader-Willi Syndrome (PWS)?

Prader-Willi syndrome is caused by genetic changes on an "unstable" region of chromosome 15 that affects the regulation of gene expression, or how genes turn on and off. This part of the chromosome is called unstable because it is prone to being shuffled around by the cell's genetic machinery before the chromosome is passed on from parent to child.

The genetic changes that cause Prader-Willi syndrome occur in a portion of the chromosome, referred to as the Prader-Willi critical region (PWCR), around the time of conception or during early fetal development.1 This region was identified in 1990 using genetic DNA probes. Although Prader-Willi syndrome is genetic, it usually is not inherited and generally develops due to deletions or partial deletions on chromosome 15.

Specific changes to the chromosome can include the following:

- **Deletions.** A section of a chromosome may be lost or deleted, along with the functions that this section supported. About 65% to 75% of Prader-Willi syndrome cases result from the loss of function of several genes in one region of the father's chromosome 15, due to deletion. The corresponding mother's genes on chromosome 15 are always inactive and thus cannot make up for the deletion on the father's chromosome 15. The missing paternal genes normally play a fundamental role in regulating hunger and fullness.

- **Maternal uniparental disomy**. A cell usually contains one set of chromosomes from the father and another set from the mother. In ordinary cases, a child has two chromosome 15s, one from each parent. In 20% to 30% of Prader-Willi syndrome cases, the child has two chromosome 15s from the mother and none from the father. Because genes located in the PWCR are normally inactive in the chromosome that comes from the mother, the child's lack of active genes in this region leads to Prader-Willi syndrome.

- **An imprinting center defect.** Genes in the PWCR on the chromosome that came from the mother are normally inactivated, due to a process known as "imprinting" that affects whether the cell is able to "read" a gene or not. In less than 5% of Prader-Willi syndrome cases, the chromosome 15 inherited from the father is imprinted in the same way as the mother's. This can be caused by a small deletion in a region of the father's chromosome that controls the imprinting process, called the imprinting center. In these cases, both of the child's copies of chromosome 15 have inactive PWCRs, leading to Prader-Willi syndrome.[2]

What Are the Treatments for Prader-Willi Syndrome (PWS)?

Parents can enroll infants with PWS in early intervention programs. However, even if a PWS diagnosis is delayed, treatments are valuable at any age.

The types of treatment depend on the individual's symptoms. The healthcare provider may recommend the following:

- **Use of special nipples or tubes for feeding difficulties.** Difficulty in sucking is one of the most common symptoms of newborns with Prader-Willi syndrome. Special nipples or tubes are used for several months to feed newborns and infants who are unable to suck properly, to make sure that the infant is fed adequately and grows. To ensure that the child is growing properly, the health care provider will monitor height, weight, and body mass index (BMI) monthly during infancy.

- **Strict supervision of daily food intake.** Once overeating starts between ages 2 and 4 years, supervision will help to minimize food hoarding and stealing and prevent rapid weight gain and severe obesity. Parents should lock refrigerators and all cabinets containing food. No medications have proven beneficial in reducing food-seeking behavior. A well-balanced, low-calorie diet and regular exercise are essential and must be maintained for the rest of the individual's life. People with PWS rarely need more than 1,000 to 1,200 calories per day. Height, weight, and BMI should be monitored every 6 months during the first 10 years of life after infancy and once a year after age 10 for the rest of the person's life to make sure he or she is maintaining a healthy weight. Ongoing consultation with a dietitian to guarantee adequate vitamin and mineral intake, including calcium and vitamin D, might be needed.

- **Growth Hormone (GH) therapy.** GH therapy has been demonstrated to increase height, lean body mass, and mobility; decrease fat mass; and improve movement and flexibility in individuals with PWS from infancy through adulthood. When given early in life, it also may prevent or reduce behavioral difficulties. Additionally, GH therapy can help improve speech, improve abstract reasoning, and often allow information to be processed more quickly. It also has been shown to improve sleep quality and resting energy expenditure. GH therapy usually is started during infancy or at diagnosis with PWS. This therapy often continues during adulthood at 20% to 25% of the recommended dose for children.

- **Treatment of eye problems by a pediatric ophthalmologist.** Many infants have trouble getting their eyes to focus together. These infants should be referred to a pediatric ophthalmologist who has expertise in working with infants with disabilities.

- **Treatment of curvature of the spine by an orthopedist.** An orthopedist should evaluate and treat, if necessary, curvature of the spine (scoliosis). Treatment will be the same as that for people with scoliosis who do not have PWS.

- **Sleep studies and treatment.** Sleep disorders are common with PWS. Treating a sleep disorder can help improve the quality of sleep. The same treatments that health care providers use with the general population can apply to individuals with PWS.

- **Physical therapy.** Muscle weakness is a serious problem among individuals with PWS. For children younger than age 3, physical therapy may increase muscular strength and help such children achieve developmental milestones. For older children, daily exercise will help build lean body mass.

- **Behavioral therapy.** People with PWS have difficulty controlling their emotions. Using behavioral therapy can help.

Stubbornness, anger, and obsessive-compulsive behavior, including obsession with food, should be handled with behavioral management programs using firm limit-setting strategies. Structure and routines also are advised.

- **Medications.** Medications, especially serotonin reuptake inhibitors (SRIs), may reduce obsessive-compulsive symptoms. SRIs also may help manage psychosis.

- **Early interventions / Special needs programs.** Individuals with PWS have varying degrees of intellectual difficulty and learning disabilities. Early intervention programs, including speech therapy for delays in acquiring language and for difficulties with pronunciation, should begin as early as possible and continue throughout childhood. Special education is almost always necessary for school-age children. Groups that offer training in social skills may also prove beneficial. An individual aide is often useful in helping PWS children focus on schoolwork.

- **Sex hormone treatments and/or corrective surgery.** These treatments are used to treat small genitals (penis, scrotum, clitoris).

- **Replacement of sex hormones.** Replacement of sex hormones during puberty may result in development of adequate secondary sex characteristics (e.g., breasts, pubic hair, a deeper voice).

- **Placement in group homes during adulthood.** Group homes offer necessary structure and supervision for adults with PWS, helping them avoid compulsive eating, severe obesity, and other health problems.

Section 19.6

Triple X Syndrome

This section includes text excerpted from "47 XXX syndrome,"
Genetic and Rare Diseases Information Center (GARD), National
Institutes of Health (NIH), March 16, 2016.

What Is Triple X Syndrome?

47 XXX syndrome, also called trisomy X or triple X syndrome, is characterized by the presence of an additional (third) X chromosome in each of a female's cells (which normally have two X chromosomes). An extra copy of the X chromosome is associated with tall stature, learning problems, and other features in some girls and women. Seizures or kidney abnormalities occur in about ten percent of affected females. 47 XXX syndrome is usually caused by a random event during the formation of reproductive cells (eggs and sperm). An error in cell division called nondisjunction can result in reproductive cells with an abnormal number of chromosomes. Treatment typically focuses on specific symptoms, if present. Some females with 47 XXX syndrome have an extra X chromosome in only some of their cells; this is called 46,XX/47,XXX mosaicism.

What Are the Signs and Symptoms of 47 XXX Syndrome?

Many women with 47 XXX syndrome have no symptoms or only mild symptoms. In other cases, symptoms may be more pronounced. Females with 47 XXX syndrome may be taller than average, but the condition usually does not cause unusual physical features. Minor physical findings can be present in some individuals and may include epicanthal folds, hypertelorism (widely spaced eyes), upslanting palpebral fissures, clinodactyly, overlapping digits (fingers or toes), pes planus (flat foot), and pectus excavatum. The condition is associated with an increased risk of learning disabilities and delayed development of speech and language skills. Delayed development of motor skills (such as sitting and walking), weak muscle tone (hypotonia), and behavioral and emotional difficulties are also possible, but these characteristics vary widely among affected girls and women. Seizures or kidney abnormalities occur in about ten percent of affected females. Most females with the condition have normal sexual development and are able to conceive children.

Is 47 XXX Syndrome Inherited?

Most cases of 47 XXX syndrome are not inherited. The chromosomal change usually occurs as a random event during the formation of reproductive cells (eggs and sperm). An error in cell division called nondisjunction can result in reproductive cells with an abnormal number of chromosomes. For example, an egg or sperm cell may gain an extra copy of the X chromosome as a result of nondisjunction. If one of these reproductive cells contributes to the genetic makeup of a child, the child will have an extra X chromosome in each of the body's cells. 46,XX/47,XXX mosaicism is also not inherited. It occurs as a random event during cell division in the early development of an embryo. As a result, some of an affected person's cells have two X chromosomes (46,XX), and other cells have three X chromosomes (47,XXX).

Transmission of an abnormal number of X chromosomes from women with 47 XXX syndrome is rare, although it has been reported. Some reports suggest a <5% increased risk for a chromosomally abnormal pregnancy, and other more recent reports suggest that <1% may be more accurate. These risks are separate from the risks of having a chromosomally abnormal pregnancy due to maternal age or any other factors.

Furthermore, these risks generally apply only to women with non-mosaic 47 XXX syndrome, as mosaicism may increase the risk of passing on an abnormal number of X chromosomes and potential outcomes. Each individual with 47 XXX syndrome who is interested in learning about their own risks to have a child with a chromosome abnormality or other genetic abnormality should speak with their healthcare provider or a genetics professional.

How Is 47 XXX Syndrome Diagnosed?

47 XXX syndrome may first be suspected based on the presence of certain developmental, behavioral or learning disabilities in an individual. The diagnosis can be confirmed with chromosomal analysis (karyotyping), which can be performed on a blood sample. This test

would reveal the presence of an extra X chromosome in body cells. 47 XXX syndrome may also be identified before birth (prenatally), based on chromosomal analysis performed on a sample taken during an amniocentesis or chorionic villus sampling (CVS) procedure. However, in these cases, confirmation testing with a test called FISH is recommended in order to evaluate the fetus for mosaicism (when only a percentage of the cells have the extra X chromosome).

How Might 47 XXX Syndrome Be Treated?

There is no cure for 47 XXX syndrome, and there is no way to remove the extra X chromosome that is present in an affected individual's cells. Management of the condition varies and depends on several factors including the age at diagnosis, the specific symptoms that are present, and the overall severity of the disorder in the affected individual. Early intervention services are typically recommended for infants and children that are diagnosed with the condition. Specific recommendations include developmental assessment by four months of age to evaluate muscle tone and strength; language and speech assessment by 12 months of age; pre-reading assessment during preschool years; and an assessment of additional learning disabilities as well as social and emotional problems. Evidence suggests that children with 47 XXX syndrome are very responsive to early intervention services and treatment. Some services that affected children may take part in include speech therapy, occupational therapy, physical therapy, and developmental therapy and counseling.

It is also recommended that infants and children with 47 XXX syndrome receive kidney and heart evaluations to detect possible abnormalities. Adolescent and adult women who have late periods, menstrual abnormalities, or fertility issues should be evaluated for primary ovarian failure (POF). Additional treatment for this disorder depends on the specific signs and symptoms present in the affected individual.

Section 19.7

Turner Syndrome

This section includes text excerpted from "Learning about Turner Syndrome," National Human Genome Research Institute (NHGRI), National Institutes of Health (NIH), September 24, 2013.

What Is Turner Syndrome?

Turner syndrome is a chromosomal condition that alters development in females. Women with this condition tend to be shorter than average and are usually unable to conceive a child (infertile) because of an absence of ovarian function. Other features of this condition that can vary among women who have Turner syndrome include: extra skin on the neck (webbed neck), puffiness or swelling (lymphedema) of the hands and feet, skeletal abnormalities, heart defects and kidney problems.

This condition occurs in about 1 in 2,500 female births worldwide, but is much more common among pregnancies that do not survive to term (miscarriages and stillbirths).

Turner syndrome is a chromosomal condition related to the X chromosome.

Researchers have not yet determined which genes on the X chromosome are responsible for most signs and symptoms of Turner syndrome. They have, however, identified one gene called SHOX that is important for bone development and growth. Missing one copy of this gene likely causes short stature and skeletal abnormalities in women with Turner syndrome.

What Are the Symptoms of Turner Syndrome?

Girls who have Turner syndrome are shorter than average. They often have normal height for the first three years of life, but then have a slow growth rate. At puberty they do not have the usual growth spurt.

Non-functioning ovaries are another symptom of Turner syndrome. Normally a girl's ovaries begin to produce sex hormones (estrogen and progesterone) at puberty. This does not happen in most girls who have Turner syndrome. They do not start their periods or develop breasts without hormone treatment at the age of puberty.

Even though many women who have Turner have non-functioning ovaries and are infertile, their vagina and womb are totally normal.

In early childhood, girls who have Turner syndrome may have frequent middle ear infections. Recurrent infections can lead to hearing loss in some cases.

Girls with Turner Syndrome are usually of normal intelligence with good verbal skills and reading skills. Some girls, however, have problems with math, memory skills and fine-finger movements.

How Is Turner Syndrome Diagnosed?

A diagnosis of Turner syndrome may be suspected when there are a number of typical physical features observed such as webbed neck, a broad chest and widely spaced nipples. Sometimes diagnosis is made at birth because of heart problems, an unusually wide neck or swelling of the hands and feet.

The two main clinical features of Turner syndrome are short stature and the lack of the development of the ovaries.

Many girls are diagnosed in early childhood when a slow growth rate and other features are identified. Diagnosis sometimes takes place later when puberty does not occur.

Turner syndrome may be suspected in pregnancy during an ultrasound test. This can be confirmed by prenatal testing chorionic villous sampling or amniocentesis to obtain cells from the unborn baby for chromosomal analysis. If a diagnosis is confirmed prenatally, the baby may be under the care of a specialist pediatrician immediately after birth.

Diagnosis is confirmed by a blood test, called a karyotype. This is used to analyze the chromosomal composition of the female.

What Is the Treatment for Turner Syndrome?

During childhood and adolescence, girls may be under the care of a pediatric endocrinologist, who is a specialist in childhood conditions of the hormones and metabolism.

Growth hormone injections are beneficial in some individuals with Turner syndrome. Injections often begin in early childhood and may increase final adult height by a few inches.

Estrogen replacement therapy is usually started at the time of normal puberty, around 12 years to start breast development. Estrogen and progesterone are given a little later to begin a monthly 'period,' which is necessary to keep the womb healthy. Estrogen is also given to prevent osteoporosis.

Babies born with a heart murmur or narrowing of the aorta may need surgery to correct the problem. A heart expert (cardiologist) will assess and follow up any treatment necessary.

Girls who have Turner syndrome are more likely to get middle ear infections. Repeated infections may lead to hearing loss and should be evaluated by the pediatrician. An ear, nose, and throat specialist (ENT) may be involved in caring for this health issue.

High blood pressure is quite common in women who have Turner syndrome. In some cases, the elevated blood pressure is due to narrowing of the aorta or a kidney abnormality. However, most of the time, no specific cause for the elevation is identified. Blood pressure should be checked routinely and, if necessary, treated with medication. Women who have Turner syndrome have a slightly higher risk of having an underactive thyroid or developing diabetes. This should also be monitored during routine health maintenance visits and treated if necessary.

Regular health checks are very important. Special clinics for the care of girls and women who have Turner syndrome are available in some areas, with access to a variety of specialists. Early preventive care and treatment is very important.

Almost all women are infertile, but pregnancy with donor embryos may be possible.

Having appropriate medical treatment and support allows a woman with Turner syndrome to lead a normal, healthy, and happy life.

Is Turner Syndrome Inherited?

Turner syndrome is not usually inherited in families. Turner syndrome occurs when one of the two X chromosomes normally found in women is missing or incomplete. Although the exact cause of Turner syndrome is not known, it appears to occur as a result of a random error during the formation of either the eggs or sperm.

Humans have 46 chromosomes, which contain all of a person's genes and DNA (Deoxyribonucleic acid). Two of these chromosomes, the sex chromosomes, determine a person's gender. Both of the sex chromosomes in females are called X chromosomes. (This is written as XX.) Males have an X and a Y chromosome (written as XY). The two sex chromosomes help a person develop fertility and the sexual characteristics of their gender.

In Turner syndrome, the girl does not have the usual pair of two complete X chromosomes. The most common scenario is that the girl has only one X chromosome in her cells. Some girls with Turner syndrome do have two X chromosomes, but one of the X chromosomes is incomplete. In another scenario, the girl has some cells in her body with two X chromosomes, but other cells have only one. This is called mosaicism.

Section 19.8

22q11.2 Deletion Syndrome

This section includes text excerpted from "22q11.2 Deletion Syndrome," Genetics Home Reference (GHR), National Institutes of Health (NIH), April 12, 2016.

What is 22q11.2 Deletion Syndrome?

22q11.2 deletion syndrome (which is also known by several other names, listed below) is a disorder caused by the deletion of a small piece of chromosome 22. The deletion occurs near the middle of the chromosome at a location designated q11.2.

22q11.2 deletion syndrome has many possible signs and symptoms that can affect almost any part of the body. The features of this syndrome vary widely, even among affected members of the same family. Common signs and symptoms include heart abnormalities that are often present from birth, an opening in the roof of the mouth (a cleft palate), and distinctive facial features. People with 22q11.2 deletion syndrome often experience recurrent infections caused by problems with the immune system, and some develop autoimmune disorders such as rheumatoid arthritis and Graves disease in which the immune system attacks the body's own tissues and organs. Affected individuals may also have breathing problems, kidney abnormalities, low levels of calcium in the blood (which can result in seizures), a decrease in blood platelets (thrombocytopenia), significant feeding difficulties, gastrointestinal problems, and hearing loss. Skeletal differences are possible, including mild short stature, and less frequently, abnormalities of the spinal bones.

Many children with 22q11.2 deletion syndrome have developmental delays, including delayed growth and speech development, and learning disabilities. Later in life, they are at an increased risk of developing mental illnesses such as schizophrenia, depression, anxiety, and bipolar disorder. Additionally, affected children are more likely than children without 22q11.2 deletion syndrome to have attention deficit hyperactivity disorder (ADHD) and developmental conditions such as autism spectrum disorders that affect communication and social interaction.

Because the signs and symptoms of 22q11.2 deletion syndrome are so varied, different groupings of features were once described as separate conditions. Doctors named these conditions DiGeorge syndrome, velocardiofacial syndrome (also called Shprintzen syndrome), and conotruncal anomaly face syndrome. In addition, some children with the 22q11.2 deletion were diagnosed with the autosomal dominant form of Opitz G/BBB syndrome and Cayler cardiofacial syndrome. Once the genetic basis for these disorders was identified, doctors determined that they were all part of a single syndrome with many possible signs and symptoms. To avoid confusion, this condition is usually called 22q11.2 deletion syndrome, a description based on its underlying genetic cause.

What are the Symptoms of 22q11.2 Deletion Syndrome?

22q11.2 deletion syndrome affects an estimated 1 in 4,000 people. However, the condition may actually be more common than this estimate because doctors and researchers suspect it is underdiagnosed due to its variable features. The condition may not be identified in people with mild signs and symptoms, or it may be mistaken for other disorders with overlapping features.

Other Names for this Condition

- 22q11.2DS
- autosomal dominant Opitz G/BBB syndrome
- CATCH22
- Cayler cardiofacial syndrome
- conotruncal anomaly face syndrome (CTAF)
- deletion 22q11.2 syndrome
- DiGeorge syndrome

- Sedlackova syndrome
- Shprintzen syndrome
- VCFS
- velocardiofacial syndrome

Section 19.9

Williams Syndrome (WS)

This section includes text excerpted from "NINDS Williams Syndrome Information Page," National Institute of Neurological Disorders and Stroke (NINDS), June 30, 2015.

What is Williams Syndrome?

Williams Syndrome (WS) is a rare genetic disorder characterized by mild to moderate delays in cognitive development or learning difficulties, a distinctive facial appearance, and a unique personality that combines over-friendliness and high levels of empathy with anxiety. The most significant medical problem associated with WS is cardiovascular disease caused by narrowed arteries. WS is also associated with elevated blood calcium levels in infancy. A random genetic mutation (deletion of a small piece of chromosome 7), rather than inheritance, most often causes the disorder.

However, individuals who have WS have a 50 percent chance of passing it on if they decide to have children. The characteristic facial features of WS include puffiness around the eyes, a short nose with a broad nasal tip, wide mouth, full cheeks, full lips, and a small chin. People with WS are also likely to have a long neck, sloping shoulders, short stature, limited mobility in their joints, and curvature of the spine. Some individuals with WS have a star-like pattern in the iris of their eyes. Infants with WS are often irritable and colicky, with feeding problems that keep them from gaining weight. Chronic abdominal pain is common in adolescents and adults. By age 30, the majority of individuals with WS have diabetes or pre-diabetes and mild to moderate sensorineural hearing loss (a form of deafness due to disturbed function of the auditory nerve).

For some people, hearing loss may begin as early as late childhood. WS also is associated with a characteristic "cognitive profile" of mental strengths and weaknesses composed of strengths in verbal short-term memory and language, combined with severe weakness in visuospatial construction (the skills used to copy patterns, draw, or write). Within language, the strongest skills are typically in concrete, practical vocabulary, which in many cases is in the low average to average range for the general population. Abstract or conceptual-relational vocabulary is much more limited. Most older children and adults with WS speak fluently and use good grammar. More than 50% of children with WS have attention deficit disorders (ADD or ADHD), and about 50% have specific phobias, such as a fear of loud noises. The majority of individuals with WS worry excessively.

Is There Any Treatment?

There is no cure for Williams syndrome, nor is there a standard course of treatment. Because WS is an uncommon and complex disorder, multidisciplinary clinics have been established at several centers in the United States. Treatments are based on an individual's particular symptoms. People with WS require regular cardiovascular monitoring for potential medical problems, such as symptomatic narrowing of the blood vessels, high blood pressure, and heart failure.

What Is the Prognosis?

The prognosis for individuals with WS varies. Some degree of impaired intellect is found in most people with the disorder. Some adults are able to function independently, complete academic or vocational school, and live in supervised homes or on their own; most live with a caregiver. Parents can increase the likelihood that their child will be able to live semi-independently by teaching self-help skills early. Early intervention and individualized educational programs designed with the distinct cognitive and personality profiles of WS in mind also help individuals maximize their potential. Medical complications associated with the disorder may shorten the lifespans of some individuals with WS.

What Research Is Being Done?

The National Institutes of Health (NIH), and the National Institute of Neurological Disorders and Stroke (NINDS), have funded many of the research studies exploring the genetic and neurobiological origins of WS. In the early 1990s, researchers located and identified the genetic mutation responsible for the disorder: the deletion of a small section of chromosome 7 that contains approximately 25 genes. NINDS continues to support WS researchers including, for example, groups that are attempting to link specific genes with the corresponding facial, cognitive, personality, and neurological characteristics of WS.

Chapter 20

Emotional Disturbance

What Is Emotional Disturbance?

The term "emotional disturbance" is used in this chapter because that is the term used in the nation's special education law, the Individuals with Disabilities Education Act (IDEA).

IDEA defines emotional disturbance as follows:

"...a condition exhibiting one or more of the following characteristics over a long period of time and to a marked degree that adversely affects a child's educational performance:

1. An inability to learn that cannot be explained by intellectual, sensory, or health factors

2. An inability to build or maintain satisfactory interpersonal relationships with peers and teachers

3. Inappropriate types of behavior or feelings under normal circumstances

4. A general pervasive mood of unhappiness or depression

5. A tendency to develop physical symptoms or fears associated with personal or school problems"

This chapter includes text excerpted from "Emotional Disturbance," Center for Parent Information and Resources (CPIR), March 2015.

As defined by IDEA, emotional disturbance includes schizophrenia but does not apply to children who are socially maladjusted, unless it is determined that they have an emotional disturbance.

Characteristics

As is evident in IDEA's definition, emotional disturbances can affect an individual in areas beyond the emotional. Depending on the specific mental disorder involved, a person's physical, social, or cognitive skills may also be affected. The National Alliance on Mental Illness (NAMI) puts this very well:

Mental illnesses are medical conditions that disrupt a person's thinking, feeling, mood, ability to relate to others and daily functioning. Just as diabetes is a disorder of the pancreas, mental illnesses are medical conditions that often result in a diminished capacity for coping with the ordinary demands of life.

Some of the characteristics and behaviors seen in children who have an emotional disturbance include:

- Hyperactivity (short attention span, impulsiveness)

- Aggression or self-injurious behavior (acting out, fighting)

- Withdrawal (not interacting socially with others, excessive fear or anxiety)

- Immaturity (inappropriate crying, temper tantrums, poor coping skills)

- Learning difficulties (academically performing below grade level)

Children with the most serious emotional disturbances may exhibit distorted thinking, excessive anxiety, bizarre motor acts, and abnormal mood swings.

Many children who do not have emotional disturbance may display some of these same behaviors at various times during their development. However, when children have an emotional disturbance, these behaviors continue over long periods of time. Their behavior signals that they are not coping with their environment or peers.

Causes

No one knows the actual cause or causes of emotional disturbance, although several factors—heredity, brain disorder, diet, stress, and family functioning—have been suggested and vigorously researched. A great deal of research goes on every day, but to date, researchers have not found that any of these factors are the direct cause of behavioral or emotional problems.

According to NAMI, mental illnesses can affect persons of any age, race, religion, or income. Further:

Mental illnesses are not the result of personal weakness, lack of character, or poor upbringing. Mental illnesses are treatable. Most people diagnosed with a serious mental illness can experience relief from their symptoms by actively participating in an individual treatment plan.

Frequency

According to the Centers for Disease Control and Prevention (CDC), approximately 8.3 million children (14.5%) aged 4–17 years have parents who've talked with a healthcare provider or school staff about the child's emotional or behavioral difficulties. Nearly 2.9 million children have been prescribed medication for these difficulties.

Help for School-Aged Children

IDEA requires that special education and related services be made available free of charge to every eligible child with a disability, including preschoolers (ages 3-21). These services are specially designed to address the child's individual needs associated with the disability—in this case, emotional disturbance, as defined by IDEA (and further specified by states). In the 2003-2004 school year, more than 484,000 children and youth with emotional disturbance received these services to address their individual needs related to emotional disturbance.

Determining a child's eligibility for special education and related services begins with a full and individual evaluation of the child. Under IDEA, this evaluation is provided free of charge in public schools.

A Look at Specific Emotional Disturbances

As mentioned, emotional disturbance is a commonly used umbrella term for a number of different mental disorders. Let's take a brief look at some of the most common of these.

Anxiety Disorders

We all experience anxiety from time to time, but for many people, including children, anxiety can be excessive, persistent, seemingly uncontrollable, and overwhelming. An irrational fear of everyday situations may be involved. This high level of anxiety is a definite warning sign that a person may have an anxiety disorder.

As with the term emotional disturbance, "anxiety disorder" is an umbrella term that actually refers to several distinct disabilities that share the core characteristic of irrational fear: generalized anxiety disorder (GAD), obsessive-compulsive disorder (OCD), panic disorder, posttraumatic stress disorder (PTSD), social anxiety disorder (also called social phobia), and specific phobias.

According to the Anxiety Disorders Association of America, anxiety disorders are the most common psychiatric illnesses affecting children and adults. They are also highly treatable. Unfortunately, only about 1/3 of those affected receive treatment.

Bipolar Disorder

Also known as manic-depressive illness, bipolar disorder is a serious medical condition that causes dramatic mood swings from overly "high" and/or irritable to sad and hopeless, and then back again, often with periods of normal mood in between. Severe changes in energy and behavior go along with these changes in mood.

For most people with bipolar disorder, these mood swings and related symptoms can be stabilized over time using an approach that combines medication and psychosocial treatment.

Conduct Disorder

Conduct disorder refers to a group of behavioral and emotional problems in youngsters. Children and adolescents with this disorder have great difficulty following rules and behaving in a socially acceptable way. This may include some of the following behaviors:

- aggression to people and animals
- destruction of property
- deceitfulness, lying, or stealing
- truancy or other serious violations of rules

Although conduct disorder is one of the most difficult behavior disorders to treat, young people often benefit from a range of services that include:

- training for parents on how to handle child or adolescent behavior

- family therapy

- training in problem solving skills for children or adolescents

- community-based services that focus on the young person within the context of family and community influences

Eating Disorders

Eating disorders are characterized by extremes in eating behavior—either too much or too little—or feelings of extreme distress or concern about body weight or shape. Females are much more likely than males to develop an eating disorder.

Anorexia nervosa and *bulimia nervosa* are the two most common types of eating disorders. Anorexia nervosa is characterized by self-starvation and dramatic loss of weight. Bulimia nervosa involves a cycle of binge eating, then self-induced vomiting or purging. Both of these disorders are potentially life-threatening.

Binge eating is also considered an eating disorder. It's characterized by eating excessive amounts of food, while feeling unable to control how much or what is eaten. Unlike with bulimia, people who binge eat usually do not purge afterward by vomiting or using laxatives.

According to the National Eating Disorders Association (NEDA):

"The most effective and long-lasting treatment for an eating disorder is some form of psychotherapy or counseling, coupled with careful attention to medical and nutritional needs. Some medications have been shown to be helpful. Ideally, whatever treatment is offered should be tailored to the individual, and this will vary according to both the severity of the disorder and the patient's individual problems, needs, and strengths."

Obsessive-Compulsive Disorder

Often referred to as OCD, obsessive-compulsive disorder is actually considered an anxiety disorder. OCD is characterized by recurrent, unwanted thoughts (obsessions), and/or repetitive behaviors (compulsions). Repetitive behaviors (handwashing, counting, checking, or cleaning) are often performed with the hope of preventing obsessive thoughts or making them go away. Performing these so-called "rituals," however, provides only temporary relief, and not performing them markedly increases anxiety.

A large body of scientific evidence suggests that OCD results from a chemical imbalance in the brain. Treatment for most people with OCD should include one or more of the following:

- therapist trained in behavior therapy
- Cognitive Behavior Therapy (CBT)
- medication (usually an antidepressant)

Psychotic Disorders

"Psychotic disorders" is another umbrella term used to refer to severe mental disorders that cause abnormal thinking and perceptions. Two of the main symptoms are delusions and hallucinations. Delusions are false beliefs, such as thinking that someone is plotting against you. Hallucinations are false perceptions, such as hearing, seeing, or feeling something that is not there. Schizophrenia is one type of psychotic disorder. There are others as well.

Treatment for psychotic disorders will differ from person to person, depending on the specific disorder involved. Most are treated with a combination of medications and psychotherapy (a type of counseling).

More about School

As mentioned, emotional disturbance is one of the categories of disability specified in IDEA. This means that a child with an emotional disturbance may be eligible for special education and related services in public school. These services can be of tremendous help to students who have an emotional disturbance.

Typically, educational programs for children with an emotional disturbance need to include attention to providing emotional and behavioral support as well as helping them to master academics, develop social skills, and increase self-awareness, self-control, and self-esteem. A large body of research exists regarding methods of providing students with **positive behavioral support** (PBS) in the school environment, so that problem behaviors are minimized and positive, appropriate behaviors are fostered. It is also important to know that, within the school setting:

For a child whose **behavior** impedes learning (including the learning of others), the team developing the child's Individualized Education Program (IEP) needs to consider, if appropriate, strategies to address that behavior, including positive behavioral interventions, strategies, and supports.

Students eligible for special education services under the category of emotional disturbance may have IEPs that include **psychological or counseling services**. These are important related services available under IDEA and are to be provided by a qualified social worker, psychologist, guidance counselor, or other qualified personnel.

Other Considerations

Children and adolescents with an emotional disturbance should receive services based on their individual needs, and everyone involved in their education or care needs to be well-informed about the care that they are receiving. It's important to coordinate services between home, school, and community, keeping the communication channels open between all parties involved.

Chapter 21

Epilepsy

Epilepsy is a seizure disorder. According to the Epilepsy Foundation of America, a seizure happens when a brief, strong surge of electrical activity affects part or all of the brain. Seizures can last from a few seconds to a few minutes. They can have different symptoms, too, from convulsions and loss of consciousness, to signs such as blank staring, lip smacking, or jerking movements of arms and legs.

Some people can have a seizure and yet not have epilepsy. For example, many young children have convulsions from fevers. Other types of seizures not classified as epilepsy include those caused by an imbalance of body fluids or chemicals or by alcohol or drug withdrawal. Thus, a single seizure does not mean that the person has epilepsy. Generally speaking, the diagnosis of epilepsy is made when a person has two or more unprovoked seizures.

Incidence

About three million Americans have epilepsy. **Of the 200,000 new cases diagnosed each year, nearly 45,000 are children and adolescents.** Epilepsy affects people in all nations and of all races. Its incidence is greater in African American and socially disadvantaged populations.

This chapter includes text excerpted from "Epilepsy," Center for Parent Information and Resources (CPIR), July 2015.

Characteristics

Although the symptoms listed below do not necessarily mean that a person has epilepsy, it is wise to consult a doctor if you or a member of your family experiences one or more of them:

- "Blackouts" or periods of confused memory

- Episodes of staring or unexplained periods of unresponsiveness

- Involuntary movement of arms and legs

- "Fainting spells" with incontinence or followed by excessive fatigue

- Odd sounds, distorted perceptions, or episodic feelings of fear that cannot be explained

Doctors have described more than 30 different types of seizures. These are divided into two major categories—**generalized seizures** and **partial seizures** (also known as focal seizures).

Generalized Seizures: This type of seizure involves both sides of the brain from the beginning of the seizure. The best known subtype of generalized seizures is the **grand mal** seizure. In a grand mal seizure, the person's arms and legs stiffen (the tonic phase), and then begin to jerk (the clonic phase). That's why the grand mal seizure is also known as a generalized tonic clonic seizure.

Grand mal seizures typically last 1-2 minutes and are followed by a period of confusion and then deep sleep. The person will not remember what happened during the seizure.

You may also have heard of the **petit mal** seizure, which is an older term for another type of generalized seizure. It's now called an absence seizure, because during the seizure, the person stares blankly off into space and doesn't seem to be aware of his or her surroundings. The person may also blink rapidly and seem to chew. Absence seizures typically last from 2-15 seconds and may not be noticed by others. Afterwards, the person will resume whatever he or she was doing at the time of the seizure, without any memory of the event.

Partial Seizures: Partial seizures are so named because they involve only one hemisphere of the brain. They may be simple partial seizures (in which the person jerks and may have odd sensations and perceptions, but doesn't lose consciousness) or complex partial seizures (in which consciousness is impaired or lost). Complex partial seizures often involve periods of "automatic behavior" and altered consciousness. This is typified by purposeful-looking behavior, such as buttoning or unbuttoning a shirt. Such behavior, however, is unconscious, may be repetitive, and is usually not remembered afterwards.

Diagnosis

Diagnosing epilepsy is a **multi-step process.** According to the Epilepsy Foundation of America:

...the doctor's main tool...is a careful medical history with as much information as possible about what the seizures looked like and what happened just before they began. The doctor will also perform a thorough physical examination, especially of the nervous system, as well as analysis of blood and other bodily fluids.

The doctor may also order an electroencephalograph **(EEG)** of the patient's brain activity, which may show patterns that help the doctor decide whether or not someone has epilepsy. Other tests may also be used—such as the **CT** (computerized tomography) or **MRI** (magnetic resonance imaging)—in order to look for any growths, scars, or other physical conditions in the brain that may be causing the seizures. Which tests and how many of them are ordered may vary, depending on how much each test reveals.

Treatment

Anti-epileptic medication is the most common treatment for epilepsy. It's effective in stopping seizures in 70% of patients. Interestingly, it's not uncommon for doctors to wait a while before prescribing an anti-seizure medication, especially if the patient is a young child. Unless the EEG of the patient's brain is clearly abnormal, doctors may suggest waiting until a second or even third seizure occurs. Why? Because studies show that an otherwise normal child who has had a single seizure has a relatively low (15%) risk of a second one.

When anti-epileptic medications are not effective in stopping a person's seizures, other treatment options may be discussed. These include:

- surgery to remove the areas of the brain that are producing the seizures

- stimulation of the vagus nerve (a large nerve in the neck), where short bursts of electrical energy are directed into the brain via the vagus nerve

- a ketogenic diet (one that is very high in fats and low in carbo-hydrates), which makes the body burn fat for energy instead of glucose

According to the Epilepsy Foundation of America, 10% of new patients cannot bring their seizures disorder under control despite optimal medical management.

Educational and Developmental Considerations

It's not unusual for seizures to interfere with a child's development and learning. For example, if a student has the type of seizure characterized by periods of fixed staring, he or she is likely to miss parts of what the teacher is saying. If teachers—or other caregivers such as babysitters, daycare providers, preschool teachers, K-12 personnel—observe such an episode, it's important that they document and report it promptly to parents (and the school nurse, if appropriate).

Because epilepsy can affect a child's learning and development (even babies), families will want to learn more about the systems of help that are available. Much of that help comes from the nation's special education law, the Individuals with Disabilities Education Act (IDEA), which makes available these two sets of services:

- Early intervention: A system of services to help infants and toddlers with disabilities (before their 3rd birthday) and their families

- Special education and related services: Services available through the public school system for school-aged children, including preschoolers (ages 3-21)

In both of these systems, eligible children receive special services designed to address the developmental, functional, and educational needs resulting from their disability.

To access early intervention services for a child up to his or her 3rd birthday, ask your child's pediatrician for a referral. You can also call the local hospital's maternity ward or pediatric ward, and ask for the contact information of the local early intervention program.

To access special education services for a school-aged child, get in touch with your local public school system. Calling the elementary school in your neighborhood is an excellent place to start. Ask to have your child evaluated to see if he or she is eligible for services.

More about Services under IDEA

The process of finding a child eligible for early intervention or special education and related services under IDEA begins with a **comprehensive and individual evaluation of the child** in order to:

- establish that the child does, indeed, have a disability

- get a detailed picture of how the disability affects the child functionally, developmentally, and academically

- document the child's special needs related to the disability

This evaluation is provided free of charge through either the early intervention system (for infants and toddlers under the age of 3) or through the local school system (for children ages 3-21). Under IDEA, children with epilepsy are usually found eligible for services under the category of "Other Health Impairment" (OHI). We've included IDEA's definition of OHI below.

IDEA's Definition Of "Other Health Impairment"

The nation's special education law specifically mentions epilepsy in its definition of "Other Health Impairment," a category under which children may be found eligible for special education and related services. Here's IDEA's definition.

(9) Other health impairment means having limited strength, vitality, or alertness, including a heightened alertness to environmental stimuli, that results in limited alertness with respect to the educational environment, that—

(i) Is due to chronic or acute health problems such as asthma, attention deficit disorder or attention deficit hyperactivity disorder, diabetes, epilepsy, a heart condition, hemophilia, lead poisoning, leukemia, nephritis, rheumatic fever, sickle cell anemia, and Tourette syndrome; and

(ii) Adversely affects a child's educational performance. [34 CFR §300.8(c)(9)]

Babies and toddlers: When a baby or toddler is found eligible for early intervention, parents meet with the early intervention staff, and together they develop what is known as an Individualized Family Service Plan (IFSP). The IFSP will describe the child's unique needs as well as the services the child will receive to address those needs. The IFSP will also emphasize the unique needs of the family, so that parents and other family members will know how to help their young child with epilepsy. Early intervention services may be provided on a sliding-fee basis, meaning that the costs to the family will depend upon their income.

School-aged children: When a child is found eligible for special education and related services, school staff and parents meet and develop what is known as an Individualized Education Program (IEP). This document is very important in the educational life of a child with epilepsy, because it details the nature of the child's needs and the services that the public school system will provide free of charge to address those needs.

Succeeding at School

Special education and related services can be very helpful to children with epilepsy attending public school. Because the disorder affects memory and concentration, accommodations in the classroom and during testing are key to students' academic success. Some common accommodations and services provided to students with epilepsy are listed at the end of this section.

Related services may be every bit as important for children with epilepsy, especially **school health services and school nurse services**—which can provide the child's medication during school hours or give first aid instruction on seizure management to the student's teachers, for example.

Depending on the child's unique needs, other related services may also be necessary so that the student benefits from his or her special education program—for example, counseling services. Children and youth with epilepsy must deal with the psychological and social aspects of the condition. These include public misperceptions and fear of seizures, loss of self-control during the seizure episode, and compliance with medications. Counseling services may help students with epilepsy address the complexities of living with this disorder. The school can also help by providing epilepsy education programs for staff and students, including information on how to recognize a seizure and what to do if a seizure occurs.

It is important that the **teachers and school staff are informed about the child's condition**, possible effects of medication, and what to do in case a seizure occurs at school. Most parents find that a friendly conversation with the teacher(s) at the beginning of the school year is the best way to handle the situation. Even if a child has seizures that are largely controlled by medication, it is still best to notify the school staff about the condition.

School personnel and the family should **work together to monitor the effectiveness of medication** as well as any side effects. If a child's physical or intellectual skills seem to change, it is important to tell the doctor. There may also be hearing or perception problems caused by changes in the brain. Written observations of both the family and school staff will be helpful in discussions with the child's doctor.

Accommodations in the Classroom

The accommodations that a child with epilepsy receives are determined by his or her IEP team (which includes the parents). Here are some possibilities to consider.

To address memory deficits

- Provide written or pictorial instructions
- Use voice recordings of verbal instructions
- Have a peer buddy take notes for the student or permit tape recording
- Divide large tasks into smaller steps
- Provide a checklist of assignments and a calendar with due dates
- Decrease memory demands during classwork and testing (e.g., use recognition rather than recall tasks)

To address health concerns

- Be flexible about time missed from school to seek treatment or adjust to new medications
- Provide extra time for assignments and a modified workload (fatigue is a common side effect of seizures and medications)
- Replace fluorescent lighting with full spectrum lighting
- Provide private area to rest or recover from a seizure

Chapter 22

Fetal Alcohol Spectrum Disorders (FASDs)

Chapter Contents

Section 22.1

Facts about
Fetal Alcohol Spectrum Disorders

This section includes text excerpted from "Fetal Alcohol Spectrum
Disorders (FASDs)," Centers for Disease Control and
Prevention (CDC), April 16, 2015.

Fetal Alcohol Spectrum Disorders (FASDs)

Fetal alcohol spectrum disorders (FASDs) are a group of conditions that can occur in a person whose mother drank alcohol during pregnancy. These effects can include physical problems and problems with behavior and learning. Often, a person with an FASD has a mix of these problems.

Cause and Prevention

FASDs are caused by a woman drinking alcohol during pregnancy. Alcohol in the mother's blood passes to the baby through the umbilical cord. When a woman drinks alcohol, so does her baby.

There is no known safe amount of alcohol during pregnancy or when trying to get pregnant. There is also no safe time to drink during pregnancy. Alcohol can cause problems for a developing baby throughout pregnancy, including before a woman knows she's pregnant. All types of alcohol are equally harmful, including all wines and beer.

To prevent FASDs, a woman should not drink alcohol while she is pregnant, or when she might get pregnant. This is because a woman could get pregnant and not know for up to four to six weeks. In the United States, nearly half of pregnancies are unplanned.

If a woman is drinking alcohol during pregnancy, it is never too late to stop drinking. Because brain growth takes place throughout pregnancy, the sooner a woman stops drinking the safer it will be for her and her baby.

FASDs are completely preventable if a woman does not drink alcohol during pregnancy—so why take the risk?

Signs and Symptoms

FASDs refer to the whole range of effects that can happen to a person whose mother drank alcohol during pregnancy. These conditions can affect each person in different ways, and can range from mild to severe.

A person with an FASD might have:

- Abnormal facial features, such as a smooth ridge between the nose and upper lip (this ridge is called the philtrum)
- Small head size
- Shorter-than-average height
- Low body weight
- Poor coordination
- Hyperactive behavior
- Difficulty with attention
- Poor memory
- Difficulty in school (especially with math)
- Learning disabilities
- Speech and language delays
- Intellectual disability or low intelligence quotient (IQ)
- Poor reasoning and judgment skills
- Sleep and sucking problems as a baby
- Vision or hearing problems
- Problems with the heart, kidneys, or bones

Types of FASDs

Different terms are used to describe FASDs, depending on the type of symptoms.

- **Fetal Alcohol Syndrome (FAS):** FAS represents the most involved end of the FASD spectrum. Fetal death is the most extreme outcome from drinking alcohol during pregnancy. People with FAS might have abnormal facial features, growth problems, and central nervous system (CNS) problems. People

221

with FAS can have problems with learning, memory, attention span, communication, vision, or hearing. They might have a mix of these problems. People with FAS often have a hard time in school and trouble getting along with others.

- **Alcohol-Related Neurodevelopmental Disorder (ARND):** People with ARND might have intellectual disabilities and problems with behavior and learning. They might do poorly in school and have difficulties with math, memory, attention, judgment, and poor impulse control.

- **Alcohol-Related Birth Defects (ARBD):** People with ARBD might have problems with the heart, kidneys, or bones or with hearing. They might have a mix of these.

The term fetal alcohol effects (FAE) was previously used to describe intellectual disabilities and problems with behavior and learning in a person whose mother drank alcohol during pregnancy. In 1996, the Institute of Medicine (IOM) replaced FAE with the terms alcohol-related neurodevelopmental disorder (ARND) and alcohol-related birth defects (ARBD).

Diagnosis

The term FASDs is not meant for use as a clinical diagnosis. Centers for Disease Control and Prevention (CDC) worked with a group of experts and organizations to review the research and develop guidelines for diagnosing FAS. The guidelines were developed for FAS only. CDC and its partners are working to put together diagnostic criteria for other FASDs, such as ARND.

Diagnosing FAS can be hard because there is no medical test, like a blood test, for it. And other disorders, such as ADHD (attention-deficit/hyperactivity disorder) and Williams syndrome, have some symptoms like FAS.

To diagnose FAS, doctors look for:

- Abnormal facial features (e.g., smooth ridge between nose and upper lip)

- Lower-than-average height, weight, or both

- Central nervous system problems (e.g., small head size, problems with attention and hyperactivity, poor coordination)

- Prenatal alcohol exposure; although confirmation is not required to make a diagnosis

Treatment

FASDs last a lifetime. There is no cure for FASDs, but research shows that early intervention treatment services can improve a child's development.

There are many types of treatment options, including medication to help with some symptoms, behavior and education therapy, parent training, and other alternative approaches. No one treatment is right for every child. Good treatment plans will include close monitoring, follow-ups, and changes as needed along the way.

Also, "protective factors" can help reduce the effects of FASDs and help people with these conditions reach their full potential.

Protective factors include:

- Diagnosis before six years of age

- Loving, nurturing, and stable home environment during the school years

- Absence of violence

- Involvement in special education and social services

Get Help

If you or the doctor thinks there could be a problem, **ask the doctor for a referral to a specialist** (someone who knows about FASDs), such as a developmental pediatrician, child psychologist, or clinical geneticist. In some cities, there are clinics whose staffs have special training in diagnosing and treating children with FASDs. To find doctors and clinics in your area, visit the National and State Resource Directory from the National Organization on Fetal Alcohol Syndrome (NOFAS).

At the same time, as you ask the doctor for a referral to a specialist, **call your state's public early childhood system** to request a free evaluation to find out if your child qualifies for intervention services. This is sometimes called a *Child Find* evaluation. You do not need to wait for a doctor's referral or a medical diagnosis to make this call.

Where to call for a free evaluation from the state depends on your child's age:

- **If your child is younger than 3 years old**, contact your local early intervention system

- **If your child is 3 years old or older**, contact your local public school system

Even if your child is not old enough for kindergarten or enrolled in a public school, call your local elementary school or board of education and ask to speak with someone who can help you have your child evaluated.

Section 22.2

Alcohol Use in Pregnancy

This section contains text excerpted from the following sources: Text in this section beginning with the heading "Alcohol Use and Pregnancy," is excerpted from "Fetal Alcohol Spectrum Disorders (FASDs)," Centers for Disease Control and Prevention (CDC), April 17, 2014; Text beginning with the heading "A Study on Alcohol Use during Pregnancy and Developmental Outcomes" is excerpted from "Fetal Alcohol Spectrum Disorders (FASDs)," Centers for Disease Control and Prevention (CDC), August 20, 2013.

Alcohol Use and Pregnancy

There is no known safe amount of alcohol use during pregnancy or while trying to get pregnant. There is also no safe time during pregnancy to drink. All types of alcohol are equally harmful, including all wines and beer. When a pregnant woman drinks alcohol, so does her baby.

Women also should not drink alcohol if they are sexually active and do not use effective contraception (birth control). This is because a woman might get pregnant and expose her baby to alcohol before she knows she is pregnant. Nearly half of all pregnancies in the United States are unplanned. Most women will not know they are pregnant for up to four to six weeks.

Fetal alcohol spectrum disorders (FASDs) are completely preventable if a woman does not drink alcohol during pregnancy. Why take the risk?

Why Alcohol Is Dangerous?

Alcohol in the mother's blood passes to the baby through the umbilical cord. Drinking alcohol during pregnancy can cause miscarriage, stillbirth, and a range of lifelong physical, behavioral, and intellectual disabilities. These disabilities are known as fetal alcohol spectrum disorders (FASDs). Children with FASDs might have the following characteristics and behaviors:

- Abnormal facial features, such as a smooth ridge between the nose and upper lip (this ridge is called the philtrum)
- Small head size
- Shorter-than-average height
- Low body weight
- Poor coordination
- Hyperactive behavior
- Difficulty with attention
- Poor memory
- Difficulty in school (especially with math)
- Learning disabilities
- Speech and language delays
- Intellectual disability or low IQ (intelligence quotient)
- Poor reasoning and judgment skills
- Sleep and sucking problems as a baby
- Vision or hearing problems
- Problems with the heart, kidney, or bones

How Much Alcohol Is Dangerous?

There is no known safe amount of alcohol to drink while pregnant.

When Alcohol Is Dangerous?

There is no safe time to drink alcohol during pregnancy. Alcohol can cause problems for the developing baby throughout pregnancy, including before a woman knows she is pregnant. Drinking alcohol in the first three months of pregnancy can cause the baby to have abnormal facial features. Growth and central nervous system problems (e.g., low birthweight, behavioral problems) can occur from drinking alcohol anytime during pregnancy. The baby's brain is developing throughout pregnancy and can be affected by exposure to alcohol at any time.

If a woman is drinking alcohol during pregnancy, it is never too late to stop. The sooner a woman stops drinking, the better it will be for both her baby and herself.

Get Help!

If you are pregnant or trying to get pregnant and cannot stop drinking, get help! Contact your healthcare provider, local Alcoholics Anonymous, or local alcohol treatment center.

A Study on Alcohol Use during Pregnancy and Developmental Outcomes

The journal Alcoholism: Clinical and Experimental Research published a meta-analysis of multiple studies examining how drinking patterns of women during pregnancy (such as low-to-moderate alcohol use or binge drinking) can affect the development of their children. This topic is an area of public health concern, particularly due to contradicting media reports. The results of this review highlight the importance of avoiding alcohol use, especially binge drinking, during pregnancy. It provides evidence that there is no known safe amount of alcohol to drink while pregnant.

Findings from This Study

- Based on eight studies that included over 10,000 children aged 6 months to 14 years, the authors found that any binge drinking during pregnancy was associated with the child having problems with cognition

- Based on three high-quality studies of approximately 11,900 children aged 9 months to 5 years, the authors found that moderate drinking during pregnancy was associated with the child having behavior problems

- The authors found no significant impact of alcohol use during pregnancy on other outcomes of child development that were studied, such as academic performance or language development

- Findings of this meta-analysis support previous findings suggesting harmful effects of binge drinking during pregnancy on child cognition

- Drinking alcohol during pregnancy at low levels (less than daily drinking) might increase the chance of child behavior problems

About This Study

Researchers collected and analyzed information from previous studies to look at whether low-to-moderate alcohol use or binge drinking by women during pregnancy could affect the later development of their children. This is the first meta-analysis of studies of low-to-moderate alcohol use or binge drinking during pregnancy and later cognitive outcomes.

Section 22.3

Conditions Associated with FASD

This section includes text excerpted from "Fetal Alcohol Spectrum Disorders (FASDs)," Centers for Disease Control and Prevention (CDC), April 5, 2016.

Secondary Conditions

Fetal alcohol spectrum disorders (FASDs) often lead to other disorders, called "secondary conditions." Secondary conditions are problems that a person is not born with, but might get as a result of having an FASD. These conditions can be improved or prevented with appropriate treatments for children and adults with FASDs and their families.

Following are some of the secondary conditions that have been found to be associated with FASDs.

Mental Health Problems

Several studies have shown an increased risk for cognitive disorders (e.g., problems with memory), mental illness, or psychological problems among people with FASDs.

The most frequently diagnosed disorders are:

- Attention problems, including attention-deficit/hyperactivity disorder (ADHD)

- Conduct disorder (aggression toward others and serious violations of rules, laws, and social norms)

- Alcohol or drug dependence

- Depression

Other psychiatric problems, such as anxiety disorders, eating disorders, and posttraumatic stress disorder, have also been reported for some patients.

Disrupted School Experience

Children with FASDs are at a higher risk for being suspended, expelled, or dropping out of school. Difficulty getting along with other children, poor relationships with teachers, and truancy are some of the reasons that lead to their removal from the school setting. Many children with FASDs remain in school but have negative experiences because of their behavioral challenges.

In a 2004 study, disrupted school experience was reported for 14% of school children and 61% of adolescents and adults with FASDs. About 53% of the adolescents with FASDs had been suspended from school, 29% had been expelled, and 25% had dropped out.

Trouble with the Law

Teenagers and adults with FASDs are at a higher risk for having interactions with police, authorities, or the judicial system. Difficulty controlling anger and frustration, combined with problems understanding the motives of others, result in many people with FASDs being involved in violent or explosive situations. People with FASDs can be very easy to persuade and manipulate, which can lead to their taking part in illegal acts without being aware of it. Trouble with the law is reported overall for 14% of children and 60% of adolescents and adults with FASDs.

Inappropriate Sexual Behavior

People with FASDs are at higher risk for showing inappropriate sexual behavior, such as inappropriate advances and inappropriate touching. If the person with an FASD is also a victim of violence, the risk of participating in sexually inappropriate behavior increases. Inappropriate sexual behaviors increase slightly with age from 39% in children to 48% in adolescents and 52% in adults with FASDs.

Alcohol and Drug Problems

Studies suggest that more than a third of people with FASDs have had problems with alcohol or drugs, with more than half of them requiring inpatient treatment.

Dependent Living and Problems with Employment over 21 Years

Adults with FASDs generally have difficulty sustaining employment or living independently in their communities.

Chapter 23

Gerstmann Syndrome

What Is Gerstmann Syndrome?

Gerstmann syndrome is a cognitive impairment that results from damage to a specific area of the brain—the left parietal lobe in the region of the angular gyrus. It may occur after a stroke or in association with damage to the parietal lobe. It is characterized by four primary symptoms: a writing disability (agraphia or dysgraphia), a lack of understanding of the rules for calculation or arithmetic (acalculia or dyscalculia), an inability to distinguish right from left, and an inability to identify fingers (finger agnosia). The disorder should not be confused with *Gerstmann-Sträussler-Scheinker disease*, a type of transmissible spongiform encephalopathy.

In addition to exhibiting the above symptoms, many adults also experience aphasia, (difficulty in expressing oneself when speaking, in understanding speech, or in reading and writing).

There are few reports of the syndrome, sometimes called *developmental Gerstmann syndrome*, in children. The cause is not known. Most cases are identified when children reach school age, a time when they are challenged with writing and math exercises. Generally, children with the disorder exhibit poor handwriting and spelling skills, and difficulty with math functions, including adding, subtracting, multiplying, and dividing. An inability to differentiate right from left

This chapter includes text excerpted from "NINDS Gerstmann's Syndrome Information Page," National Institute of Neurological Disorders and Stroke (NINDS), July 2, 2008. Reviewed June 2016.

and to discriminate among individual fingers may also be apparent. In addition to the four primary symptoms, many children also suffer from constructional apraxia, an inability to copy simple drawings. Frequently, there is also an impairment in reading. Children with a high level of intellectual functioning as well as those with brain damage may be affected with the disorder.

Is There Any Treatment?

There is no cure for Gerstmann syndrome. Treatment is symptomatic and supportive. Occupational and speech therapies may help diminish the dysgraphia and apraxia. In addition, calculators and word processors may help school children cope with the symptoms of the disorder.

What Is the Prognosis?

In adults, many of the symptoms diminish over time. Although it has been suggested that in children symptoms may diminish over time, it appears likely that most children probably do not overcome their deficits, but learn to adjust to them.

What Research Is Being Done?

The NINDS supports research on disorders that result from damage to the brain such as dysgraphia. The NINDS and other components of the National Institutes of Health (NIH) also support research on learning disabilities. Current research avenues focus on developing techniques to diagnose and treat learning disabilities and increase understanding of the biological basis of them.

Chapter 24

Hearing Disabilities

Chapter Contents

Section 24.1

Facts about Hearing Disabilities

This section includes text excerpted from "Hearing Loss in Children," Centers for Disease Control and Prevention (CDC), October 23, 2015.

Hearing Loss

A hearing loss can happen when any part of the ear is not working in the usual way. This includes the outer ear, middle ear, inner ear, hearing (acoustic) nerve, and auditory system.

Signs and Symptoms

The signs and symptoms of hearing loss are different for each child. If you think that your child might have hearing loss, ask the child's doctor for a hearing screening as soon as possible. Don't wait!

Even if a child has passed a hearing screening before, it is important to look out for the following signs.

Signs in Babies

- Does not startle at loud noises.

- Does not turn to the source of a sound after 6 months of age.

- Does not say single words, such as "dada" or "mama" by 1 year of age.

- Turns head when he or she sees you but not if you only call out his or her name. This sometimes is mistaken for not paying attention or just ignoring, but could be the result of a partial or complete hearing loss.

- Seems to hear some sounds but not others.

Signs in Children

- Speech is delayed.

- Speech is not clear.

- Does not follow directions. This sometimes is mistaken for not paying attention or just ignoring, but could be the result of a partial or complete hearing loss.

- Often says, "Huh?"

- Turns the TV volume up too high.

Babies and children should reach milestones in how they play, learn, communicate, and act. A delay in any of these milestones could be a sign of hearing loss or other developmental problem.

Screening and Diagnosis

Hearing screening can tell if a child might have hearing loss. Hearing screening is easy and is not painful. In fact, babies are often asleep while being screened. It takes a very short time—usually only a few minutes.

Babies

All babies should have a hearing screening no later than one month of age. Most babies have their hearing screened while still in the hospital. If a baby does not pass a hearing screening, it's very important to get a full hearing test as soon as possible, but no later than 3 months of age.

Children

Children should have their hearing tested before they enter school or any time there is a concern about the child's hearing. Children who do not pass the hearing screening need to get a full hearing test as soon as possible.

Treatments and Intervention Services

No single treatment or intervention is the answer for every person or family. Good treatment plans will include close monitoring, follow-ups and any changes needed along the way. There are many different types of communication options for children with hearing loss and for their families. Some of these options include:

- Learning other ways to communicate, such as sign language

- Technology to help with communication, such as hearing aids and cochlear implants

- Medicine and surgery to correct some types of hearing loss

- Family support services

Causes and Risk Factors

Hearing loss can happen any time during life–from before birth to adulthood.

Following are some of the things that can increase the chance that a child will have hearing loss:

- A genetic cause: About 1 out of 2 cases of hearing loss in babies is due to genetic causes. Some babies with a genetic cause for their hearing loss might have family members who also have a hearing loss. About 1 out of 3 babies with genetic hearing loss have a "syndrome." This means they have other conditions in addition to the hearing loss, such as Down syndrome or Usher syndrome.

- For about 1 out of 4 cases of hearing loss in babies is due to maternal infections during pregnancy, complications after birth, and head trauma. For example, the child:

  - Was exposed to infection, such as cytomegalovirus (CMV) infection, before birth

  - Spent 5 days or more in a hospital neonatal intensive care unit (NICU) or had complications while in the NICU

  - Needed a special procedure like a blood transfusion to treat bad jaundice

  - Has head, face or ears shaped or formed in a different way than usual

  - Has a condition like a neurological disorder that may be associated with hearing loss

  - Had an infection around the brain and spinal cord called meningitis

  - Received a bad injury to the head that required a hospital stay

- For about 1 out of 4 babies born with hearing loss, the cause is unknown.

Prevention

Following are tips for parents to help prevent hearing loss in their children:

- Have a healthy pregnancy.

- Learn how to prevent cytomegalovirus (CMV) infection during pregnancy.

- Make sure your child gets all the regular childhood vaccines.

- Keep your child away from high noise levels, such as from very loud toys.

Get Help

- If you think that your child might have hearing loss, ask the child's doctor for a **hearing screening** as soon as possible. Don't wait!

- If your child does not pass a hearing screening, ask the child's doctor for a **full hearing test** as soon as possible.

- If your child has hearing loss, talk to the child's doctor about **treatment and intervention services**.

Hearing loss can affect a child's ability to develop speech, language, and social skills. The earlier children with hearing loss start getting services, the more likely they are to reach their full potential. If you are a parent and you suspect your child has hearing loss, trust your instincts and speak with your child's doctor.

Section 24.2

Early Intervention and Special Education for Hearing Impairment

This section includes text excerpted from "Hearing Loss in
Children," Centers for Disease Control and Prevention (CDC),
February 18, 2015.

Treatment and Intervention Services

No single treatment or intervention is the answer for every child
or family. Good intervention plans will include close monitoring, follow-ups and any changes needed along the way. There are many different options for children with hearing loss and their families.
Some of the treatment and intervention options include:

- Working with a professional (or team) who can help a child and
  family learn to communicate.

- Getting a hearing device, such as a hearing aid.

- Joining support groups.

- Taking advantage of other resources available to children with a
  hearing loss and their families.

Early Intervention and Special Education

Early Intervention (0–3 years)

Hearing loss can affect a child's ability to develop speech, language,
and social skills. The earlier a child who is deaf or hard-of-hearing
starts getting services, the more likely the child's speech, language,
and social skills will reach their full potential.

Early intervention program services help young children with hearing loss learn language skills and other important skills. Research
shows that early intervention services can greatly improve a child's
development.

Babies that are diagnosed with hearing loss should begin to get intervention services as soon as possible, but **no later than 6 months of age**.

There are many services available through the Individuals with Disabilities Education Improvement Act 2004 (IDEA 2004). Services for children from birth through 36 months of age are called Early Intervention or Part C services. Even if your child has not been diagnosed with a hearing loss, he or she may be eligible for early intervention treatment services. The IDEA 2004 says that children under the age of three years (36 months) who are at risk of having developmental delays may be eligible for services. These services are provided through an early intervention system in your state. Through this system, you can ask for an evaluation.

Special Education (3–22 years)

Special education is instruction specifically designed to address the educational and related developmental needs of older children with disabilities, or those who are experiencing developmental delays. Services for these children are provided through the public school system. These services are available through the Individuals with Disabilities Education Improvement Act 2004, Part B.

Early Hearing Detection and Intervention (EHDI) Program

Every state has an Early Hearing Detection and Intervention (EHDI) program. EHDI works to identify infants and children with hearing loss. EHDI also promotes timely follow-up testing and services or interventions for any family whose child has a hearing loss. If your child has a hearing loss or if you have any concerns about your child's hearing, call toll free 1-800-CDC-INFO or contact your local EHDI Program coordinator to find available services in your state.

Technology

Many people who are deaf or hard-of-hearing have some hearing. The amount of hearing a deaf or hard-of-hearing person has is called "residual hearing." Technology does not "cure" hearing loss, but may help a child with hearing loss to make the most of their residual hearing. For those parents who choose to have their child use technology, there are many options, including:

- Hearing aids
- Cochlear implants
- Bone-anchored hearing aids
- Other assistive devices

Hearing Aids

Hearing aids make sounds louder. They can be worn by people of any age, including infants. Babies with hearing loss may understand sounds better using hearing aids. This may give them the chance to learn speech skills at a young age.

There are many styles of hearing aids. They can help many types of hearing losses. A young child is usually fitted with behind-the-ear style hearing aids because they are better suited to growing ears.

Cochlear Implants

A cochlear implant may help many children with severe to profound hearing loss—even very young children. It gives that child a way to hear when a hearing aid is not enough. Unlike a hearing aid, cochlear implants do not make sounds louder. A cochlear implant sends sound signals directly to the hearing nerve.

A cochlear implant has two main parts—the parts that are placed inside the ear during surgery, and the parts that are worn outside the ear after surgery. The parts outside the ear send sounds to the parts inside the ear.

Centers for Disease Control and Prevention (CDC) and the U.S. Food and Drug Administration (FDA) carried out studies in 2002 and 2006 to learn more about a possible link between cochlear implants and bacterial meningitis in children with cochlear implants.

Bone-Anchored Hearing Aids

This type of hearing aid can be considered when a child has either a conductive, mixed or unilateral hearing loss and is specifically suitable for children who cannot otherwise wear 'in the ear' or 'behind the ear' hearing aids.

Other Assistive Devices

Besides hearing aids, there are other devices that help people with hearing loss. Following are some examples of other assistive devices:

• FM System

An FM system is a kind of device that helps people with hearing loss hear in background noise. FM stands for frequency modulation. It is the same type of signal used for radios. FM systems send sound from a microphone used by someone speaking to a person wearing the receiver. This system is sometimes used with hearing aids. An extra piece is attached to the hearing aid that works with the FM system.

- Captioning

Many television programs, videos, and DVDs are captioned. Television sets made after 1993 are made to show the captioning. You don't have to buy anything special. Captions show the conversation spoken in soundtrack of a program on the bottom of the television screen.

- Other devices

There are many other devices available for children with hearing loss. Some of these include:

- Text messaging
- Telephone amplifiers
- Flashing and vibrating alarms
- Audio loop systems
- Infrared listening devices
- Portable sound amplifiers
- TTY (Text Telephone or teletypewriter)

Medical and Surgical

Medications or surgery may also help make the most of a person's hearing. This is especially true for a conductive hearing loss, or one that involves a part of the outer or middle ear that is not working in the usual way.

One type of conductive hearing loss can be caused by a chronic ear infection. A chronic ear infection is a build-up of fluid behind the eardrum in the middle ear space. Most ear infections are managed with medication or careful monitoring. Infections that don't go away with medication can be treated with a simple surgery that involves putting a tiny tube into the eardrum to drain the fluid out.

Another type of conductive hearing loss is caused by either the outer and or middle ear not forming correctly while the baby was growing in the mother's womb. Both the outer and middle ear need to work together in order for sound to be sent correctly to the inner ear. If any of these parts did not form correctly, there might be a hearing loss in that ear. This problem may be improved and perhaps even corrected with surgery. An ear, nose, and throat doctor (otolaryngologist) is the health care professional who usually takes care of this problem.

Placing a cochlear implant or bone-anchored hearing aid will also require a surgery.

Learning Language

Without extra help, children with hearing loss have problems learning language. These children can then be at risk for other delays. Families who have children with hearing loss often need to change their communication habits or learn special skills (such as sign language) to help their children learn language. These skills can be used together with hearing aids, cochlear implants, and other devices that help children hear.

Family Support Services

For many parents, their child's hearing loss is unexpected. Parents sometimes need time and support to adapt to the child's hearing loss.

Parents of children with recently identified hearing loss can seek different kinds of support. Support is anything that helps a family and may include advice, information, having the chance to get to know other parents that have a child with hearing loss, locating a deaf mentor, finding childcare or transportation, giving parents time for personal relaxation or just a supportive listener.

Section 24.3

Language and Communication Tools for Hearing Impairment

This section includes text excerpted from "Hearing Loss in Children," Centers for Disease Control and Prevention (CDC), February 18, 2015.

Learning Language

People with hearing loss and their families often need special skills to be able to learn language and communicate. These skills can be used together with hearing aids, cochlear implants, and other devices that help people hear. There are several approaches that can help, each emphasizing different language learning skills.

Some families choose a single approach because that's what works best for them. Other people choose skills from two or more approaches because that's what works best for them.

Following are language approaches, and the skills that are sometimes included in each of them:

- **Auditory-Oral**

  Natural Gestures, Listening, Speech (Lip) Reading, Spoken Speech

- **Auditory-Verbal**

  Listening, Spoken Speech

- **Bilingual**

  American Sign Language and English

- **Cued Speech**

  Cueing, Speech (Lip) Reading

- **Total Communication**

Conceptually Accurate Signed English (CASE), Signing Exact English (SEE), Finger Spelling, Listening, Manually Coded English (MCE), Natural Gestures, Speech (Lip) Reading, Spoken Speech.

Communication Tools

American Sign Language

American Sign Language (ASL) is a language itself. While English and Spanish are spoken languages, ASL is a visual language.

ASL is a complete language. People communicate using hand shapes, direction and motion of the hands, body language, and facial expressions. ASL has its own grammar, word order, and sentence structure. People can share feelings, jokes, and complete ideas using ASL.

Like any other language, ASL must be learned. People can take ASL classes and start teaching their baby even while they are still learning it. A baby can learn ASL as a first language. Also, experts in ASL can work with families to help them learn ASL.

Children can use many other skills with ASL. Finger spelling is one skill that is almost always used with ASL. Finger spelling is used to spell out words that don't have a sign—such as names of people and places.

Manually Coded English (MCE)

Manually Coded English (MCE) is made up of signs that are a visual code for spoken English. MCE is a code for a language—the English language. Many of the signs (hand shapes and hand motions) in MCE are borrowed from American Sign Language (ASL). But unlike ASL, the grammar, word order, and sentence structure of MCE are similar to the English language.

Children and adults can use many other communication tools along with MCE. One that is commonly used is finger spelling, which is used to spell out words that don't have a sign in MCE—such as names of people and places.

Conceptually Accurate Signed English (CASE)

Conceptually Accurate Signed English (CASE) (sometimes called Pidgin Signed English (PSE)) has developed between people who use American Sign Language (ASL), and people who use Manually Coded English (MCE), using signs based on ASL and MCE. This helps them understand each other better. CASE is flexible, and can be changed depending on the people using it.

Other communication tools can be used with CASE. Often, finger spelling is used in combination with CASE. Finger spelling is used to spell out words that don't have a sign, such as names of people and places.

Cued Speech

Cued Speech helps people who are deaf or hard-of-hearing better understand spoken languages.

When watching a person's mouth, many speech sounds look the same on the face even though the sounds heard are not the same. For instance, the words "mat," "bat," and "pat," look the same on the face even though they sound very different. When "cueing" English, the person communicating uses eight hand shapes and four places near the mouth to help the person looking tell the difference between speech sounds. Cued Speech allows the person to make out sounds and words when they are using other building blocks, such as speech reading (lip reading) or auditory training (listening).

Finger Spelling

With Finger Spelling the person uses hands and fingers to spell out words. Hand shapes represent the letters in the alphabet. Finger Spelling is used with many other communication methods; it is almost never used by itself. It is most often used with American Sign Language (ASL), Conceptually Accurate Signed English (CASE), and Manually Coded English (MCE) to spell out words that don't have a sign, such as the names of places or people.

Natural Gestures

"Natural Gestures"—or body language—are actions that people normally do to help others understand a message. For example, if a parent wants to ask a toddler if he or she wants to be picked up, the parent might stretch out her arms and ask, "Up?" For an older child, the parent might motion with her arms as she calls the child to come inside. Or, the parent might put a first finger over her mouth and nose to show that the child needs to be quiet.

Babies will begin to use this building block naturally if they can see what others are doing. This building block is not taught, it just comes naturally. It is always used with other building blocks.

Listening / Auditory Training

Most people who are deaf or hard-of-hearing have some hearing. This is called "residual hearing." Some people rely or learn how to maximize their resideral hearing (auditory training). This building block is often used in combination with other building blocks (such as hearing aids, cochlear implants, and other assistive devices).

Listening might seem easy to a person with hearing. But for a person with hearing loss, Listening is often hard without proper training. Like all other tools, the skill of Listening must be learned. Often a speech-language pathologist (a professional trained to teach people how to use speech and language) will work with the person with hearing loss and the family.

Spoken Speech

People can use speech to express themselves. Speech is a skill that many people take for granted. Learning to speak is a skill that can help build language.

Speech or learning to speak is often used in combination with hearing aids, cochlear implants, and other assistive devices that help people maximize their residual hearing. A person with some residual hearing may find it easier to learn speech than a person with no residual hearing. Since speech can only be used by a person to express him or herself other building blocks, such hearing with a hearing aid, must be added in order to help the person understands what is being said so they can communicate with others.

Speaking may seem easy to a person with hearing. But for a person with hearing loss, speaking is often hard without proper training. Like all other communication tools, the skill of speaking must be learned. Often a speech-language pathologist (a professional trained to teach people how to use speech and language) will work with the person with hearing loss and the family.

Speech Reading

Speech Reading (or lip reading) helps a person with hearing loss understand speech. The person watches the movements of a speaker's mouth and face, and understands what the speaker is saying. About 40% of the sounds in the English language can be seen on the lips of a speaker in good conditions, such as a well-lit room where the child can see the speaker's face. But some words can't be read. For example: "bop," "mop," and "pop," look exactly alike when spoken. (You can see this for yourself in a mirror). A good speech reader might be able to see only 4 to 5 words in a 12-word sentence.

Children often use speech reading in combination with other tools, such as auditory training (listening), cued speech, and others. But it can't be successful alone. Babies will naturally begin using this building block if they can see the speaker's mouth and face. But as a child gets older, he or she will still need some training.

Sometimes, when talking with a person who is deaf or hard-of-hearing, people will exaggerate their mouth movements or talk very loudly. Exaggerated mouth movements and a loud voice can make speech reading very hard. It is important to talk in a normal way and look directly at your child's face and make sure he or she is watching you.

Chapter 25

Pervasive Developmental Disorders (PDD)

Chapter Contents

Section 25.1

Facts about Developmental Disabilities

This section includes text excerpted from "Developmental Disabilities," Centers for Disease Control and Prevention (CDC), September 22, 2015.

Developmental disabilities are a group of conditions due to an impairment in physical, learning, language, or behavior areas. These conditions begin during the developmental period, may impact day-to-day functioning, and usually last throughout a person's lifetime.

Developmental Milestones

Skills such as taking a first step, smiling for the first time, and waving "bye-bye" are called developmental milestones. Children reach milestones in how they play, learn, speak, behave, and move (for example, crawling and walking).

Children develop at their own pace, so it's impossible to tell exactly when a child will learn a given skill. However, the developmental milestones give a general idea of the changes to expect as a child gets older.

As a parent, you know your child best. If your child is not meeting the milestones for his or her age, or if you think there could be a problem with your child's development, talk with your child's doctor or health care provider and share your concerns. Don't wait.

If You're Concerned

If your child is not meeting the milestones for his or her age, or you are concerned about your child's development, talk with your child's doctor and share your concerns. Don't wait!

Developmental Monitoring and Screening

A child's growth and development are followed through a partnership between parents and health care professionals. At each well-child visit, the doctor looks for developmental delays or problems and talks with the parents about any concerns the parents might have. This is called *developmental monitoring.*

Any problems noticed during developmental monitoring should be followed up with *developmental screening.* Developmental screening is a short test to tell if a child is learning basic skills when he or she should, or if there are delays.

If a child has a developmental delay, it is important to get help as soon as possible. Early identification and intervention can have a significant impact on a child's ability to learn new skills, as well as reduce the need for costly interventions over time.

Causes and Risk Factors

Developmental disabilities begin anytime during the developmental period and usually last throughout a person's lifetime. Most developmental disabilities begin before a baby is born, but some can happen after birth because of injury, infection, or other factors.

Most developmental disabilities are thought to be caused by a complex mix of factors. These factors include genetics; parental health and behaviors (such as smoking and drinking) during pregnancy; complications during birth; infections the mother might have during pregnancy or the baby might have very early in life; and exposure of the mother or child to high levels of environmental toxins, such as lead. For some developmental disabilities, such as fetal alcohol syndrome, which is caused by drinking alcohol during pregnancy, we know the cause. But for most, we don't.

Following are some examples of what we know about specific developmental disabilities:

- At least 25% of hearing loss among babies is due to maternal infections during pregnancy, such as cytomegalovirus (CMV) infection; complications after birth; and head trauma.

- Some of the most common known causes of intellectual disability include fetal alcohol syndrome; genetic and chromosomal conditions, such as Down syndrome and fragile X syndrome; and certain infections during pregnancy, such as toxoplasmosis.

- Children who have a sibling are at a higher risk of also having an autism spectrum disorder.

- Low birthweight, premature birth, multiple birth, and infections during pregnancy are associated with an increased risk for many developmental disabilities.

251

- Untreated newborn jaundice (high levels of bilirubin in the blood during the first few days after birth) can cause a type of brain damage known as kernicterus. Children with kernicterus are more likely to have cerebral palsy, hearing and vision problems, and problems with their teeth. Early detection and treatment of newborn jaundice can prevent kernicterus.

The Study to Explore Early Development (SEED) is a multiyear study funded by CDC. It is currently the largest study in the United States to help identify factors that may put children at risk for autism spectrum disorders and other developmental disabilities.

Who Is Affected?

Developmental disabilities occur among all racial, ethnic, and socioeconomic groups. Recent estimates in the United States show that about one in six, or about 15%, of children aged 3 through 17 years have a one or more developmental disabilities, such as:

- ADHD
- autism spectrum disorder
- cerebral palsy
- hearing loss
- intellectual disability
- learning disability
- vision impairment
- and other developmental delays.

For over a decade, CDC's Autism and Developmental Disabilities Monitoring (ADDM) Network has been tracking the number and characteristics of children with autism spectrum disorder, cerebral palsy, and intellectual disability in several diverse communities throughout the United States.

Living with a Developmental Disability

Children and adults with disabilities need health care and health programs for the same reasons anyone else does—to stay well, active, and a part of the community.

Having a disability does not mean a person is not healthy or that he or she cannot be healthy. Being healthy means the same thing for all of us—getting and staying well so we can lead full, active lives. That includes having the tools and information to make healthy choices and knowing how to prevent illness. Some health conditions, such as asthma, gastrointestinal symptoms, eczema and skin allergies, and migraine headaches, have been found to be more common among children with developmental disabilities. Thus, it is especially important for children with developmental disabilities to see a health care provider regularly.

CDC does not study education or treatment programs for people with developmental disabilities, nor does it provide direct services to people with developmental disabilities or to their families. However, CDC has put together a list of resources for people affected by developmental disabilities.

Section 25.2

What Are Pervasive Development Disorders (PDD)?

This section includes text excerpted from "NINDS Pervasive Developmental Disorders Information Page," National Institute of Neurological Disorders and Stroke (NINDS), February 1, 2016.

Overview

The diagnostic category of pervasive developmental disorders (PDD) refers to a group of disorders characterized by delays in the development of socialization and communication skills. Parents may note symptoms as early as infancy, although the typical age of onset is before three years of age. Symptoms may include problems with using and understanding language; difficulty relating to people, objects, and events; unusual play with toys and other objects; difficulty with changes in routine or familiar surroundings, and repetitive body movements or behavior patterns. Autism (a developmental brain disorder characterized by impaired social interaction and communication skills, and a limited range of activities and interests) is the most characteristic and best studied PDD. Other types of PDD include Asperger Syndrome, Childhood Disintegrative Disorder, and Rett Syndrome. Children with PDD vary widely in abilities, intelligence, and behaviors. Some children do not speak at all, others speak in limited phrases or conversations, and some have relatively normal language development. Repetitive play skills and limited social skills are generally evident. Unusual responses to sensory information, such as loud noises and lights, are also common.

Is There Any Treatment?

There is no known cure for PDD. Medications are used to address specific behavioral problems; therapy for children with PDD should be specialized according to need. Some children with PDD benefit from specialized classrooms in which the class size is small and instruction is given on a one-to-one basis. Others function well in standard special education classes or regular classes with additional support.

What Is the Prognosis?

Early intervention including appropriate and specialized educational programs and support services plays a critical role in improving the outcome of individuals with PDD. PDD is not fatal and does not affect normal life expectancy.

What Research Is Being Done?

The National Institute of Neurological Disorders and Stroke (NINDS) conducts and supports research on developmental disabilities, including PDD. Much of this research focuses on understanding the neurological basis of PDD and on developing techniques to diagnose, treat, prevent, and ultimately cure this and similar disorders.

Section 25.3

Autism Spectrum Disorder (ASD)

This section includes text excerpted from "Autism Spectrum
Disorder Fact Sheet," National Institute of Neurological
Disorders and Stroke (NINDS), February 1, 2016.

What Is Autism Spectrum Disorder?

Autism spectrum disorder (ASD) refers to a group of complex neurodevelopment disorders characterized by repetitive and characteristic
patterns of behavior and difficulties with social communication and
interaction. The symptoms are present from early childhood and affect
daily functioning.

The term "spectrum" refers to the wide range of symptoms, skills,
and levels of disability in functioning that can occur in people with
ASD. Some children and adults with ASD are fully able to perform
all activities of daily living while others require substantial support
to perform basic activities. The *Diagnostic and Statistical Manual of
Mental Disorders* (DSM-5, published in 2013) includes Asperger syndrome, childhood disintegrative disorder, and pervasive developmental
disorders not otherwise specified (PDD-NOS) as part of ASD rather
than as separate disorders. A diagnosis of ASD includes an assessment
of intellectual disability and language impairment.

ASD occurs in every racial and ethnic group, and across all socioeconomic levels. However, boys are significantly more likely to develop
ASD than girls. The latest analysis from the Centers for Disease Control and Prevention estimates that 1 in 68 children has ASD.

What Are Some Common Signs of ASD?

Even as infants, children with ASD may seem different, especially
when compared to other children their own age. They may become
overly focused on certain objects, rarely make eye contact, and fail to
engage in typical babbling with their parents. In other cases, children
may develop normally until the second or even third year of life, but
then start to withdraw and become indifferent to social engagement.

255

The severity of ASD can vary greatly and is based on the degree to which social communication, insistence of sameness of activities and surroundings, and repetitive patterns of behavior affect the daily functioning of the individual.

Social Impairment and Communication Difficulties

Many people with ASD find social interactions difficult. The mutual give-and-take nature of typical communication and interaction is often particularly challenging. Children with ASD may fail to respond to their names, avoid eye contact with other people, and only interact with others to achieve specific goals. Often children with ASD do not understand how to play or engage with other children and may prefer to be alone. People with ASD may find it difficult to understand other people's feelings or talk about their own feelings.

People with ASD may have very different verbal abilities ranging from no speech at all to speech that is fluent, but awkward and inappropriate. Some children with ASD may have delayed speech and language skills, may repeat phrases, and give unrelated answers to questions. In addition, people with ASD can have a hard time using and understanding non-verbal cues such as gestures, body language, or tone of voice. For example, young children with ASD might not understand what it means to wave goodbye. People with ASD may also speak in flat, robot-like or a sing-song voice about a narrow range of favorite topics, with little regard for the interests of the person to whom they are speaking.

Repetitive and Characteristic Behaviors

Many children with ASD engage in repetitive movements or unusual behaviors such as flapping their arms, rocking from side to side, or twirling. They may become preoccupied with parts of objects like the wheels on a toy truck. Children may also become obsessively interested in a particular topic such as airplanes or memorizing train schedules. Many people with ASD seem to thrive so much on routine that changes to the daily patterns of life—like an unexpected stop on the way home from school—can be very challenging. Some children may even get angry or have emotional outbursts, especially when placed in a new or overly stimulating environment.

What Disorders Are Related to ASD?

Certain known genetic disorders are associated with an increased risk for autism, including fragile X syndrome (which causes intellectual disability) and tuberous sclerosis (which causes benign tumors to grow in the brain and other vital organs)—each of which results from a mutation in a single, but different, gene. Recently, researchers have discovered other genetic mutations in children diagnosed with autism, including some that have not yet been designated as named syndromes. While each of these disorders is rare, in aggregate, they may account for 20 percent or more of all autism cases.

People with ASD also have a higher than average risk of having epilepsy. Children whose language skills regress early in life—before age 3—appear to have a risk of developing epilepsy or seizure-like brain activity. About 20 to 30 percent of children with ASD develop epilepsy by the time they reach adulthood. Additionally, people with both ASD and intellectual disability have the greatest risk of developing seizure disorder.

How Is ASD Diagnosed?

ASD symptoms can vary greatly from person to person depending on the severity of the disorder. Symptoms may even go unrecognized for young children who have mild ASD or less debilitating handicaps. Very early indicators that require evaluation by an expert include:

- no babbling or pointing by age one

- no single words by age 16 months or two-word phrases by age two

- no response to name

- loss of language or social skills previously acquired

- poor eye contact

- excessive lining up of toys or objects

- no smiling or social responsiveness

Later indicators include:

- impaired ability to make friends with peers

- impaired ability to initiate or sustain a conversation with others

- absence or impairment of imaginative and social play

- repetitive or unusual use of language

- abnormally intense or focused interest

- preoccupation with certain objects or subjects

- inflexible adherence to specific routines or rituals

Health care providers will often use a questionnaire or other screening instrument to gather information about a child's development and behavior. Some screening instruments rely solely on parent observations, while others rely on a combination of parent and doctor observations. If screening instruments indicate the possibility of ASD, a more comprehensive evaluation is usually indicated.

A comprehensive evaluation requires a multidisciplinary team, including a psychologist, neurologist, psychiatrist, speech therapist, and other professionals who diagnose and treat children with ASD. The team members will conduct a thorough neurological assessment and in-depth cognitive and language testing. Because hearing problems can cause behaviors that could be mistaken for ASD, children with delayed speech development should also have their hearing tested.

What Causes ASD?

Scientists believe that both genetics and environment likely play a role in ASD. There is great concern that rates of autism have been increasing in recent decades without full explanation as to why. Researchers have identified a number of genes associated with the disorder. Imaging studies of people with ASD have found differences in the development of several regions of the brain. Studies suggest that ASD could be a result of disruptions in normal brain growth very early in development. These disruptions may be the result of defects in genes that control brain development and regulate how brain cells communicate with each other. Autism is more common in children born prematurely. Environmental factors may also play a role in gene function and development, but no specific environmental causes have yet been identified. The theory that parental practices are responsible for ASD has long been disproved. Multiple studies have shown that vaccination to prevent childhood infectious diseases does not increase the risk of autism in the population.

What Role Do Genes Play?

Twin and family studies strongly suggest that some people have a genetic predisposition to autism. Identical twin studies show that if one twin is affected, then the other will be affected between 36 to 95 percent of the time. There are a number of studies in progress to determine the specific genetic factors associated with the development of ASD. In families with one child with ASD, the risk of having a second child with the disorder also increases. Many of the genes found to be associated with autism are involved in the function of the chemical connections between brain neurons (synapses). Researchers are looking for clues about which genes contribute to increased susceptibility. In some cases, parents and other relatives of a child with ASD show mild impairments in social communication skills or engage in repetitive behaviors. Evidence also suggests that emotional disorders such as bipolar disorder and schizophrenia occur more frequently than average in the families of people with ASD.

In addition to genetic variations that are inherited and are present in nearly all of a person's cells, recent research has also shown that *de novo*, or spontaneous, gene mutations can influence the risk of developing autism spectrum disorder. *De novo* mutations are changes in sequences of deoxyribonucleic acid or DNA, the hereditary material in humans, which can occur spontaneously in a parent's sperm or egg cell or during fertilization. The mutation then occurs in each cell as the fertilized egg divides. These mutations may affect single genes or they may be changes called copy number variations, in which stretches of DNA containing multiple genes are deleted or duplicated. Recent studies have shown that people with ASD tend to have more copy number *de novo* gene mutations than those without the disorder, suggesting that for some the risk of developing ASD is not the result of mutations in individual genes but rather spontaneous coding mutations across many genes. *De novo* mutations may explain genetic disorders in which an affected child has the mutation in each cell but the parents do not and there is no family pattern to the disorder. Autism risk also increases in children born to older parents. There is still much research to be done to determine the potential role of environmental factors on spontaneous mutations and how that influences ASD risk.

Do Symptoms of Autism Change over Time?

For many children, symptoms improve with age and behavioral treatment. During adolescence, some children with ASD may become depressed or experience behavioral problems, and their treatment may need some modification as they transition to adulthood. People with ASD usually continue to need services and supports as they get older, but depending on severity of the disorder, people with ASD may be able to work successfully and live independently or within a supportive environment.

How Is Autism Treated?

There is no cure for ASD. Therapies and behavioral interventions are designed to remedy specific symptoms and can substantially improve those symptoms. The ideal treatment plan coordinates therapies and interventions that meet the specific needs of the individual. Most health care professionals agree that the earlier the intervention, the better.

Educational/behavioral interventions: Early behavioral/educational interventions have been very successful in many children with ASD. In these interventions therapists use highly structured and intensive skill-oriented training sessions to help children develop social and language skills, such as applied behavioral analysis, which encourages positive behaviors and discourages negative ones. In addition, family counseling for the parents and siblings of children with ASD often helps families cope with the particular challenges of living with a child with ASD.

Medications: While medication can't cure ASD or even treat its main symptoms, there are some that can help with related symptoms such as anxiety, depression, and obsessive-compulsive disorder. Antipsychotic medications are used to treat severe behavioral problems. Seizures can be treated with one or more anticonvulsant drugs. Medication used to treat people with attention deficit disorder can be used effectively to help decrease impulsivity and hyperactivity in people with ASD. Parents, caregivers, and people with autism should use caution before adopting any unproven treatments.

Section 25.4

Asperger Syndrome

This section includes text excerpted from "Asperger Syndrome," Genetic and Rare Diseases Information Center (GARD), June 8, 2015.

What Is Asperger Syndrome?

Asperger syndrome (AS) is an autism spectrum disorder, a type of neurological condition characterized by impaired language and communication skills, and repetitive or restrictive thought and behavior patterns. Unlike many people with autism, those with AS retain their early language skills. Features of AS include an obsessive interest in a particular object or topic; high vocabulary; formal speech patterns; repetitive routines or habits; inappropriate social and emotional behavior; impaired non-verbal communication; and uncoordinated motor skills. AS is likely caused by a combination of genetic and environmental influences. While autism spectrum disorders including AS sometimes run in families, no specific inheritance pattern has been recognized.

Is Asperger Syndrome Inherited?

Autism spectrum disorders including Asperger syndrome sometimes "run in families," but no specific inheritance pattern has been recognized. The condition is likely caused by a combination of genetic and environmental factors, which means that not all people with a genetic predisposition will be affected. A consultation with a genetics professional is recommended for those with specific questions about genetic risks to themselves or family members.

What Is the Long-Term Outlook for People with Asperger Syndrome?

Asperger syndrome (AS) is considered to be a life-long disorder, but the long-term outlook (prognosis) varies among affected people. With proper support, education, and treatment, people with AS can learn to cope with their disabilities and can enjoy a good quality of life. While features of the disorder may diminish over time, many people continue to struggle with social interactions and personal relationships. Many adults with AS are able to work successfully in mainstream jobs, although they may continue to need encouragement and moral support to maintain an independent life.

Section 25.5

Rett Syndrome

This section includes text excerpted from "Rett Syndrome," Genetics Home Reference (GHR), National Institutes of Health (NIH), April 26, 2016.

What Is Rett Syndrome?

Rett syndrome is a brain disorder that occurs almost exclusively in girls. The most common form of the condition is known as classic Rett syndrome. After birth, girls with classic Rett syndrome have 6 to 18 months of apparently normal development before developing severe problems with language and communication, learning, coordination, and other brain functions. Early in childhood, affected girls lose purposeful use of their hands and begin making repeated hand wringing, washing, or clapping motions. They tend to grow more slowly than other children and have a small head size (microcephaly). Other signs and symptoms that can develop include breathing abnormalities, seizures, an abnormal side-to-side curvature of the spine (scoliosis), and sleep disturbances.

Researchers have described several variant or atypical forms of Rett syndrome, which can be milder or more severe than the classic form.

Frequency

This condition affects an estimated 1 in 8,500 females.

Genetic Changes

Classic Rett syndrome and some variant forms of the condition are caused by mutations in the *MECP2* gene. This gene provides instructions for making a protein (MeCP2) that is critical for normal brain function. Although the exact function of the MeCP2 protein is unclear, it is likely involved in maintaining connections (synapses) between nerve cells (neurons). It may also be necessary for the normal function of other types of brain cells.

The MeCP2 protein is thought to help regulate the activity of genes in the brain. This protein may also control the production of different versions of certain proteins in brain cells. Mutations in the MECP2 gene alter the MeCP2 protein or result in the production of less protein, which appears to disrupt the normal function of neurons and other cells in the brain. Specifically, studies suggest that changes in the MeCP2 protein may reduce the activity of certain neurons and impair their ability to communicate with one another. It is unclear how these changes lead to the specific features of Rett syndrome.

Several conditions with signs and symptoms overlapping those of Rett syndrome have been found to result from mutations in other genes. These conditions, including *FOXG1* syndrome, were previously thought to be variant forms of Rett syndrome. However, doctors and researchers have identified some important differences between the conditions, so they are now usually considered to be separate disorders.

Inheritance Pattern

In more than 99 percent of people with Rett syndrome, there is no history of the disorder in their family. Many of these cases result from new mutations in the *MECP2* gene.

A few families with more than one affected family member have been described. These cases helped researchers determine that classic Rett syndrome and variants caused by *MECP2* gene mutations have an X-linked dominant pattern of inheritance. A condition is considered X-linked if the mutated gene that causes the disorder is located on the X chromosome, one of the two sex chromosomes. The inheritance is dominant if one copy of the altered gene in each cell is sufficient to cause the condition.

Males with mutations in the *MECP2* gene often die in infancy. However, a small number of males with a genetic change involving *MECP2* have developed signs and symptoms similar to those of Rett syndrome, including intellectual disability, seizures, and movement problems. In males, this condition is described as MECP2-related severe neonatal encephalopathy.

Diagnosis and Management

These resources address the diagnosis or management of Rett syndrome:

- Boston Children's Hospital
- Cleveland Clinic

Other Names for this Condition

- Autism-dementia-ataxia-loss of purposeful hand use syndrome
- Rett disorder
- Rett disorder
- Rett syndrome
- RTS
- RTT

Chapter 26

Specific Language Impairment

What Is Specific Language Impairment?

Specific language impairment (SLI) is a language disorder that delays the mastery of language skills in children who have no hearing loss or other developmental delays. SLI is also called developmental language disorder, language delay, or developmental dysphasia. It is one of the most common childhood learning disabilities, affecting approximately 7 to 8 percent of children in kindergarten. The impact of SLI persists into adulthood.

What Causes Specific Language Impairment?

The cause of SLI is unknown, but recent discoveries suggest it has a strong genetic link. Children with SLI are more likely than those without SLI to have parents and siblings who also have had difficulties and delays in speaking. In fact, 50 to 70 percent of children with SLI have at least one other family member with the disorder.

This chapter includes text excerpted from "Specific Language Impairment," National Institute on Deafness and Other Communication Disorders (NIDCD), April 24, 2015.

What Are the Symptoms of Specific Language Impairment?

Children with SLI are often late to talk and may not produce any words until they are 2 years old. At age 3, they may talk, but may not be understood. As they grow older, children with SLI will struggle to learn new words and make conversation. Having difficulty using verbs is a hallmark of SLI. Typical errors that a 5-year-old child with SLI would make include dropping the "s" from the end of present-tense verbs, dropping past tense, and asking questions without the usual "be" or "do" verbs. For example, instead of saying "She rides the horse," a child with SLI will say, "She ride the horse." Instead of saying "He ate the cookie," a child with SLI will say, "He eat the cookie." Instead of saying "Why does he like me?", a child with SLI will ask, "Why he like me?"

How Is Specific Language Impairment Diagnosed in Children?

The first person to suspect a child might have SLI is often a parent or preschool or school teacher. A number of speech-language professionals might be involved in the diagnosis, including a speech-language pathologist (a health professional trained to evaluate and treat children with speech or language problems). Language skills are tested using assessment tools that evaluate how well the child constructs sentences and keeps words in their proper order, the number of words in his or her vocabulary, and the quality of his or her spoken language. There are a number of tests commercially available that can specifically diagnose SLI. Some of the tests use interactions between the child and puppets and other toys to focus on specific rules of grammar, especially the misuse of verb tenses. These tests can be used with children between 3 and 8 years of age and are especially useful for identifying children with SLI once they enter school.

What Treatments Are Available for Specific Language Impairment?

Because SLI affects reading it also affects learning. If it is not treated early, it can affect a child's performance in school. Since the early signs of SLI are often present in children as young as 3 years old, the preschool years can be used to prepare them for kindergarten with special programs designed to enrich language development. This kind of classroom program might enlist normally developing children to act as role models for children with SLI and feature activities that encourage role-playing and sharing time, as well as hands-on lessons to explore new, interesting vocabulary. Some parents also might want their child to see a speech-language pathologist, who can assess their child's needs, engage him or her in structured activities, and recommend home materials for at-home enrichment.

What Kinds of Research Are Being Conducted?

The National Institute on Deafness and Other Communication Disorders (NIDCD) supports a wide variety of research to understand the genetic underpinnings of SLI, the nature of the language deficits that cause it, and better ways to diagnose and treat children with it.

- **Genetic research:** An NIDCD-supported investigator recently has identified a mutation in a gene on chromosome 6, called the KIAA0319 gene, that appears to play a key role in SLI. The mutation plays a supporting role in other learning disabilities, such as dyslexia, some cases of autism, and speech sound disorders (conditions in which speech sounds are either not produced or produced or used incorrectly). This finding lends support to the idea that difficulties in learning language may be coming from the same genes that influence difficulties with reading and understanding printed text. Other potentially influential genes also are being explored.

- **Bilingual research:** The standardized tests that speech-language pathologists use in schools to screen for language impairments are based on typical language development milestones in English. Because bilingual children are more likely to score in the at-risk range on these tests, it becomes difficult to distinguish between children who are struggling to learn a new language and children with true language impairments. After studying a large group of Hispanic children who speak English as a second language, NIDCD-funded researchers have developed a dual language diagnostic test to identify bilingual children with language impairments. It's now being tested in a group of children 4 to 6 years old, and will eventually be expanded to children 7 to 9 years old. The same research team is also trying out an intervention program with a small group of bilingual first graders with SLI to find techniques and strategies to help them succeed academically.

- **Diagnostic research:** Children with SLI have significant communication problems, which are also characteristic of most children with autism spectrum disorders (ASD). Impairments in understanding and the onset of spoken language are common in both groups. No one knows yet if there are early developmental signs that could signal or predict language difficulties and might potentially allow for early identification and intervention with these children. The NIDCD is currently funding researchers looking for risk markers associated with SLI and ASD that could signal later problems in speech and communication. In a group of children 6 months to 1 year old who, because of family history, are at risk for SLI or ASD, the investigators are collecting data using behavioral, eye-tracking, and neurophysiological measures, as well as general measures of cognitive and brain development. They will then follow these children until they are 3 years old to see if there are indicators that are specific to SLI or ASD or that could predict the development of either disorder. Findings from this research could have a major influence in developing new approaches to early screening and diagnosis for SLI and ASD.

Chapter 27

Tourette Syndrome (TS)

Chapter Contents

Section 27.1

Tourette Syndrome: Overview

This section includes text excerpted from "Tourette Syndrome Fact Sheet," National Institute of Neurological Disorders and Stroke (NINDS), April 16, 2014.

What Is Tourette Syndrome?

Tourette syndrome (TS) is a neurological disorder characterized by repetitive, stereotyped, involuntary movements and vocalizations called tics. The disorder is named for Dr. Georges Gilles de la Tourette, the pioneering French neurologist who in 1885 first described the condition in an 86-year-old French noblewoman.

The early symptoms of TS are typically noticed first in childhood, with the average onset between the ages of 3 and 9 years. TS occurs in people from all ethnic groups; males are affected about three to four times more often than females. It is estimated that 200,000 Americans have the most severe form of TS, and as many as one in 100 exhibit milder and less complex symptoms such as chronic motor or vocal tics. Although TS can be a chronic condition with symptoms lasting a lifetime, most people with the condition experience their worst tic symptoms in their early teens, with improvement occurring in the late teens and continuing into adulthood.

What Are the Symptoms?

Tics are classified as either simple or complex. Simple motor tics are sudden, brief, repetitive movements that involve a limited number of muscle groups. Some of the more common simple tics include eye blinking and other eye movements, facial grimacing, shoulder shrugging, and head or shoulder jerking. Simple vocalizations might include repetitive throat-clearing, sniffing, or grunting sounds. Complex tics are distinct, coordinated patterns of movements involving several muscle groups. Complex motor tics might include facial grimacing combined with a head twist and a shoulder shrug. Other complex motor tics may actually appear purposeful, including sniffing or touching objects, hopping, jumping, bending, or twisting. Simple vocal tics may include throat-clearing, sniffing/snorting, grunting, or barking. More complex vocal tics include words or phrases. Perhaps the most dramatic and disabling tics include motor movements that result in self-harm such as punching oneself in the face or vocal tics including coprolalia (uttering socially inappropriate words such as swearing) or echolalia (repeating the words or phrases of others). However, coprolalia is only present in a small number (10 to 15 percent) of individuals with TS. Some tics are preceded by an urge or sensation in the affected muscle group, commonly called a premonitory urge. Some with TS will describe a need to complete a tic in a certain way or a certain number of times in order to relieve the urge or decrease the sensation.

Tics are often worse with excitement or anxiety and better during calm, focused activities. Certain physical experiences can trigger or worsen tics, for example tight collars may trigger neck tics, or hearing another person sniff or throat-clear may trigger similar sounds. Tics do not go away during sleep but are often significantly diminished.

What Is the Course of Tourette Syndrome?

Tics come and go over time, varying in type, frequency, location, and severity. The first symptoms usually occur in the head and neck area and may progress to include muscles of the trunk and extremities. Motor tics generally precede the development of vocal tics and simple tics often precede complex tics. Most patients experience peak tic severity before the mid-teen years with improvement for the majority of patients in the late teen years and early adulthood. Approximately 10-15 percent of those affected have a progressive or disabling course that lasts into adulthood.

Can People with TS Control Their Tics?

Although the symptoms of TS are involuntary, some people can sometimes suppress, camouflage, or otherwise manage their tics in an effort to minimize their impact on functioning. However, people with TS often report a substantial buildup in tension when suppressing their tics to the point where they feel that the tic must be expressed (against their will). Tics in response to an environmental trigger can appear to be voluntary or purposeful but are not.

What Causes Tourette Syndrome?

Although the cause of TS is unknown, current research points to abnormalities in certain brain regions (including the basal ganglia,

271

frontal lobes, and cortex), the circuits that interconnect these regions, and the neurotransmitters (dopamine, serotonin, and norepinephrine) responsible for communication among nerve cells. Given the often complex presentation of TS, the cause of the disorder is likely to be equally complex.

What Disorders Are Associated with Tourette Syndrome?

Many individuals with TS experience additional neurobehavioral problems that often cause more impairment than the tics themselves. These include inattention, hyperactivity and impulsivity (attention deficit hyperactivity disorder—ADHD); problems with reading, writing, and arithmetic; and obsessive-compulsive symptoms such as intrusive thoughts/worries and repetitive behaviors. For example, worries about dirt and germs may be associated with repetitive hand-washing, and concerns about bad things happening may be associated with ritualistic behaviors such as counting, repeating, or ordering and arranging. People with TS have also reported problems with depression or anxiety disorders, as well as other difficulties with living, that may or may not be directly related to TS. In addition, although most individuals with TS experience a significant decline in motor and vocal tics in late adolescence and early adulthood, the associated neurobehavioral conditions may persist. Given the range of potential complications, people with TS are best served by receiving medical care that provides a comprehensive treatment plan.

How Is Tourette Syndrome Diagnosed?

TS is a diagnosis that doctors make after verifying that the patient has had both motor and vocal tics for at least 1 year. The existence of other neurological or psychiatric conditions can also help doctors arrive at a diagnosis. Common tics are not often misdiagnosed by knowledgeable clinicians. However, atypical symptoms or atypical presentations (for example, onset of symptoms in adulthood) may require specific specialty expertise for diagnosis. There are no blood, laboratory, or imaging tests needed for diagnosis. In rare cases, neuroimaging studies, such as magnetic resonance imaging (MRI) or computerized tomography (CT), electroencephalogram (EEG) studies, or certain blood tests may be used to rule out other conditions that might be confused with TS when the history or clinical examination is atypical.

It is not uncommon for patients to obtain a formal diagnosis of TS only after symptoms have been present for some time. The reasons for this are many. For families and physicians unfamiliar with TS, mild and even moderate tic symptoms may be considered inconsequential, part of a developmental phase, or the result of another condition. For example, parents may think that eye blinking is related to vision problems or that sniffing is related to seasonal allergies. Many patients are self-diagnosed after they, their parents, other relatives, or friends read or hear about TS from others.

How Is Tourette Syndrome Treated?

Because tic symptoms often do not cause impairment, the majority of people with TS require no medication for tic suppression. However, effective medications are available for those whose symptoms interfere with functioning. Neuroleptics (drugs that may be used to treat psychotic and non-psychotic disorders) are the most consistently useful medications for tic suppression; a number are available but some are more effective than others (for example, haloperidol and pimozide).

Unfortunately, there is no one medication that is helpful to all people with TS, nor does any medication completely eliminate symptoms. In addition, all medications have side effects. Many neuroleptic side effects can be managed by initiating treatment slowly and reducing the dose when side effects occur. The most common side effects of neuroleptics include sedation, weight gain, and cognitive dulling. Neurological side effects such as tremor, dystonic reactions (twisting movements or postures), parkinsonian-like symptoms, and other dyskinetic (involuntary) movements are less common and are readily managed with dose reduction.

Discontinuing neuroleptics after long-term use must be done slowly to avoid rebound increases in tics and withdrawal dyskinesias. One form of dyskinesia called tardive dyskinesia is a movement disorder distinct from TS that may result from the chronic use of neuroleptics. The risk of this side effect can be reduced by using lower doses of neuroleptics for shorter periods of time.

Other medications may also be useful for reducing tic severity, but most have not been as extensively studied or shown to be as consistently useful as neuroleptics. Additional medications with demonstrated efficacy include alpha-adrenergic agonists such as clonidine and guanfacine. These medications are used primarily for hypertension but are also used in the treatment of tics. The most common side effect from these medications that precludes their use is sedation. However, given the lower side effect risk associated with these medications, they are often used as first-line agents before proceeding to treatment with neuroleptics.

Effective medications are also available to treat some of the associated neurobehavioral disorders that can occur in patients with TS. Recent research shows that stimulant medications such as methylphenidate and dextroamphetamine can lessen ADHD symptoms in people with TS without causing tics to become more severe. However, the product labeling for stimulants currently contraindicates the use of these drugs in children with tics/TS and those with a family history of tics. Scientists hope that future studies will include a thorough discussion of the risks and benefits of stimulants in those with TS or a family history of TS and will clarify this issue. For obsessive-compulsive symptoms that significantly disrupt daily functioning, the serotonin reuptake inhibitors (clomipramine, fluoxetine, fluvoxamine, paroxetine, and sertraline) have been proven effective in some patients.

Behavioral treatments such as awareness training and competing response training can also be used to reduce tics. A recent NIH-funded, multi-center randomized control trial called Cognitive Behavioral Intervention for Tics, or CBIT, showed that training to voluntarily move in response to a premonitory urge can reduce tic symptoms. Other behavioral therapies, such as biofeedback or supportive therapy, have not been shown to reduce tic symptoms. However, supportive therapy can help a person with TS better cope with the disorder and deal with the secondary social and emotional problems that sometimes occur.

Is Tourette Syndrome Inherited?

Evidence from twin and family studies suggests that TS is an inherited disorder. Although early family studies suggested an autosomal dominant mode of inheritance (an autosomal dominant disorder is one in which only one copy of the defective gene, inherited from one parent, is necessary to produce the disorder), more recent studies suggest that the pattern of inheritance is much more complex. Although there may be a few genes with substantial effects, it is also possible that many genes with smaller effects and environmental factors may play a role in the development of TS.

Genetic studies also suggest that some forms of ADHD and OCD are genetically related to TS, but there is less evidence for a genetic relationship between TS and other neurobehavioral problems that commonly co-occur with TS. It is important for families to understand that genetic predisposition may not necessarily result in full-blown

TS; instead, it may express itself as a milder tic disorder or as obsessive-compulsive behaviors. It is also possible that the gene-carrying offspring will not develop any TS symptoms.

The gender of the person also plays an important role in TS gene expression. At-risk males are more likely to have tics and at-risk females are more likely to have obsessive-compulsive symptoms.

Genetic counseling of individuals with TS should include a full review of all potentially hereditary conditions in the family.

What Is the Prognosis?

Although there is no cure for TS, the condition in many individuals improves in the late teens and early 20s. As a result, some may actually become symptom-free or no longer need medication for tic suppression. Although the disorder is generally lifelong and chronic, it is not a degenerative condition. Individuals with TS have a normal life expectancy. TS does not impair intelligence. Although tic symptoms tend to decrease with age, it is possible that neurobehavioral disorders such as ADHD, OCD, depression, generalized anxiety, panic attacks, and mood swings can persist and cause impairment in adult life.

What Is the Best Educational Setting for Children with Tourette Syndrome?

Although students with TS often function well in the regular classroom, ADHD, learning disabilities, obsessive-compulsive symptoms, and frequent tics can greatly interfere with academic performance or social adjustment. After a comprehensive assessment, students should be placed in an educational setting that meets their individual needs. Students may require tutoring, smaller or special classes, and in some cases special schools.

All students with TS need a tolerant and compassionate setting that both encourages them to work to their full potential and is flexible enough to accommodate their special needs. This setting may include a private study area, exams outside the regular classroom, or even oral exams when the child's symptoms interfere with his or her ability to write. Untimed testing reduces stress for students with TS.

What Research Is Being Done?

Within the Federal government, the National Institute of Neurological Disorders and Stroke (NINDS), a part of the National Institutes of

Health (NIH), is responsible for supporting and conducting research on the brain and nervous system. The NINDS and other NIH components, such as the National Institute of Mental Health, the Eunice Kennedy Shriver National Institute of Child Health and Human Development, the National Institute on Drug Abuse, and the National Institute on Deafness and Other Communication Disorders, support research of relevance to TS, either at NIH laboratories or through grants to major research institutions across the country. Another component of the Department of Health and Human Services, the Centers for Disease Control and Prevention, funds professional education programs as well as TS research.

Knowledge about TS comes from studies across a number of medical and scientific disciplines, including genetics, neuroimaging, neuropathology, clinical trials (medication and non-medication), epidemiology, neurophysiology, neuroimmunology, and descriptive/diagnostic clinical science.

Genetic studies. Currently, NIH-funded investigators are conducting a variety of large-scale genetic studies. Rapid advances in the technology of gene discovery will allow for genome-wide screening approaches in TS, and finding a gene or genes for TS would be a major step toward understanding genetic risk factors. In addition, understanding the genetics of TS genes may strengthen clinical diagnosis, improve genetic counseling, lead to the clarification of pathophysiology, and provide clues for more effective therapies.

Neuroimaging studies. Advances in imaging technology and an increase in trained investigators have led to an increasing use of novel and powerful techniques to identify brain regions, circuitry, and neurochemical factors important in TS and related conditions.

Neuropathology. There has been an increase in the number and quality of donated postmortem brains from TS patients available for research purposes. This increase, coupled with advances in neuropathological techniques, has led to initial findings with implications for neuroimaging studies and animal models of TS.

Clinical trials. A number of clinical trials in TS have recently been completed or are currently underway. These include studies of stimulant treatment of ADHD in TS and behavioral treatments for reducing tic severity in children and adults. Smaller trials of novel approaches to treatment such as dopamine agonists and glutamatergic medications also show promise.

Epidemiology and clinical science. Careful epidemiological studies now estimate the prevalence of TS to be substantially higher than previously thought with a wider range of clinical severity. Furthermore, clinical studies are providing new findings regarding TS and co-existing conditions. These include subtyping studies of TS and OCD, an examination of the link between ADHD and learning problems in children with TS, a new appreciation of sensory tics, and the role of co-existing disorders in rage attacks. One of the most important and controversial areas of TS science involves the relationship between TS and autoimmune brain injury associated with group A beta-hemolytic streptococcal infections or other infectious processes. There are a number of epidemiological and clinical investigations currently underway in this intriguing area.

Section 27.2

Tourette Syndrome: Other Concerns and Conditions

This section includes text excerpted from "Tourette Syndrome (TS)," Centers for Disease Control and Prevention (CDC), November 30, 2015.

Other Concerns and Conditions

Tourette syndrome (TS) often occurs with other related conditions (also called co-occurring conditions). These conditions can include attention deficit hyperactivity disorder (ADHD), obsessive-compulsive disorder (OCD), and other behavioral or conduct problems. People with TS and related conditions can be at higher risk for learning, behavioral, and social problems.

The symptoms of other disorders can complicate the diagnosis and treatment of TS and create extra challenges for people with TS and their families, educators, and health professionals.

Findings from a national Centers for Disease Control and Prevention (CDC) study indicated that 86% of children who had been diagnosed with TS also had been diagnosed with at least one additional mental health, behavioral, or developmental condition based on parent report.

Among children with TS:

- 63% had ADHD

- 26% had behavioral problems, such as oppositional defiant disorder (ODD) or conduct disorder (CD)

- 49% had anxiety problems

- 25% had depression

- 35% had an autism spectrum disorder

- 47% had a learning disability

- 29% had a speech or language problem

- 30% had a developmental delay

- 12% had an intellectual disability

Because co-occurring conditions are so common among people with TS, it is important for doctors to assess every child with TS for other conditions and problems.

Attention Deficit Hyperactivity Disorder (ADHD)

In this national CDC study, ADHD was the most common co-occurring condition among children with TS. Of children who had been diagnosed with TS, 63% also had been diagnosed with ADHD.

Children with ADHD have trouble paying attention and controlling impulsive behaviors. They might act without thinking about what the result will be and, in some cases, they are also overly active. It is normal for children to have trouble focusing and behaving at one time or another. However, these behaviors continue beyond early childhood (0-5 years of age) among children with ADHD. Symptoms of ADHD can continue and can cause difficulty at school, at home, or with friends.

Obsessive-Compulsive Behaviors

People with obsessive-compulsive behaviors have unwanted thoughts (obsessions) that they feel a need to respond to (compulsions). Obsessive-compulsive behaviors and obsessive-compulsive disorder (OCD) have been shown to occur among more than one-third of people with TS. Sometimes it is difficult to tell the difference between complex tics that a child with TS may have and obsessive-compulsive behaviors.

Behavior or Conduct Problems

Findings from the CDC study indicated that behavior or conduct problems, such as oppositional defiant disorder (ODD) or conduct disorder (CD), had been diagnosed among 26% of children with TS.

Oppositional Defiant Disorder (ODD)

People with ODD show negative, defiant and hostile behaviors toward adults or authority figures. ODD usually starts before a child is 8 years of age, but no later than early adolescence. Symptoms might occur most often with people the individual knows well, such as family members or a regular care provider. The behaviors associated with ODD are present beyond what might be expected for the person's age, and result in major problems in school, at home, or with peers.

Examples of ODD behaviors include:

- Losing one's temper a lot
- Arguing with adults or refusing to comply with adults' rules or requests
- Getting angry or being resentful or vindictive often
- Annoying others on purpose or easily becoming annoyed with others
- Blaming other people often for one's own mistakes or misbehavior

Conduct Disorder (CD)

People with CD have aggression toward others and break rules, laws, and social norms. Increased injuries and difficulty with friends also are common among people with CD. In addition, the symptoms of CD happen in more than one area in the person's life (for example, at home, in the community, and at school).

CD is severe and highly disruptive to a person's life and to others in his or her life. It also is very challenging to treat. If a person has CD it is important to get a diagnosis and treatment plan from a mental health professional as soon as possible.

Rage

Some people with TS have anger that is out of control, or episodes of "rage." Rage is not a disorder that can be diagnosed. Symptoms of rage might include extreme verbal or physical aggression. Examples of verbal aggression include extreme yelling, screaming, and cursing. Examples of physical aggression include extreme shoving, kicking, hitting, biting, and throwing objects. Rage symptoms are more likely to occur among those with other behavioral disorders such as ADHD, ODD, or CD.

Among people with TS, symptoms of rage are more likely to occur at home than outside the home. Treatment of rage can include learning how to relax, social skills training, and therapy. Some of these methods will help individuals and families better understand what can cause the rage, how to avoid encouraging these behaviors, and how to use appropriate discipline for these behaviors. In addition, treating other behavioral disorders that the person might have, such as ADHD, ODD, or CD can help to reduce symptoms of rage.

Anxiety

There are many different types of anxiety disorders with many different causes and symptoms. These include generalized anxiety disorder, OCD, panic disorder, post-traumatic stress disorder, separation anxiety, and different types of phobias. Separation anxiety is most common among young children. These children feel very worried when they are apart from their parents.

Depression

Everyone feels worried, anxious, sad, or stressed from time to time. However, if these feelings do not go away and they interfere with daily life (for example, keeping a child home from school or other activities, or keeping an adult from working or attending social activities), a person might have depression. Having either a depressed mood or a loss of interest or pleasure for at least 2 weeks might mean that someone has depression. Children and teens with depression might be irritable instead of sad.

To be diagnosed with depression, other symptoms also must be present, such as:

- Changes in eating habits or weight gain or loss.

- Changes in sleep habits.

- Changes in activity level (others notice increased activity or that the person has slowed down).

- Less energy.

- Feelings of worthlessness or guilt.

- Difficulty thinking, concentrating, or making decisions.

- Repeated thoughts of death.

- Thoughts or plans about suicide, or a suicide attempt.

Depression can be treated with counseling and medication.

Other Health Concerns

Children with TS can also have other health conditions that require care. Findings from the recent CDC study found that 43% of children who had been diagnosed with TS also had been diagnosed with at least one additional chronic health condition.

Among children with TS:

- 28% had asthma

- 13% had hearing or vision problems

- 12% had a bone, joint, or muscle problems

- 9% had suffered a brain injury or concussion

The rates of asthma and hearing or vision problems were similar to children with TS, but bone, joint, or muscle problems as well as brain injury or concussion were higher for children with TS. Children with TS were also less likely to receive effective coordination of care or have a medical home, which means a primary care setting where a team of providers provides health care and preventive services.

Educational Concerns

As a group, people with TS have levels of intelligence similar to those of people without TS. However, people with TS might be more likely to have learning differences, a learning disability, or a developmental delay that affects their ability to learn.

Many people with TS have problems with writing, organizing, and paying attention. People with TS might have problems processing what they hear or see. This can affect the person's ability to learn by listening to or watching a teacher. Or, the person might have problems with their other senses (such as how things feel, smell, taste, and movement) that affects learning and behavior. Children with TS might have trouble with social skills that affect their ability to interact with others.

As a result of these challenges, children with TS might need extra help in school. Many times, these concerns can be addressed with accommodations and behavioral interventions (for example, help with social skills).

Accommodations can include things such as providing a different testing location or extra testing time, providing tips on how to be more organized, giving the child less homework, or letting the child use a computer to take notes in class. Children also might need behavioral interventions, therapy, or they may need to learn strategies to help with stress, paying attention, or other symptoms.

Chapter 28

Traumatic Brain Injury (TBI)

Chapter Contents

Section 28.1

Basics of Traumatic Brain Injury

This chapter includes text excerpted from "Report to Congress on
Traumatic Brain Injury in the United States: Epidemiology
and Rehabilitation," Centers for Disease Control
and Prevention (CDC), 2015.

Introduction

A traumatic brain injury (TBI) is an injury that disrupts the normal function of the brain. It can be caused by a bump, blow, or jolt to the head or a penetrating head injury. Explosive blasts can also cause TBI, particularly among those who serve in the U.S. military. In 2010, the Centers for Disease Control and Prevention (CDC) estimated that TBIs accounted for approximately 2.5 million emergency department (ED) visits, hospitalizations, and deaths in the United States, either as an isolated injury or in combination with other injuries. Of these persons, approximately 87% (2,213,826) were treated in and released from EDs, another 11% (283,630) were hospitalized and discharged, and approximately 2% (52,844) died. However, these numbers underestimate the occurrence of TBIs. They do not account for those persons who did not receive medical care, had outpatient or office-based visits, or those who received care at a federal facility, such as persons serving in the U.S. military or those seeking care at a Veterans Affairs hospital. Those who serve in the U.S. military are at significant risk for TBI as Department of Defense data revealed that from 2000 through 2011 235,046 service members (or 4.2% of the 5,603,720 who served in the Army, Air Force, Navy, and Marine Corps) were diagnosed with a TBI.

Definition of Traumatic Brain Injury (TBI)

CDC defines TBI as a disruption in the normal function of the brain that can be caused by a bump, blow, or jolt to the head or a penetrating head injury. Explosive blasts can also cause TBI, particularly among those who serve in the U.S. military. Observing one of the following clinical signs constitutes an alteration in brain function:

- Any period of loss of or decreased consciousness;

- Any loss of memory for events immediately before (retrograde amnesia) or after the injury (post- traumatic amnesia);

- Neurologic deficits such as muscle weakness, loss of balance and coordination, disruption of vision, change in speech and language, or sensory loss;

- Any alteration in mental state at the time of the injury such as confusion, disorientation, slowed thinking, or difficulty with concentration.

Not all bumps, blows, or jolts to the head result in TBI. Additionally, not all persons who experience a TBI will have behavioral effects or a TBI-related disability. However, the combination of several factors—trauma from the head striking or being struck by an object, an object penetrating the brain, acceleration/deceleration movement of the brain not caused by direct trauma to the brain, and the presentation of signs and symptoms of TBI either immediately or shortly after the suspected event—is sufficient to classify a person as having sustained a TBI.

Characteristics of Traumatic Brain Injury (TBI)

Classification of TBI based on patterns and types of injury is important to ensure proper treatment and long-term therapy. However, the complexity of TBI and limitations of available assessment tools make this challenging. A primary brain injury occurs immediately after impact and is a direct result of mechanical trauma. Depending on the injury mechanism and severity, the initial event might cause direct, primary physical alterations of the brain tissue. A secondary brain injury can occur hours or days after the initial traumatic event and can arise from complications initiated by the primary injury such as inflammation, cell receptor-mediated dysfunction, free radical and oxidative damage, and calcium or other ion-mediated cell damage. Cerebral edema, or brain swelling, is a common secondary brain injury and a frequent cause of brain death in persons with severe TBI.

As in other tissue injuries, an inflammatory reaction to TBI can occur. Inflammation is involved in the repair of brain tissue after injury, but it also can contribute to secondary brain damage. Secondary injury also might result from other systemic events related to multiple injuries in other organs or body parts.

TBI can appear as a focal (localized) or diffuse (widespread) injury. Some persons exhibit both. A focal injury results when bleeding, bruising, or a penetrating injury is isolated to a portion of the brain. A diffuse brain injury occurs when brain tissue suffers more widespread damage, often resulting from acceleration and deceleration forces. Impact of the head against another object can cause focal brain injury under the skull at the site of impact and at a site on the opposite side of the head. The most common form of TBI is caused by a combination of impact and acceleration/deceleration forces, such as those occurring in high-speed motor vehicle crashes.

Certain regions of the brain are particularly vulnerable to the external forces that cause TBI. External forces that initiate brain movement can stretch and disrupt the integrity of brain tissue and cause the brain to impact bony protuberances within the skull. The frontotemporal lobes of the brain are particularly susceptible to this phenomenon because these regions are situated above bony surfaces in the skull where brain tissue can be easily injured with impact or forceful movement. For this reason it has been hypothesized that the susceptibility of the frontotemporal lobes are the basis for the cognitive and behavioral symptoms commonly experienced after a TBI.

Section 28.2

Consequences of Traumatic Brain Injury

This chapter includes text excerpted from "Report to Congress on Traumatic Brain Injury in the United States: Epidemiology and Rehabilitation," Centers for Disease Control and Prevention (CDC), 2015.

Health and Other Effects of Traumatic Brain Injury (TBI)

TBIs can lead to a spectrum of secondary conditions that might result in long-term impairment, unctional limitation, disability, and reduced quality of life. Health effects associated with TBI can be broadly categorized into cognitive, behavioral/emotional, motor, and somatic symptoms. Given the high frequency of frontal lobe injury, cognitive impairment is the hallmark injury of TBI; however, combinations of these health effects are frequently experienced. The evolution of secondary symptoms following TBI will vary across persons and is dependent on the injury location, injury severity, and medical history before the injury. Although not an exhaustive list of potential TBI-related health effects, common cognitive, behavioral/emotional, motor, sensory, and somatic signs and symptoms associated with TBI are presented in Table 28.1.

Psychological and neurologic disorders also can develop following TBI, which also might contribute to varying degrees of long-term impairment, functional limitation, or disability. These include mood disorders, (e.g., depression), and post-traumatic epilepsy. Post-traumatic stress disorder (PTSD) and dementia also are conditions of concern for persons affected by TBI. Considerable gaps in understanding exist with regard to the overlap and specific relations among TBI and these conditions.

Table 28.1. Health Effects Associated with TBI

Category	Description
Cognitive	Deficits in: attention; learning and memory; executive functions like planning and decision-making; language and communication; reaction time; reasoning and judgment
Behavioral/ Emotional	Delusions; hallucinations; severe mood disturbance; sustained irrational behavior; agitation; aggression; confusion; impulsivity; social inappropriateness
Motor	Changes in muscle tone; paralysis; impaired coordination; changes in balance, or trouble walking
Sensory	Changes in vision and hearing; sensitivity to light
Somatic signs and symptoms	Headache; fatigue; sleep disturbance; dizziness; chronic pain

Adverse health effects also affect work-related behaviors, and these include difficulties with social interactions, organizational obstacles caused by an acquired disability, health and safety concerns, and challenges with work attitude, skills, behavior, and performance. For working-aged adults, the return to work, school, and other pre-injury activities after TBI are key elements for life satisfaction. Failure to achieve a self-perceived productive role in society after TBI comes at personal and economic cost to injured persons, their families, and society. However, gainful employment for a person affected by TBI has positively influenced outcomes and contributed to self-reported life satisfaction.

Burden of Traumatic Brain Injury (TBI)

Incidence and Epidemiology

Each year, approximately 30 million injury-related emergency department (ED) visits, hospitalizations, and deaths occur in the United States. Of the injury hospitalizations, approximately 16% included TBI as a primary or secondary diagnosis. Of the injury deaths, approximately one-third included a TBI as a direct or underlying cause of death. In 2010, CDC estimated that TBIs accounted for approximately 2.5 million ED visits, hospitalizations, and deaths in the United States, either as an isolated injury or in combination with other injuries. Of these persons, approximately 87% (2,213,826) were treated in and released from EDs, another 11% (283,630) were hospitalized and discharged, and approximately 2% (52,844) died. These figures, however, underestimate the occurrence of TBIs, as they do not account for those persons who did not receive medical care, had outpatient or office-based visits, or those who received care at a federal facility (i.e., persons serving in the U.S. military or seeking care at a Veterans Affairs hospital). Department of Defense data revealed that from 2000 through 2011 235,046 service members (or 4.2% of the 5,603,720 who served in the Army, Air Force, Navy, and Marine Corps) were diagnosed with a TBI.

In the United States, children aged 0–4 years, adolescents aged 15–19 years, and older adults aged ≥75 years are the groups most likely to have a TBI-related ED visit or hospitalization. Adults aged ≥75 years have the highest rates of TBI-related hospitalizations and deaths among all age groups. Overall, males account for approximately 59% of all reported TBI-related medical visits in the United States.

As shown in Table 28.2, during 2002−2010, the leading causes of TBI-related ED visits were falls, being struck by or against an object, and motor-vehicle traffic crashes. The leading causes of TBI-related hospitalizations were falls, motor-vehicle traffic incidents, and assaults. For TBI-related deaths, the leading causes were motor-vehicle traffic incidents, suicides, and falls. The proportion of TBIs occurring during sports and recreation-related activities is undetermined because of limitations of the data source. However, according to the National Electronic Injury Surveillance System–All Injury Program, during 2001–2009 (CDC, 2011) the activities associated with the greatest estimated number of TBI-related ED visits were bicycling, football, playground activities, basketball, and soccer among persons younger than 19 years.

Table 28.2. Estimated Average Annual Numbers of Traumatic Brain Injury-Related Emergency Department (ED) Visits, Hospitalizations, and Deaths, by External Cause, United States, 2002–2010

Mechanism of injury	ED visits	Hospitalizations	Deaths
Falls	6,58,668	66,291	10,944
Struck by or against an object	3,04,797	6,808	372
Motor vehicle traffic	2,32,240	53,391	14,795
Assault/Homicide	1,79,408	15,032	5,665
Self-inflicted/ Suicide	*	*	14,713
Other	1,22,667	25,478	4,990
Unknown	97,018	1,13,172	0

* Estimates not reported because of small numbers.

Incidence of TBI-related Disability

In the United States availability of data related to the incidence of TBI-related disability is limited. The few national-level estimates that have been reported are based on extrapolations of state-level data from South Carolina and Colorado. These extrapolations suggest that 3.2 million–5.3 million persons were living with a TBI-related disability at the time of those studies.

Unique Considerations for Specific Populations

TBI can pose challenges for all persons, regardless of age, sex, geography, military status, or other distinguishing characteristics. Although the risk factors, health effects, and long-term implications of TBI vary for each person, some persons require special considerations (e.g., pediatric and older adult age groups, residents of rural geographical areas, military service members and veterans, and incarcerated populations).

Children (Aged 0–19 Years)

Approximately 145,000 children and adolescents aged 0–19 years are estimated to be living with substantial and long-lasting limitations in social, behavioral, physical, or cognitive functioning following a TBI. However, these numbers likely underestimate the true consequences of pediatric TBI, given the underreporting of mild TBI (mTBI) or concussion, and abusive head trauma.

A TBI experienced by a child can contribute to physical impairments, lowered cognitive and academic skills relative to developmental expectations, and deficits in behavior, socialization, and adaptive functioning, depending on the presence of factors that influence outcomes. Some studies suggest that even children with mild injuries are at risk for disability. Children with a TBI can experience specific impairments in language, memory, problem-solving, perceptual-motor skills, attention, and executive function.

In pediatric populations, some effects of a TBI may not be present initially, but can emerge later in a child's development. This delay of onset can manifest itself in later academic failure, chronic behavior problems, social isolation, and difficulty with employment, relationships, and, in some cases, difficulty with the law. Unlike other injuries with chronic consequences, the physical effects of TBI in children are often difficult to recognize. For this reason, common behavioral manifestations of TBI in children and adolescents, such as lack of inhibition, difficulty reading social cues, and emotional ability, might be mistakenly attributed to other causes ranging from lack of motivation and laziness to bad parenting.

Older Adults (75 Years)

Current studies estimate that approximately 775,000 older adults live with long-term disability associated with TBI. The TBI sequelae of older adults are often attributed to the aging process rather than an injury, preventing affected seniors from being accurately diagnosed and treated. Older adults affected by TBI have a higher risk for mortality and worse functional outcomes following injury than younger patients with similar injuries, regardless of initial TBI severity. The societal and medical-care costs of TBI also are more extensive for older adults than younger patients. When compared with younger patients, older adults had longer hospital stays and slower rates of functional improvement during inpatient rehabilitation. Preexisting medical conditions, also were found to increase the length of stay among older adults in outpatient rehabilitation.

Cognitive Rehabilitation

The Cognitive Rehabilitation (CR) Task Force of the American Congress of Rehabilitation Medicine (ACRM) Brain Injury Interdisciplinary Special Interest Group evaluated 370 studies and found that CR is effective during the post-acute period—even 1 year or more after injury. Further analysis of the scientific literature suggests that CR is effective in patients with moderate and severe TBI. However, an Institute of Medicine (IOM) committee concluded that the evidence was insufficient to provide practice guidelines, particularly with respect to selecting the most effective treatments for a specific person (IOM, 2011). The insufficiency of the evidence was largely attributed to limitations in research designs for rehabilitation evaluation studies. And yet, empirical support for CR is growing with the strongest level of evidence for the following interventions:

- Direct attention training accompanied by metacognitive training to promote development of compensatory strategies and generalization;

- Interventions to address functional communication deficits and memory strategies for mild memory impairments;

- Meta-cognitive strategies for executive function deficits; and

- Comprehensive holistic neuropsychological rehabilitation.

Preliminary evidence supports the effectiveness of group-based rehabilitation treatment of pragmatic communication disorders. However, research that demonstrates the effectiveness of cognitively based treatments for listening, speaking, reading, and writing, in social, educational, occupational, and community settings is lacking.

Chapter 29

Visual Impairment

Blindness

Have you ever put on a blindfold and pretended that you couldn't see? You probably bumped into things and got confused about which way you were going. But if you had to, you could get adjusted and learn to live without your sight.

Lots of people have done just that. They have found ways to learn, play, and work, even though they have trouble seeing or can't see at all.

How Seeing Happens?

Your eyes and your brain work together to see. The eye is made up of many different parts, including the cornea, iris, lens, and retina. These parts all work together to focus on light and images. Your eyes then use special nerves to send what you see to your brain, so your brain can process and recognize what you're seeing. In eyes that work correctly, this process happens almost instantly.

When this doesn't work the way it should, a person may be visually impaired, or blind. The problem may affect one eye or both eyes.

When you think of being blind, you might imagine total darkness. But most people who are blind can still see a little light or shadows. They just can't see things clearly. People who have some sight, but still need a lot of help, are sometimes called "legally blind."

Text in this chapter is excerpted from "Blindness," © 1995–2016. The Nemours Foundation/KidsHealth®. Reprinted with permission.

What Causes Blindness?

Vision problems can develop before a baby is born. Sometimes, parts of the eyes don't form the way they should. A kid's eyes might look fine, but the brain has trouble processing the information they send. The optic nerve sends pictures to the brain, so if the nerve doesn't form correctly, the baby's brain won't receive the messages needed for sight.

Blindness can be genetic (or inherited), which means that this problem gets passed down to a kid from parents through genes.

Blindness also can be caused by an accident, if something hurts the eye. That's why it's so important to protect your eyes when you play certain sports, such as hockey.

Some illnesses, such as diabetes, can damage a person's vision over time. Other eye diseases, such as cataracts, can cause vision problems or blindness, but they usually affect older people.

What Does the Doctor Do?

A kid who has serious trouble with vision might see an ophthalmologist, a doctor who specializes in eye problems. Even babies might see an ophthalmologist if their parents think they might be having trouble seeing.

At the doctor visit, the doctor will talk with the parents and the kid (if the kid is old enough to describe what's going on). A doctor might use an eye chart to find out how well the kid can see. You've probably seen these charts that contain letters of different sizes. It's a way of testing how well a person can see. Someone with really good vision would be able to read certain letters from 20 feet (6 meters) away.

Eyesight this good is called 20/20 vision, although some people can see even better than that. The numbers change depending on how clearly a person can see. The larger or closer something needs to be in order for it to be seen, the worse a person's vision is.

Many times, glasses or contact lenses are all that's needed to help kids see better. But if glasses and contact lenses can't make someone's vision any better—and the person needs to get really close to something to see it—he or she may be considered blind. For instance, someone with good vision might be able to see an object from 200 feet (61 meters) away, but someone is considered blind if he or she needs to be 20 feet (6 meters) away to see the same object.

Babies and little kids won't be able to use the eye chart, but doctors can check their vision by doing special vision tests or something as simple as putting a toy in front of the child to see if he or she can focus on it.

The ophthalmologist also will examine the kid's eyes using special medication and lighting that allows him or her to see into the eyeballs.

The ophthalmologist will look at each part of the eye to check for problems, such as a cataract (cloudiness of the eye's lens). Once the doctor knows what's causing the vision problem, he or she can begin planning how to treat it.

In some cases, an operation can help improve a kid's vision. For example, if a kid has a cataract, doctors may do surgery to remove it.

Is Learning Different?

A baby who is blind can still learn and develop normally. But the baby's parents will need the help of specialists who know how to help blind children. It's often a great idea for the child to attend special learning programs designed just for little kids who have trouble seeing. These programs would make the most of the senses that the kid does have, such as touch, hearing, smell, and taste.

Touch comes in handy when a child is older and wants to read books. Kids who are visually impaired can learn to read by using a special system called braille. Braille is a way of expressing letters, words, and thoughts. To read braille, a person feels a series of little bumps that are associated with letters in the alphabet. For instance, "A" is represented as one bump. Computer programs and other devices that can "see" turn the words on a page into braille.

Hearing is another important sense if a kid has vision problems. Some devices can read out loud what's written on a page. With special equipment, a visually impaired kid can read almost anything. These kinds of technologies can be helpful in learning. Kids who are blind might attend a special school, or they might attend regular classes, aided by special devices and specialists.

Hot Dog!

Kids who have vision problems will get help from their parents, doctors, and teachers. When they are older, some of them may get a hand—or should we say a paw?—from a guide dog. These helper dogs are trained to be a blind person's eyes. That means the dog learns to be very alert to surroundings so he or she can be a good guide for the person.

Not only are these dogs great friends, they give blind people independence, so they can accomplish what they want to accomplish.

Many blind people have gone on to do amazing things in many different fields, including music, the arts, and even sports. Serious vision problems didn't stop runner Marla Runyan. She was the first legally blind person to ever qualify for the Olympics.

Part Four

Learning Disabilities and the Educational Process

Chapter 30

Decoding Learning Disabilities

An Expert's View on Learning Disabilities

Reading Disability Expert Brett Miller Addresses Learning in Class, at Home, and in Science

Much of what we do in our early schooling and into our adult lives depends on being able to read, write, and do basic mathematics. Children with learning disabilities can face significant academic and emotional challenges as they struggle to master these skills.

Learning disabilities are caused by differences in brain function that affect how a person's brain processes information. They are not an indication of a person's intelligence; people with learning disabilities are just as bright as other people. While learning disabilities can last a person's lifetime, they may be lessened with the right educational supports.

Brett Miller, Ph.D., oversees the *Eunice Kennedy Shriver* National Institute Child Health Human Development (NICHD)-funded research portfolio focused on learning disabilities. The program's aim is to understand how children learn to read, write, and do math, why some children struggle so mightily to acquire these skills, and what can be done to help them.

This chapter includes text excerpted from "Decoding Learning Disabilities," *Eunice Kennedy Shriver* National Institute Child Health and Human Development (NICHD), December 29, 2015.

How Common Are Learning Disabilities?

Learning disabilities are one of the more prevalent disability conditions. It is estimated that between 12 percent and 20 percent of individuals have some type of learning disability. Dyslexia is the most common learning disability.

How Do Learning Disabilities Fit into the Mission of NICHD?

The *Eunice Kennedy Shriver* National Institute Child Health Human Development (NICHD) mission includes ensuring that individuals develop into healthy and productive people free from disease and disability, including learning disabilities. The mission also talks about rehabilitation for individuals who have a disability.

Teaching Children with Learning Disabilities

Brett Miller Gives an Example of NICHD-Funded Research on Learning Disabilities?

A study that came out of an investment in the Learning Disabilities Research Centers provided some results. This study picked up kids at the end of fifth grade who were more than one year behind in their reading level. They were given explicit, systematic, and direct instruction in reading for 1, 2, or 3 years. That is, the children were directly and explicitly taught the component reading skills—including the rules of phonics—building their reading skill from the ground up. They also were given plenty of opportunity to practice their reading and to more generally enhance their understanding of the text.

Children who made good progress within the first year transitioned to less intensive interventions. Those who continued to struggle got a second year of even more intensive intervention: smaller group instruction, and more direct and explicit instruction. And those who continued to have difficulty went into a third year of intervention that was even more intensive than the first two years.

They found that the children who have three years of intensive intervention show really robust growth in reading comprehension and in word-level reading. And so this is a success story.

The flip side is that while gains are shown, they weren't able to reduce the gap between the reading levels of these children and their peers. Their peers also continued to develop their reading skill, and so the gap remained.

Does This Study Have Implications for Teaching Children with Learning Disabilities?

This and other studies suggest that children with learning disabilities need direct, explicit, and systematic instruction, when talking about reading or mathematics.

These children will likely need more time to build their skills and receive instruction in smaller groups so that they get more focused attention—it can be a small group, it can be one on one—depending upon the needs of the child and how significant their learning challenges are.

It is known know that the most efficient and effective interventions are for the youngest learners. Starting young helps reduce the impact the disability has on their broader academic development.

When Should These Interventions Begin?

The risk factors are identifiable when kids roll into kindergarten and even before that. For instance, if a parent has a learning disability, the child is at increased risk for having a learning disability.

If a child has a higher risk of having reading difficulties going into preschool or kindergarten, their performance can be monitored and very explicit, direct, and systematic instruction can be given early on. Fortunately, this type of instruction not only benefits those who struggle, but also benefits those who don't, so it's effective for all kids.

Can This Intervention Be within the Context of the Entire Class?

This is exactly the hope and intent.

The Science of Learning Disabilities

What Do Brain Imaging Studies Tell Us?

Brain imaging studies give us a window into understanding reading and reading disabilities. For the kids who develop typically with reading compared to those who don't, we see more focal activation in areas on the left hemisphere of the brain and activation of parts of the left hemisphere that relate to improved word reading.

Kids who struggle with reading show more disperse activation in the left hemisphere. But if they successfully respond to a reading intervention, they show a brain activation pattern that looks much more like individuals who don't struggle to read.

This is a remarkable example of what we call neuroplasticity; that is, you give an intervention in the classroom, and when the intervention is successful, you see changes in the structure and function of the brain.

Are There Genes Associated with Learning Disabilities?

Learning disabilities are complex conditions, and there's no single gene that causes a learning disability or a reading disability. At this point, we've identified about nine dyslexia susceptibility genes. If you have one of these genes, it doesn't mean that you'll have dyslexia; it means that you're at higher risk for having dyslexia. This is one piece of information that could help in ascertaining who would be at risk for problems.

Are There New Technologies to Help People with Learning Disabilities?

There are a number of resources now that individuals with learning disabilities have available to them to help support their learning. For example, there is software that reads books to a person. There are efforts to have more books recorded. Recorded books have the benefit of reading that sounds more natural and with appropriate intonation, as opposed to the reading software. But it's not practical to record every book, so reading will still be a necessary skill.

For individuals who have problems with writing, there are tools to help structure sentences and organize paragraphs and longer papers.

After Graduation

What Tips Are Suggested for Parents to Help Their Children?

If you're a parent of a younger child, you can create a language-rich environment by talking with and reading with your child. This can help your child understand language structure—where to pause, how to allow someone else to talk—and improve his or her vocabulary.

You should read books to your child every day, giving them the story, vocabulary, background, and an understanding of how text is structured, how reading flows from left to right [in English], and how the pages are turned. You can ask children questions to encourage them to think about what you've been reading and what's coming next in the story.

For children with a math disability [dyscalculia], you can point out numbers in your environment. When you're going to the grocery store or doing everyday tasks, you can incorporate opportunities to learn about numbers. For example, where you see three apples, you can count them. You're taking advantage of these opportunities to immerse your child in language and mathematical reasoning–rich environments.

For children in school, create a positive environment where you celebrate successes and work with the challenges. It's important for parents to be role models who read and are engaged in their own life-long learning. You can show children the calculations or measurements that you're doing, like showing them how you do the bills or measuring length of objects with a tape measure. You can have writing activities like doing diaries, blogs, or other activities that are engaging and fun for your children.

What Do We Know about Helping Children Who Have Learning Disabilities Achieve and Thrive beyond School?

The skills that will help individuals with learning disabilities transition into adult employment or postsecondary education include knowing their challenges and being able to advocate for themselves to get the resources to succeed. In college, that might mean getting more time to take tests or getting software to read text more efficiently.

Are There Personality Characteristics Associated with Success That Parents Could Help Promote?

Talking about grit, the idea is to stick with it, and persevere. The effort you put toward a task is going to be important in order to succeed. And it helps to be lighthearted and to realize that everyone faces challenges in life and to stay positive.

Chapter 31

Understanding Your Child's Right to Special Education Services

Chapter Contents

Section 31.1

Individuals with Disabilities Education Act (IDEA)

This section includes text excerpted from "Individuals with Disabilities Education Act (IDEA)," Disability.gov, May 20, 2014.

Two of the main laws that help fund special education and protect the rights of students with disabilities are the Individuals with Disabilities Education Act (IDEA) and Section 504 of the Rehabilitation Act (often just called "Section 504."). The IDEA was originally passed in 1975 to make sure that children with disabilities have the opportunity to receive a free, appropriate public education, just like other children. IDEA requires that special education and related services be made available to every eligible child with a disability. Section 504, on the other hand, is a civil rights law that protects children with disabilities from discrimination.

Every year, millions of children receive services under the IDEA. This law governs how states and public agencies provide early intervention, and special education and related services to more than 6.5 million eligible infants, toddlers, children and youth with disabilities. Infants and toddlers (birth-2) with disabilities and their families receive early intervention services under IDEA Part C. Children and youth (ages 3-21) receive special education and related services under IDEA Part B. A couple of good places to help parents better understand this law are the Center for Parent Information and Resources and the National Center on Learning Disabilities' "An Overview of IDEA Parent Guide."

If your child does not receive special education services under IDEA, he or she does not have the protections that are available under the IDEA statute. School districts are required to provide a "free and appropriate public education" (FAPE) to each qualified student with a disability who is in the school district's jurisdiction. Under Section 504, FAPE means regular or special education and related aids and services that meet the student's individual educational needs.

The National Education Association (NEA) also has a fact sheet that explains the different protections of these laws.

The services that IDEA requires can be very important in helping children and youth with disabilities develop, learn, and succeed in school. Under the law, states are responsible for meeting the needs of eligible children with disabilities. To find out if a child is eligible for services, he or she must first be evaluated. This evaluation is free and can determine if a child has a disability, as defined by IDEA, and what special education and related services he or she may need.

Special education is instruction that is specially designed to meet the specific needs of a child with a disability. Since each child is unique, it's difficult to give an overall example of special education. Special education can be for things like travel training or vocational education, and it can take place in the classroom, in a home, in a hospital or institution, among other places. This is why you might also hear that "special education is not a place." Where it is provided depends on the child's unique needs as decided by the group of individuals (which includes the parents) that makes the placement decision. Some students with disabilities may need accommodations and other related services to help them benefit from special education. These related services may include speech-language pathology and audiology services; interpreting services; psychological services; physical and occupational therapy; therapeutic recreation; and early identification and assessment of disabilities in children. Read "Knowing Your Child's Rights" for an overview of what the IDEA requires regarding special education and related services.

Under the IDEA, special education instruction must be provided to students with disabilities in what is known as the "least restrictive environment," or LRE. IDEA's LRE provisions ensure that children with disabilities are educated with children who do not have disabilities, to the maximum extent appropriate. LRE requirements apply to students in public or private institutions or other care facilities.

There are several local organizations that help parents of children with disabilities better understand how the IDEA can help as their kids advance through the school system. Every state has at least one Parent Training and Information Center (PTI). PTIs provide parents with important information about special education so they can participate effectively in meeting the educational needs of their children. Finally, your state's department of education is an important point of entry for getting information about all the programs and services required under IDEA, and how you can help your child get the most out of their education.

Section 31.2

Section 504

This section includes text excerpted from "The Civil Rights of
Students with Hidden Disabilities under Section 504 of
the Rehabilitation Act of 1973," U.S. Department of
Education (ED), October 15, 2015.

If you are a student with a hidden disability or would like to know
more about how students with hidden disabilities are protected against
discrimination by Federal law, this section is for you.

Section 504 of the Rehabilitation Act of 1973 protects the rights
of persons with handicaps in programs and activities that receive
Federal financial assistance. Section 504 protects the rights not only
of individuals with visible disabilities but also those with disabilities
that may not be apparent.

Section 504 provides that: **"No otherwise qualified individual
with handicaps in the United States . . . shall, solely by reason
of her or his handicap, be excluded from the participation in,
be denied the benefits of, or be subjected to discrimination
under any program or activity receiving Federal financial
assistance...."**

The U.S. Department of Education (ED) enforces Section 504 in
programs and activities that receive financial assistance from ED.
Recipients of this assistance include public school districts, institutions
of higher education, and other state and local education agencies. ED
maintains an Office for Civil Rights (OCR), with ten regional offices
and a headquarters office in Washington, D.C., to enforce Section 504
and other civil rights laws that pertain to recipients of ED funds.

This section answers the following questions about the civil rights
of students with hidden disabilities and the responsibilities of ED
recipients:

- What disabilities are covered under Section 504?

- What are hidden disabilities?

- What are the responsibilities of ED recipients in preschool, elementary, secondary, and adult education?

- What are the responsibilities of ED recipients in postsecondary education?

- How can the needs of students with hidden disabilities be addressed?

Disabilities Covered Under Section 504

The ED Section 504 regulation defines an "individual with handicaps" as any person who (i) has a physical or mental impairment which substantially limits one or more major life activities, (ii) has a record of such an impairment, or (iii) is regarded as having such an impairment. The regulation further defines a physical or mental impairment as (A) any physiological disorder or condition, cosmetic disfigurement, or anatomical loss affecting one or more of the following body systems: neurological; musculoskeletal; special sense organs; respiratory, including speech organs; cardiovascular; reproductive; digestive; genitourinary; hemic and lymphatic; skin; and endocrine; or (B) any mental or psychological disorder, such as mental retardation, organic brain syndrome, emotional or mental illness, and specific learning disabilities. The definition does not set forth a list of specific diseases and conditions that constitute physical or mental impairments because of the difficulty of ensuring the comprehensiveness of any such list.

The key factor in determining whether a person is considered an "individual with handicaps" covered by Section 504 is whether the physical or mental impairment results in a substantial limitation of one or more major life activities. Major life activities, as defined in the regulation, include functions such as caring for one's self, performing manual tasks, walking, seeing, hearing, speaking, breathing, learning, and working.

The impairment must have a material effect on one's ability to perform a major life activity. For example, an individual who has a physical or mental impairment would not be considered a person with handicaps if the condition does not in any way limit the individual, or only results in some minor limitation. However, in some cases Section 504 also protects individuals who do not have a handicapping condition but are treated as though they do because they have a history of, or have been misclassified as having, a mental or physical impairment that substantially limits one or more major life activities. For example, if you have a history of a handicapping condition but no longer have the condition, or have been incorrectly classified as having such a condition, you too are protected from discrimination under Section

309

504. Frequently occurring examples of the first group are persons with histories of mental or emotional illness, heart disease, or cancer; of the second group, persons who have been misclassified as mentally retarded. Persons who are not disabled may be covered by Section 504 also if they are treated as if they are handicapped, for example, if they are infected with the human immunodeficiency virus.

What Are Hidden Disabilities?

Hidden disabilities are physical or mental impairments that are not readily apparent to others. They include such conditions and diseases as specific learning disabilities, diabetes, epilepsy, and allergy. A disability such as a limp, paralysis, total blindness or deafness is usually obvious to others. But hidden disabilities such as low vision, poor hearing, heart disease, or chronic illness may not be obvious. A chronic illness involves a recurring and long-term disability such as diabetes, heart disease, kidney and liver disease, high blood pressure, or ulcers.

Approximately four million students with disabilities are enrolled in public elementary and secondary schools in the United States. Of these 43 percent are students classified as learning disabled, 8 percent as emotionally disturbed, and 1 percent as other health impaired. These hidden disabilities often cannot be readily known without the administration of appropriate diagnostic tests.

The Responsibilities of ED Recipients in Preschool, Elementary, Secondary, and Adult Education

For coverage under Section 504, an individual with handicaps must be "qualified" for service by the school or institution receiving ED funds. For example, the ED Section 504 regulation defines a "qualified handicapped person" with respect to public preschool, elementary, secondary, or adult education services, as a person with a handicap who is:

- of an age during which persons without handicaps are provided such services;

- of any age during which it is mandatory under state law to provide such services to persons with handicaps; or

- a person for whom a state is required to provide a free appropriate public education under the Individuals with Disabilities Education Act.

Under the Section 504 regulation, a recipient that operates a public elementary or secondary a education program has a number of responsibilities toward qualified handicapped persons in its jurisdiction. These recipients must:

- Undertake annually to identify and locate all unserved handicapped children;

- Provide a "free appropriate public education" to each student with handicaps, "regardless of the nature or severity of the handicap. This means providing regular or special education and related aids and services designed to meet the individual educational needs of handicapped persons as adequately as the needs of nonhandicapped persons are met;

- Ensure that each student with handicaps is educated with nonhandicapped students to the maximum extent appropriate to the needs of the handicapped person;

- Establish nondiscriminatory evaluation and placement procedures to avoid the inappropriate education that may result from the misclassification or misplacement of students;

- Establish procedural safeguards to enable parents and guardians to participate meaningfully in decisions regarding the evaluation and placement of their children; and

- Afford handicapped children an equal opportunity to participate in nonacademic and extracurricular services and activities.

A recipient that operates a preschool education or day care program, or an adult education program may not exclude qualified handicapped persons and must take into account their needs of qualified handicapped persons in determining the aid, benefits, or services to be provided under those programs and activities.

Students with hidden disabilities frequently are not properly diagnosed. For example, a student with an undiagnosed hearing impairment may be unable to understand much of what a teacher says; a student with a learning disability may be unable to process oral or written information routinely; or a student with an emotional problem may be unable to concentrate in a regular classroom setting. As a result, these students, regardless of their intelligence, will be unable to fully demonstrate their ability or attain educational benefits equal to that of nonhandicapped students. They may be perceived by teachers and fellow students as slow, lazy, or as discipline problems.

311

Whether a child is already in school or not, if his/her parents feel the child needs special education or related services, they should get in touch with the local superintendent of schools. For example, a parent who believes his or her child has a hearing impairment or is having difficulty understanding a teacher, may request to have the child evaluated so that the child may receive appropriate education. A child with behavior problems, or one who is doing poorly academically, may have an undiagnosed hidden disability. A parent has the right to request that the school determine whether the child is handicapped and whether special education or related services are needed to provide the child an appropriate education. Once it is determined that a child needs special education or related services, the recipient school system must arrange to provide appropriate services.

The Responsibilities of ED Recipients in Postsecondary Education

The ED Section 504 regulation defines a qualified individual with handicaps for postsecondary education programs as a person with a handicap who meets the academic and technical standards requisite for admission to, or participation in, the college's education program or activity.

A college has no obligation to identify students with handicaps. In fact, Section 504 prohibits a postsecondary education recipient from making a preadmission inquiry as to whether an applicant for admission is a handicapped person. However, a postsecondary institution is required to inform applicants and other interested parties of the availability of auxiliary aids, services, and academic adjustments, and the name of the person designated to coordinate the college's efforts to carry out the requirements of Section 504. After admission (including the period between admission and enrollment), the college may make confidential inquiries as to whether a person has a handicap for the purpose of determining whether certain academic adjustments or auxiliary aids or services may be needed.

Many students with hidden disabilities, seeking college degrees, were provided with special education services during their elementary and secondary school years. It is especially important for these students to understand that postsecondary institutions also have responsibilities to protect the rights of students with disabilities. In elementary and secondary school, their school district was responsible for identifying, evaluating, and providing individualized special education and related services to meet their needs. At the postsecondary level, however, there are some important differences. The key provisions of Section 504 at the postsecondary level are highlighted below.

At the postsecondary level it is the student's responsibility to make his or her handicapping condition known and to request academic adjustments. This should be done in a timely manner. A student may choose to make his or her needs known to the Section 504 Coordinator, to an appropriate dean, to a faculty advisor, or to each professor on an individual basis.

A student who requests academic adjustments or auxiliary aids because of a handicapping condition may be requested by the institution to provide documentation of the handicap and the need for the services requested. This may be especially important to an institution attempting to understand the nature and extent of a hidden disability.

The requested documentation may include the results of medical, psychological, or emotional diagnostic tests, or other professional evaluations to verify the need for academic adjustments or auxiliary aids.

How Can the Needs of Students with Hidden Disabilities Be Addressed?

The following examples illustrate how schools can address the needs of their students with hidden disabilities.

- A student with a long-term, debilitating medical problem such as cancer, kidney disease, or diabetes may be given special consideration to accommodate the student's needs. For example, a student with cancer may need a class schedule that allows for rest and recuperation following chemotherapy.

- A student with a learning disability that affects the ability to demonstrate knowledge on a standardized test or in certain testing situations may require modified test arrangements, such as oral testing or different testing formats.

- A student with a learning disability or impaired vision that affects the ability to take notes in class may need a notetaker or tape recorder.

- A student with a chronic medical problem such as kidney or liver disease may have difficulty in walking distances or climbing stairs. Under Section 504, this student may require special parking space, sufficient time between classes, or other considerations, to conserve the student's energy for academic pursuits.

- A student with diabetes, which adversely affects the body's ability to manufacture insulin, may need a class schedule that will accommodate the student's special needs.

- An emotionally or mentally ill student may need an adjusted class schedule to allow time for regular counseling or therapy.

- A student with epilepsy who has no control over seizures, and whose seizures are stimulated by stress or tension, may need accommodation for such stressful activities as lengthy academic testing or competitive endeavors in physical education.

- A student with arthritis may have persistent pain, tenderness or swelling in one or more joints. A student experiencing arthritic pain may require a modified physical education program.

These are just a few examples of how the needs of students with hidden disabilities may be addressed. If you are a student (or a parent or guardian of a student) with a hidden disability, or represent an institution seeking to address the needs of such students, you may wish to seek further information from the Office for Civil Rights (OCR).

Section 31.3

Every Student Succeeds Act (ESSA)

This section includes text excerpted from "Every Student Succeeds Act (ESSA)," U.S. Department of Education (ED), December 10, 2015.

A New Education Law

The Every Student Succeeds Act (ESSA) was signed by President Obama on December 10, 2015, and represents good news for our nation's schools. This bipartisan measure reauthorizes the 50-year-old Elementary and Secondary Education Act (ESEA), the nation's national education law and longstanding commitment to equal opportunity for all students.

The new law builds on key areas of progress in recent years, made possible by the efforts of educators, communities, parents, and students across the country.

For example, today, high school graduation rates are at all-time highs. Dropout rates are at historic lows. And more students are going to college than ever before. These achievements provide a firm foundation for further work to expand educational opportunity and improve student outcomes under ESSA.

The previous version of the law, the No Child Left Behind (NCLB) Act, was enacted in 2002. NCLB represented a significant step forward for our nation's children in many respects, particularly as it shined a light on where students were making progress and where they needed additional support, regardless of race, income, zip code, disability, home language, or background. The law was scheduled for revision in 2007, and, over time, NCLB's prescriptive requirements became increasingly unworkable for schools and educators. Recognizing this fact, in 2010, the Obama administration joined a call from educators and families to create a better law that focused on the clear goal of fully preparing all students for success in college and careers.

Congress has now responded to that call.

ESSA reflects many of the priorities of this administration.

ESSA includes provisions that will help to ensure success for students and schools. Below are just a few. The law:

- Advances equity by upholding critical protections for America's disadvantaged and high-need students.

- Requires—for the first time—that all students in America be taught to high academic standards that will prepare them to succeed in college and careers.

- Ensures that vital information is provided to educators, families, students, and communities through annual statewide assessments that measure students' progress toward those high standards.

- Helps to support and grow local innovations—including evidence-based and place-based interventions developed by local leaders and educators—consistent with our Investing in Innovation and Promise Neighborhoods.

- Sustains and expands this administration's historic investments in increasing access to high-quality preschool.

- Maintains an expectation that there will be accountability and action to effect positive change in our lowest-performing schools, where groups of students are not making progress, and where graduation rates are low over extended periods of time.

The bipartisan bill to fix NCLB will help ensure opportunity for all of America's students:

- Holds all students to high academic standards.

- Prepares all students for success in college and career.

- Provides more kids access to high-quality preschool.

- Guarantees steps are taken to help students, and their schools, improve.

- Reduces the burden of testing while maintaining annual information for parents and students.

- Promote local innovation and invests in what works.

History of ESEA

The Elementary and Secondary Education Act (ESEA) was signed into law in 1965 by President Lyndon Baines Johnson, who believed that "full educational opportunity" should be "our first national goal." From its inception, ESEA was a civil rights law.

ESEA offered new grants to districts serving low-income students, federal grants for textbooks and library books, funding for special education centers, and scholarships for low-income college students. Additionally, the law provided federal grants to state educational agencies to improve the quality of elementary and secondary education.

NCLB and Accountability

NCLB put in place measures that exposed achievement gaps among traditionally underserved students and their peers and spurred an important national dialogue on education improvement. This focus on accountability has been critical in ensuring a quality education for all children, yet also revealed challenges in the effective implementation of this goal.

Parents, educators, and elected officials across the country recognized that a strong, updated law was necessary to expand opportunity to all students; support schools, teachers, and principals; and to strengthen our education system and economy.

In 2012, the Obama administration began granting flexibility to states regarding specific requirements of NCLB in exchange for rigorous and comprehensive state-developed plans designed to close achievement gaps, increase equity, improve the quality of instruction, and increase outcomes for all students.

Chapter 32

Early Intervention Strategies

Chapter Contents

Section 32.1

Early Intervention: An Overview

This section includes text excerpted from "Overview of Early Intervention," Center for Parent Information and Resources (CPIR), March 2014.

What Is Early Intervention?

Early intervention (EI) is a system of services that **helps babies and toddlers with developmental delays or disabilities**. Early intervention focuses on helping eligible babies and toddlers learn the basic and brand-new skills that typically develop during the first three years of life, such as:

- *physical* (reaching, rolling, crawling, and walking)
- *cognitive* (thinking, learning, solving problems)
- *communication* (talking, listening, understanding)
- *social/emotional* (playing, feeling secure and happy)
- *self-help* (eating, dressing)

Examples of early intervention services: If an infant or toddler has a disability or a developmental delay in one or more of these developmental areas, that child will likely be eligible for early intervention services. Those services will be tailored to meet the child's individual needs and may include:

- Assistive technology (devices a child might need)
- Audiology or hearing services
- Speech and language services
- Counseling and training for a family
- Medical services
- Nursing services

- Nutrition services

- Occupational therapy

- Physical therapy

- Psychological services

Services may also be provided to address the **needs and priorities of the child's family**. Family-directed services are meant to help family members understand the special needs of their child and how to enhance his or her development.

Who Is Eligible for Early Intervention?

Early intervention is intended for infants and toddlers who have a **developmental delay** or **disability**. Eligibility is determined by evaluating the child (with parents' consent) to see if the little one does, in fact, have a delay in development or a disability. Eligible children can receive early intervention services from birth through the third birthday (and sometimes beyond).

For some children, from birth

Sometimes it is known from the moment a child is born that early intervention services will be essential in helping the child grow and develop. Often this is so for children who are diagnosed at birth with a specific condition or who experience significant prematurity, very low birth weight, illness, or surgery soon after being born. Even before heading home from the hospital, this child's parents may be given a **referral** to their local early intervention office.

For others, because of delays in development

Some children have a relatively routine entry into the world, but may develop more slowly than others, experience set backs, or develop in ways that seem very different from other children. For these children, a visit with a developmental pediatrician and a thorough evaluation may lead to an early intervention referral.

Parents don't have to wait for a referral to early intervention, however. If you're concerned about your child's development, you may contact your local program directly and ask to have your child evaluated. That evaluation is provided free of charge.

However a child comes to be referred, evaluated, and determined eligible, early intervention services provide vital support so that children with developmental needs can thrive and grow.

What Is a Developmental Delay?

The term "developmental delay" is an important one in early intervention. Broadly speaking, it means that a child is delayed in some area of development. There are five areas in which development may be affected:

1. Cognitive development

2. Physical development, including vision and hearing

3. Communication development

4. Social or emotional development

5. Adaptive development

Developmental milestones

Think of all the baby skills that can fall under any one of those developmental areas! Babies and toddlers have a lot of new skills to learn, so it's always of concern when a child's development seems slow or more difficult than would normally be expected. Our developmental milestones page outlines some of the typical skills that babies and toddlers learn by certain ages. It's a good resource to consult if you're concerned that a child may have a developmental delay.

Definition of "developmental delay" defines the term for itself, including:

- describing the evaluation and assessment procedures that will be used to measure a child's development in each of the five developmental areas; and

- specifying the level of delay in functioning (or other comparable criteria) that constitutes a developmental delay in each of the five developmental areas.

What's your state's definition?

Clearly, it's important to know how your state defines "developmental delay." Find out more about that definition by visiting the Early Childhood Technical Assistance Center (ECTA) at:

www.nectac.org/~pdfs/topics/earlyid/partc_elig_table.pdf

If You Are Concerned about a Baby or Toddler's Development

It's not uncommon for parents and family members to become concerned when their beautiful baby or growing toddler doesn't seem to be developing according to the normal schedule of "baby" **milestones**.

"He hasn't rolled over yet."

"The little girl next door is already sitting up on her own!"

"She should be saying a few words by now."

Sound familiar? While it's true that children develop differently, at their own pace, and that the range of what's "normal" development is quite broad, it's hard not to worry and wonder.

What to do?

If you think that your child is not developing at the same pace or in the same way as most children his or her age, it is often a good idea to talk first to your child's pediatrician. Explain your concerns. Tell the doctor what you have observed with your child. Your child may have a disability or a developmental delay, or he or she may be at risk of having a disability or delay.

You can also get in touch with your community's early intervention program, and ask to have your little one evaluated to see if he or she has a developmental delay or disability. **This evaluation is free of charge**, won't hurt your child, and looks at his or her basic skills. Based on that evaluation, your child may be eligible for early intervention services, which will be designed to address your child's special needs or delays.

How to get in touch with your community's early intervention program?

There are several ways to connect with the EI program in your community. Try any of these suggestions:

- Contact the Pediatrics branch in a local hospital and ask where you should call to find out about early intervention services in your area.

- Ask your pediatrician for a referral to the local early intervention system.

- Visit the ECTA Center's early intervention "contacts" page, at: ectacenter.org/contact/ptccoord.asp

What to say to the early intervention contact person?

Explain that you are concerned about your child's development. Say that you think your child may need early intervention services. Explain that you would like to have your child evaluated under Part C of Individuals with Disabilities Education Act (IDEA).

Referral

Write down any information the contact person gives you. You will probably be referred to either your community's early intervention program or to what is known as *Child Find*. Child Find operates in every state to identify babies and toddlers who need early intervention services because of developmental delays or disability. You can use the Parent's Record-Keeping Worksheet to keep track of this important information. In fact, in general, it's a good idea to write down the names and phone numbers of everyone you talk to as you move through the early intervention process.

The Evaluation and Assessment Process

Service coordinator

Once connected with either Child Find or your community's early intervention program, you'll be assigned a **service coordinator** who will explain the early intervention process and help you through the next steps in that process. The service coordinator will serve as your single point of contact with the early intervention system.

Screening and/or evaluation

One of the first things that will happen is that your child will be evaluated to see if, indeed, he or she has a developmental delay or disability. (In some states, there may be a preliminary step called **screening** to see if there's cause to suspect that a baby or toddler has a disability or developmental delay.) The family's service coordinator will explain what's involved in the screening and/or evaluation and ask for your permission to proceed. You must provide your **written consent** before screening and/or evaluation may take place.

The evaluation group will be made up of qualified people who have different areas of training and experience. Together, they know about children's speech and language skills, physical abilities, hearing and vision, and other important areas of development. They know how to work with children, even very young ones, to discover if a child has a problem or is developing within normal ranges. Group members may evaluate your child together or individually. As part of the evaluation, the team will observe your child, ask your child to do things, talk to you and your child, and use other methods to gather information. These procedures will help the team find out how your child functions in the five areas of development.

Exceptions for diagnosed physical or mental conditions

It's important to note that an evaluation of your child won't be necessary if he or she is automatically eligible due to a diagnosed physical or mental condition that has a high probability of resulting in a developmental delay. Such conditions include but aren't limited to chromosomal abnormalities; genetic or congenital disorders; sensory impairments; inborn errors of metabolism; disorders reflecting disturbance of the development of the nervous system; congenital infections; severe attachment disorders; and disorders secondary to exposure to toxic substances, including fetal alcohol syndrome. Many states have policies that further specify what conditions automatically qualify an infant or toddler for early intervention (e.g., Down syndrome, Fragile X syndrome).

Determining eligibility

The results of the evaluation will be used to determine your child's eligibility for early intervention services. You and a team of professionals will meet and review all of the data, results, and reports. The people on the team will talk with you about whether your child meets the criteria under IDEA and state policy for having a developmental delay, a diagnosed physical or mental condition, or being at risk for having a substantial delay. If so, your child is generally found to be eligible for services.

Initial assessment of the child: With parental consent, indepth assessment must now be conducted to determine your child's unique needs and the early intervention services appropriate to address those needs. Initial assessment will include reviewing the results of the evaluation, personal observation of your child, and identifying his or her needs in each developmental area.

Initial assessment of the family

With approval of the family members involved, assessments of family members are also conducted to identify the resources, concerns, and priorities of the family related to enhancing the development of your child. The family-directed assessment is voluntary on the part of each family member participating in the assessment and is based on information gathered through an assessment tool and also through an interview with those family members who elect to participate.

Who pays for all this?

Under IDEA, evaluations and assessments are provided at no cost to parents. They are funded by state and federal monies.

Writing the IFSP

Having collected a great deal of information about your child and family, it's now possible for the team (including you as parents) to sit down and write an individualized plan of action for your child and family. This plan is called the **Individualized Family Service Plan (IFSP)**. It is a very important document, and you, as parents, are important members of the team that develops it. Each state has specific guidelines for the IFSP. Your service coordinator can explain what the IFSP guidelines are in your state.

Guiding principles: The IFSP is a written document that, among other things, outlines the early intervention services that your child and family will receive. One guiding principal of the IFSP is that the family is a child's greatest resource, that a young child's needs are closely tied to the needs of his or her family. The best way to support children and meet their needs is to support and build upon the individual strengths of their family. So, the **IFSP is a whole family plan** with the parents as major contributors in its development. Involvement of other team members will depend on what the child needs. These other team members could come from several agencies and may include medical people, therapists, child development specialists, social workers, and others.

What info is included in an IFSP?

Your child's IFSP must include the following:

- Your child's present physical, cognitive, communication, social/emotional, and adaptive development levels and needs.
- Family information (with your agreement), including the resources, priorities, and concerns of you, as parents, and other family members closely involved with the child.
- The major results or outcomes expected to be achieved for your child and family.
- The specific services your child will be receiving.
- Where in the natural environment (e.g., home, community) the services will be provided (if the services will not be provided in the natural environment, the IFSP must include a statement justifying why not)?
- When and where your son or daughter will receive services?
- The number of days or sessions he or she will receive each service and how long each session will last.

- Who will pay for the services?

- The name of the service coordinator overseeing the implementation of the IFSP.

- The steps to be taken to support your child's transition out of early intervention and into another program when the time comes.

The IFSP may also identify services your family may be interested in, such as financial information or information about raising a child with a disability.

Informed parental consent: The IFSP must be fully explained to you, the parents, and your suggestions must be considered. *You must give written consent for each service to be provided.* If you do not give your consent in writing, your child will not receive that service.

Reviewing and updating the IFSP: The IFSP is reviewed every six months and is updated at least once a year. This takes into account that children can learn, grow, and change quickly in just a short period of time.

Timeframes for All This

When the early intervention system receives a referral about a child with a suspected disability or developmental delay, a time clock starts running. Within **45 days**, the early intervention system must complete the critical steps discussed thus far:

- screening (if used in the state),

- initial evaluation of the child,

- initial assessments of the child and family, and

- writing the IFSP (if the child has been found eligible).

That's a tall order, but important, given how quickly children grow and change. When a baby or toddler has developmental issues, they need to be addressed as soon as possible. So—45 days, that's the timeframe from referral to completion of the IFSP for an eligible child.

Who Pays for the Services?

Whether or not you, as parents, will have to pay for any services for your child depends on the policies of your state. Check with your service coordinator. Your state's system of payments must be available in writing and given to you, so there are no surprises or unexpected bills later.

What's free to families: Under Part C of IDEA, the following services must be provided at no cost to families:

- Child Find services;

- evaluations and assessments;

- the development and review of the IFSP; and

- service coordination.

When services are not free: Depending on your state's policies, you may have to pay for certain other services. You may be charged a **"sliding-scale" fee**, meaning the fees are based on what you earn. Some services may be covered by your health insurance, by Medicaid, or by Indian Health Services. The Part C system may ask for your permission to access your public or private insurance in order to pay for the early intervention services your child receives. In most cases, the early intervention system may **not** use your health care insurance (private or public) **without your express, written consent**. If you do not give such consent, the system may **not** limit or deny you or your child services.

Every effort is made to provide services to all infants and toddlers who need help, regardless of family income. Services cannot be denied to a child just because his or her family is not able to pay for them.

Section 32.2

Response to Intervention (RTI)

This section includes text excerpted from "Assisting Students
Struggling with Reading: Response to Intervention (RTI) and
Multi-Tier Intervention in the Primary Grades," Institute
of Education Sciences (IES), U.S. Department of
Education (ED), February 2009. Reviewed June 2016.

Response to Intervention: The Multi-Tier Intervention System

Response to Intervention (RTI) is a comprehensive early detection
and prevention strategy that identifies struggling students and assists
them before they fall behind. RTI systems combine universal screening and high-quality instruction for all students with interventions
targeted at struggling students.

RTI strategies are used in both reading and math instruction. For
reading instruction in the primary grades (K–2), schools screen students at least once a year to identify students at risk for future reading
failure. Students whose screening scores indicate potential difficulties
with learning to read are provided with more intensive reading interventions. Student responses to the interventions are then measured
to determine whether they have made adequate progress and:

1. no longer need the intervention,

2. continue to need some intervention, or

3. need even more intensive intervention.

In RTI, the levels of interventions are conventionally referred to
as "tiers." RTI is typically thought of as having three tiers, with the
first tier encompassing general classroom instruction. Some states and
school districts, however, have implemented multi-tier intervention
systems with more than three tiers. Within a three-tier RTI model,
each tier is defined by specific characteristics:

*   Tier 1 instruction is generally defined as reading instruction pro-
    vided to all students in a class. Beyond this general definition,

there is no clear consensus on the meaning of the term tier 1. Instead, it is variously referred to as "evidence-based reading instruction," "high quality reading instruction," or "an instructional program...with balanced, explicit, and systematic reading instruction that fosters both code-based and text-based strategies for word identification and comprehension."

- Tier 2 interventions are provided only to students who demonstrate problems based on screening measures or weak progress from regular classroom instruction. In addition to general classroom instruction, tier 2 students receive supplemental, small group reading instruction aimed at building foundational reading skills.

- Tier 3 interventions are provided to students who do not progress after a reasonable amount of time with the tier 2 intervention and require more intensive assistance. Tier 3 (or, in districts with more than three tiers, tiers 3 and above) usually entails one-on-one tutoring with a mix of instructional interventions. Ongoing analysis of student performance data is critical in tier 3. Systematically collected data are used to identify successes and failures in instruction for individual students. If students still experience difficulty after receiving intensive services, they are evaluated for possible special education services.

Though a relatively new concept, RTI and multi-tier interventions are becoming increasingly common. This is attributed in part to the 2004 reauthorization of the Individuals with Disabilities Education Act (IDEA), which encourages states to use RTI to help prevent reading difficulties and to identify students with learning disabilities.

RTI also urges schools to use evidence-based practices in all tiers and to provide intensive services only to students who fail to benefit from a well designed, evidence-based intervention. This helps to accurately determine which students possess learning disabilities in reading since only students who do not respond to high-quality reading instruction in their general education classrooms would be considered for special education. Thus, there is the possibility—and certainly the hope—that RTI will reduce inappropriate referrals to special education, especially of ethnic minority students, low-income students, and students who received weak reading instruction.

Chapter 33

Understanding the Special Education Process: An Overview

Ten Basic Steps in Special Education

When a child is having trouble in school, it's important to find out why. The child may have a disability. By law, schools must provide special help to eligible children with disabilities. This help is called special education and related services.

There's a lot to know about the process by which children are identified as having a disability and in need of *special education* and *related services*.

This brief overview is an excellent place to start. Here, we've distilled the process into ten basic steps. Once you have the big picture of the process, it's easier to understand the many details under each step.

Step One: Child Is Identified as Possibly Needing Special Education and Related Services

There are two primary ways in which children are identified as possibly needing special education and related services: the system

This chapter includes text excerpted from "10 Basic Steps in Special Education," Center for Parent Information and Resources (CPIR), April 2014.

known as **Child Find** (which operates in each state), and by referral of a parent or school personnel.

Child Find. Each state is required by Individuals with Disabilities Education Act (IDEA) to identify, locate, and evaluate all children with disabilities in the state who need special education and related services. To do so, states conduct what are known as Child Find activities.

When a child is identified by Child Find as possibly having a disability and as needing special education, parents may be asked for permission to evaluate their child. Parents can also call the Child Find office and ask that their child be evaluated.

Referral or request for evaluation. A school professional may ask that a child be evaluated to see if he or she has a disability. Parents may also contact the child's teacher or other school professional to ask that their child be evaluated. This request may be verbal, but it's best to put it in writing.

Parental consent is needed before a child may be evaluated. Under the federal IDEA regulations, evaluation needs to be completed within 60 days after the parent gives consent. However, if a State's IDEA regulations give a different timeline for completion of the evaluation, the State's timeline is applied.

Step Two: Child Is Evaluated

Evaluation is an essential early step in the special education process for a child. It's intended to answer these questions:

- Does the child have a disability that requires the provision of special education and related services?

- What are the child's specific educational needs?

- What special education services and related services, then, are appropriate for addressing those needs?

By law, the initial evaluation of the child must be "full and individual"—which is to say, focused on that child and that child alone. The evaluation must assess the child in all areas related to the child's suspected disability.

The evaluation results will be used to decide the child's eligibility for special education and related services and to make decisions about an appropriate educational program for the child.

If the parents disagree with the evaluation, they have the right to take their child for an Independent Educational Evaluation (IEE). They can ask that the school system pay for this IEE.

Step Three: Eligibility Is Decided

A group of qualified professionals and the parents look at the child's evaluation results. Together, they decide if the child is a "child with a disability," as defined by IDEA. If the parents do not agree with the eligibility decision, they may ask for a hearing to challenge the decision.

Step Four: Child Is Found Eligible for Services

If the child is found to be a child with a disability, as defined by IDEA, he or she eligible for special education and related services. Within 30 calendar days after a child is determined eligible, a team of school professionals and the parents must meet to write an individualized education program (IEP) for the child.

Step Five: IEP Meeting Is Scheduled

The school system schedules and conducts the IEP meeting. School staff must:

- contact the participants, including the parents
- notify parents early enough to make sure they have an opportunity to attend
- schedule the meeting at a time and place agreeable to parents and the school
- tell the parents the purpose, time, and location of the meeting
- tell the parents who will be attending
- tell the parents that they may invite people to the meeting who have knowledge or special expertise about the child

Step Six: IEP Meeting Is Held and the IEP Is Written

The IEP team gathers to talk about the child's needs and write the student's IEP. Parents and the student (when appropriate) are full participating members of the team. If the child's placement (meaning, where the child will receive his or her special education and related services) is decided by a different group, the parents must be part of that group as well.

Before the school system may provide special education and related services to the child for the first time, the **parents must give consent**. The child begins to receive services as soon as possible after the IEP is written and this consent is given.

If the parents do not agree with the IEP and placement, they may discuss their concerns with other members of the IEP team and try to work out an agreement. If they still disagree, parents can ask for mediation, or the school may offer mediation. Parents may file a state complaint with the state education agency or a due process complaint, which is the first step in requesting a due process hearing, at which time mediation must be available.

Step Seven: After the IEP Is Written, Services Are Provided

The school makes sure that the child's IEP is carried out as it was written. Parents are given a copy of the IEP. Each of the child's teachers and service providers has access to the IEP and knows his or her specific responsibilities for carrying out the IEP. This includes the accommodations, modifications, and supports that must be provided to the child, in keeping with the IEP.

Step Eight: Progress Is Measured and Reported to Parents

The child's progress toward the annual goals is measured, as stated in the IEP. His or her parents are regularly informed of their child's progress and whether that progress is enough for the child to achieve the goals by the end of the year. These progress reports must be given to parents at least as often as parents are informed of their nondisabled children's progress.

Step Nine: IEP Is Reviewed

The child's IEP is reviewed by the IEP team at least once a year, or more often if the parents or school ask for a review. If necessary, the IEP is revised. Parents, as team members, must be invited to participate in these meetings. Parents can make suggestions for changes, can agree or disagree with the IEP, and agree or disagree with the placement.

If parents do not agree with the IEP and placement, they may discuss their concerns with other members of the IEP team and try to work out an agreement. There are several options, including additional testing, an independent evaluation, or asking for mediation, or a due process hearing. They may also file a complaint with the state education agency.

Step Ten: Child Is Reevaluated

At least every three years the child must be reevaluated. This evaluation is sometimes called a "triennial." Its purpose is to find out if the child continues to be a child with a disability, as defined by IDEA, and what the child's educational needs are. However, the child must be reevaluated more often if conditions warrant or if the child's parent or teacher asks for a new evaluation.

Chapter 34

Individualized Education Programs (IEPs)

What Is an Individualized Education Program (IEP)?

Kids with delayed skills or other disabilities might be eligible for special services that provide individualized education programs in public schools, free of charge to families. Understanding how to access these services can help parents be effective advocates for their kids.

The passage of the updated version of the Individuals with Disabilities Education Act (IDEA) made parents of kids with special needs even more crucial members of their child's education team.

Parents can now work with educators to develop a plan—the Individualized Education Program (IEP)—to help kids succeed in school. The IEP describes the goals the team sets for a child during the school year, as well as any special support needed to help achieve them.

Who Needs an Individualized Education Program (IEP)?

A child who has difficulty learning and functioning and has been identified as a special needs student is the perfect candidate for an IEP.

This chapter includes excerpts from "Individualized Education Programs (IEPs)," © 1995–2016. The Nemours Foundation/KidsHealth®. Reprinted with permission.

Kids struggling in school may qualify for support services, allowing them to be taught in a special way, for reasons such as:

- learning disabilities
- attention deficit hyperactivity disorder (ADHD)
- emotional disorders
- cognitive challenges
- autism
- hearing impairment
- visual impairment
- speech or language impairment
- developmental delay

How Are Services Delivered?

In most cases, the services and goals outlined in an IEP can be provided in a standard school environment. This can be done in the regular classroom (for example, a reading teacher helping a small group of children who need extra assistance while the other kids in the class work on reading with the regular teacher) or in a special resource room in the regular school. The resource room can serve a group of kids with similar needs who are brought together for help.

However, kids who need intense intervention may be taught in a special school environment. These classes have fewer students per teacher, allowing for more individualized attention.

In addition, the teacher usually has specific training in helping kids with special educational needs. The children spend most of their day in a special classroom and join the regular classes for nonacademic activities (like music and gym) or in academic activities in which they don't need extra help.

Because the goal of IDEA is to ensure that each child is educated in the least restrictive environment possible, effort is made to help kids stay in a regular classroom. However, when needs are best met in a special class, then kids might be placed in one.

The Referral and Evaluation Process

The referral process generally begins when a teacher, parent, or doctor is concerned that a child may be having trouble in the classroom, and the teacher notifies the school counselor or psychologist.

The first step is to gather specific data regarding the student's progress or academic problems. This may be done through:

- a conference with parents

- a conference with the student

- observation of the student

- analysis of the student's performance (attention, behavior, work completion, tests, classwork, homework, etc.)

This information helps school personnel determine the next step. At this point, strategies specific to the student could be used to help the child become more successful in school. If this doesn't work, the child would be tested for a specific learning disability or other impairment to help determine qualification for special services.

It's important to note, though, that the presence of a disability doesn't automatically guarantee a child will receive services. To be eligible, the disability must affect functioning at school.

To determine eligibility, a multidisciplinary team of professionals will evaluate the child based on their observations; the child's performance on standardized tests; and daily work such as tests, quizzes, classwork, and homework.

Who Is on the Team?

The professionals on the evaluation team can include:

- a psychologist

- a physical therapist

- an occupational therapist

- a speech therapist

- a special educator

- a vision or hearing specialist

- others, depending on the child's specific needs

As a parent, you can decide whether to have your child assessed. If you choose to do so, you'll be asked to sign a permission form that will detail who is involved in the process and the types of tests they use. These tests might include measures of specific school skills, such as reading or math, as well as more general developmental skills, such as speech and language. Testing does not necessarily mean that a child will receive services.

Once the team members complete their individual assessments, they develop a comprehensive evaluation report (CER) that compiles their findings, offers an educational classification, and outlines the skills and support the child will need.

The parents then have a chance to review the report before the IEP is developed. Some parents will disagree with the report, and they will have the opportunity to work together with the school to come up with a plan that best meets the child's needs.

Developing an Individualized Education Program (IEP)

The next step is an IEP meeting at which the team and parents decide what will go into the plan. In addition to the evaluation team, a regular teacher should be present to offer suggestions about how the plan can help the child's progress in the standard education curriculum.

At the meeting, the team will discuss your child's educational needs—as described in the CER—and come up with specific, measurable short-term and annual goals for each of those needs. If you attend this meeting, you can take an active role in developing the goals and determining which skills or areas will receive the most attention.

The cover page of the IEP outlines the support services your child will receive and how often they will be provided (for example, occupational therapy twice a week). Support services might include special education, speech therapy, occupational or physical therapy, counseling, audiology, medical services, nursing, vision or hearing therapy, and many others.

If the team recommends several services, the amount of time they take in the child's school schedule can seem overwhelming. To ease that load, some services may be provided on a consultative basis. In these cases, the professional consults with the teacher to come up with strategies to help the child but doesn't offer any hands-on instruction. For instance, an occupational therapist may suggest accommodations for a child with fine-motor problems that affect handwriting, and the classroom teacher would incorporate these suggestions into the handwriting lessons taught to the entire class.

Other services can be delivered right in the classroom, so the child's day isn't interrupted by therapy. The child who has difficulty with handwriting might work one on one with an occupational therapist while everyone else practices their handwriting skills. When deciding how and where services are offered, the child's comfort and dignity should be a top priority.

The IEP should be reviewed annually to update the goals and make sure the levels of service meet your child's needs. However, IEPs can be changed at any time on an as-needed basis. If you think your child needs more, fewer, or different services, you can request a meeting and bring the team together to discuss your concerns.

Your Legal Rights

Specific timelines ensure that the development of an IEP moves from referral to providing services as quickly as possible. Be sure to ask about this timeframe and get a copy of your parents' rights when your child is referred. These guidelines (sometimes called procedural safeguards) outline your rights as a parent to control what happens to your child during each step of the process.

The parents' rights also describe how you can proceed if you dis-agree with any part of the CER or the IEP—mediation and hearings both are options. You can get information about low-cost or free legal representation from the school district or, if your child is in Early Intervention (for kids ages 3 to 5), through that program.

Attorneys and paid advocates familiar with the IEP process will provide representation if you need it. You also may invite anyone who knows or works with your child whose input you feel would be helpful to join the IEP team.

A Final Word

Parents have the right to choose where their kids will be educated. This choice includes public or private elementary schools and second-ary schools, including religious schools. It also includes charter schools and homeschools.

However, it is important to understand that the rights of children with disabilities who are placed by their parents in private elemen-tary schools and secondary schools are not the same as those of kids with disabilities who are enrolled in public schools or placed by public agencies in private schools when the public school is unable to provide a free appropriate public education (FAPE).

Two major differences that parents, teachers, other school staff, private school representatives, and the kids need to know about are:

1. Children with disabilities who are placed by their parents in private schools may not get the same services they would receive in a public school.

2. Not all kids with disabilities placed by their parents in private schools will receive services.

The IEP process is complex, but it's also an effective way to address how your child learns and functions. If you have concerns, don't hesitate to ask questions about the evaluation findings or the goals recommended by the team. You know your child best and should play a central role in creating a learning plan tailored to his or her specific needs.

Chapter 35

Supports, Modifications, and Accommodations for Students

Students with Disabilities

For many students with disabilities—and for many without—**the key to success in the classroom lies in having appropriate adaptations, accommodations, and modifications made to the instruction and other classroom activities.**

Some adaptations are as simple as moving a distractible student to the front of the class or away from the pencil sharpener or the window. Other modifications may involve changing the way that material is presented or the way that students respond to show their learning.

Adaptations, accommodations, and modifications need to be individualized for students, based upon their needs and their personal learning styles and interests. It is not always obvious what adaptations, accommodations, or modifications would be beneficial for a particular student, or how changes to the curriculum, its presentation, the classroom setting, or student evaluation might be made.

This chapter includes text excerpted from "Supports, Modifications, and Accommodations for Students," Center for Parent Information and Resources (CPIR), February 2016.

A Quick Look at Terminology

You might wonder if the terms **supports**, **modifications**, and **adaptations** all mean the same thing. The simple answer is: No, not completely, but yes, for the most part. (Don't you love a clear answer?) People tend to use the terms interchangeably, to be sure, and we will do so here, for ease of reading, but distinctions can be made between the terms.

Sometimes people get confused about what it means to have a *modification* and what it means to have an *accommodation*. Usually a **modification** means *a change in what is being taught to or expected from the student*. Making an assignment easier so the student is not doing the same level of work as other students is an example of a modification.

An **accommodation** *is a change that helps a student overcome or work around the disability*. Allowing a student who has trouble writing to give his answers orally is an example of an accommodation. This student is still expected to know the same material and answer the same questions as fully as the other students, but he doesn't have to write his answers to show that he knows the information.

What is most important to know about modifications and accommodations is that both are meant to help a child to learn.

Different Types of Supports

Special Education

By definition, special education is "specially designed instruction" (§300.39). And Individuals with Disabilities Education Act (IDEA) defines that term as follows:

(3) **Specially designed instruction** means adapting, as appropriate to the needs of an eligible child under this part, the content, methodology, or delivery of instruction—(i) To address the unique needs of the child that result from the child's disability; and (ii) To ensure access of the child to the general curriculum, so that the child can meet the educational standards within the jurisdiction of the public agency that apply to all children. [(§300.39(b)(3)]

Thus, special education involves adapting the "content, methodology, or delivery of instruction." In fact, the special education field can take pride in the knowledge base and expertise it's developed in the past 30-plus years of individualizing instruction to meet the needs of students with disabilities. It's a pleasure to share some of that knowledge with you now.

Adapting Instruction

Sometimes a student may need to have changes made in class work or routines because of his or her disability. Modifications can be made to:

- **what** a child is taught
- **how** a child works at school

For example:
Jack is an eighth grade student who has learning disabilities in reading and writing. He is in a regular eighth grade class that is team-taught by a general education teacher and a special education teacher. Modifications and accommodations provided for Jack's daily school routine (and when he takes state or district-wide tests) include the following:

- Jack will have shorter reading and writing assignments.
- Jack's textbooks will be based upon the eighth grade curriculum but at his independent reading level (fourth grade).
- Jack will have test questions read/explained to him, when he asks.
- Jack will give his answers to essay-type questions by speaking, rather than writing them down.

Modifications or accommodations are most often made in the following areas:
Scheduling. For example,

- giving the student extra time to complete assignments or tests
- breaking up testing over several days

Setting. For example,

- working in a small group
- working one-on-one with the teacher

Materials. For example,

- providing audiotaped lectures or books

- giving copies of teacher's lecture notes
- using large print books, Braille, or books on digital text (such as CD, DVD, flash drive, etc.)

Instruction. For example,

- reducing the difficulty of assignments
- reducing the reading level
- using a student/peer tutor

Student Response. For example,

- allowing answers to be given orally or dictated
- using a word processor for written work
- using sign language, a communication device, Braille, or native language if it is not English.

Because adapting the content, methodology, and/or delivery of instruction is an essential element in special education and an extremely valuable support for students, it's equally essential to know as much as possible about how instruction can be adapted to address the needs of an individual student with a disability. The special education teacher who serves on the Individualized Education Program (IEP) team can contribute his or her expertise in this area, which is the essence of special education.

Related Services

One look at IDEA's definition of related services at §300.34 and it's clear that these services are supportive in nature, although not in the same way that adapting the curriculum is. Related services support children's special education and are provided when necessary to help students benefit from special education. Thus, related services must be included in the treasure chest of accommodations and supports we're exploring. That definition begins:

§300.34 Related services.

(a) **General.** Related services means transportation and such developmental, corrective, and other supportive services as are required to assist a child with a disability to benefit from special education, and includes the following.

Here's the list of related services in the law:

- speech-language pathology and audiology services

- interpreting services
- psychological services
- physical and occupational therapy
- recreation, including therapeutic recreation
- early identification and assessment of disabilities in children
- counseling services, including rehabilitation counseling
- orientation and mobility services
- medical services for diagnostic or evaluation purposes
- school health services and school nurse services
- social work services in schools

This is not an exhaustive list of possible related services. There are others (not named here or in the law) that states and schools routinely make available under the umbrella of related services. The IEP team decides which related services a child needs and specificies them in the child's IEP.

Supplementary Aids and Services

One of the most powerful types of supports available to children with disabilities are the other kinds of supports or services (other than special education and related services) that a child needs to be educated with nondisabled children to the maximum extent appropriate. Some examples of these additional services and supports, called **supplementary aids and services** in IDEA, are:

- adapted equipment—such as a special seat or a cut-out cup for drinking
- assistive technology—such as a word processor, special software, or a communication system
- training for staff, student, and/or parents
- peer tutors
- a one-on-one aide
- adapted materials—such as books on tape, large print, or high-lighted notes
- collaboration/consultation among staff, parents, and/or other professionals

The IEP team, which includes the parents, is the group that decides which supplementary aids and services a child needs to support his or her access to and participation in the school environment. The IEP team must really work together to make sure that a child gets the supplementary aids and services that he or she needs to be successful. Team members talk about the child's needs, the curriculum, and school routine, and openly explore all options to make sure the right supports for the specific child are included.

Much more can be said about these important supports and services.

Program Modifications or Supports for School Staff

If the IEP team decides that a child needs a particular modification or accommodation, this information must be included in the IEP. Supports are also available for those who work with the child, to help them help that child be successful. Supports for school staff must also be written into the IEP. Some of these supports might include:

- attending a conference or training related to the child's needs
- getting help from another staff member or administrative person
- having an aide in the classroom
- getting special equipment or teaching materials

Accommodations in Large Assessments

IDEA requires that students with disabilities take part in **state- or district-wide assessments**. These are tests that are periodically given to all students to measure achievement. It is one way that schools determine how well and how much students are learning. IDEA now states that students with disabilities should have as much involvement in the general curriculum as possible. This means that, if a child is receiving instruction in the general curriculum, he or she could take the same standardized test that the school district or state gives to nondisabled children. Accordingly, a child's IEP must include all modifications or accommodations that the child needs so that he or she can participate in state or district-wide assessments.

The IEP team can decide that a particular test is not appropriate for a child. In this case, the IEP must include:

- an explanation of why that test is not suitable for the child
- how the child will be assessed instead (often called alternate assessment).

Ask your state and/or local school district for a copy of their guidelines on the types of accommodations, modifications, and alternate assessments available to students.

Conclusion

Even a child with many needs is to be involved with nondisabled peers to the maximum extent appropriate. Just because a child has severe disabilities or needs modifications to the general curriculum does not mean that he or she may be removed from the general education class. If a child is removed from the general education class for any part of the school day, the IEP team must include in the IEP an explanation for the child's nonparticipation.

Because accommodations can be so vital to helping children with disabilities access the general curriculum, participate in school (including extracurricular and nonacademic activities), and be educated alongside their peers without disabilities, IDEA reinforces their use again and again, in its requirements, in its definitions, and in its principles. The wealth of experience that the special education field has gained over the years since IDEA was first passed by Congress is the very resource you'll want to tap for more information on what accommodations are appropriate for students, given their disability, and how to make those adaptations to support their learning.

Chapter 36

Specialized Teaching Techniques

Chapter Contents

Section 36.1

Differentiated Instruction

This section includes text excerpted from "Differentiated Instructional Strategies to Accommodate Students with Varying Needs and Learning Styles," Education Resources Information Center (ERIC), U.S. Department of Education (ED), November 18, 2013.

Introduction to Differentiated Instruction

Educators are mandated to see that all students meet the standards of their district and state. Through the use of differentiated instructional strategies, educators can meet the needs of all students and help them to meet and exceed the established standards. The objective is accomplished by choosing appropriate teaching methods to match each individual student's learning needs.

Any group of students is likely to demonstrate considerable variation in their learning characteristics and behaviors. When the group includes students with learning deficiencies or other learning disorders, the amount of variation in learning is significantly increased. The diverse learning characteristics displayed by students in today's schools make it necessary for teachers to implement a wide variety of activities in their classes. As classrooms become more culturally diverse, it becomes more imperative to differentiate instruction.

Differentiated instruction is appropriate for virtually all general education classes and is particularly beneficial to students with an array of learning challenges. Students demonstrate varying learning abilities, academic levels, learning styles, and learning preferences and need tailored instruction to meet their unique needs. Differentiated instruction recognizes the value and worth that exist in each individual; it allows students from all backgrounds and with diverse abilities to demonstrate what they know, understand, and are capable of doing.

Differentiated instruction was originated by C.A. Tomlinson in 1999, basing it primarily on Howard Gardner's concept of multiple intelligences and brain-compatible research literature. Teachers were encouraged to consider students' unique learning styles and differentiate educational activities to provide for their divergent learning styles by differentiating instruction in three areas: content, process, and product. In differentiating instruction, teachers proactively modify the curriculum, teaching methods, resources, learning activities, and student products to address the needs of individual students and small groups of students to maximize the learning opportunity for each student in the classroom.

Theoretical Basis for Differentiated Instruction

Differentiated instruction was primarily based on the theory of multiple intelligences by Howard Gardner and brain-compatible research. Gardner postulated eight different intelligences that are relatively independent but interacting cognitive capacities. The intelligences are verbal-linguistic, logical-mathematical, musical, spatial, bodily-kinesthetic, naturalistic, interpersonal, intrapersonal, and a tentative ninth one, moral intelligence. Some students demonstrate strong intelligence in one area, whereas other may demonstrate strengths in several intelligences. Each child will have his or her own unique set of intellectual strengths and weaknesses. For clarity, learning style, learning preference, and multiple intelligences are often used synonymously.

It is important, from a multiple intelligences perspective, that teachers take individual differences among students very seriously. They should gear how to teach and how to evaluate to the needs of the particular child. The bottom line is having a deep interest in children and how their minds are different from one another to help them use their minds well. Linking the multiple intelligences with a curriculum focused on understanding is an extremely powerful intellectual undertaking.

Brain-compatible instruction is related to the multiple intelligences concept but it is more solidly grounded in the neurosciences. Brain-scanning techniques allow scientists to study performance of the human brain while the subject concentrates on different types of learning tasks. It has been discovered that brains perform best when highly motivated and involved and experiencing "manageable" stress.

Three Areas of Differentiated Instruction

The core of differentiated instruction is flexibility in content, process, and product based on students' strengths, needs, and learning styles. Content is what students are to master or learn from the instruction; process is how the students must complete the learning content; and product is how the learning is demonstrated or observed. In the content area each child is taught the same curriculum but it may be quantitatively or qualitatively different. Process includes how teachers teach and how students learn. The activities provided for student learning must address differing student abilities, learning styles, and interests. Teachers must adjust their teaching style to reflect the needs of different students by finding out where students are when they come into the process and building on their prior knowledge to advance their learning. Product is the way students demonstrate what they have learned. It must reflect student learning styles and abilities. Differentiation by product, or response, must also acknowledge, respect, and value the various ways that students may respond to an activity; but unfortunately, written work is still the predominate mode used by teachers for receiving feedback.

Learning Styles and Teaching Styles

How much a student learns in a class is governed in part by that student's native ability and prior preparation but also by the compatibility of his or her learning style and the instructor's teaching style. If mismatches exist between learning styles and teaching styles students become bored and inattentive in class, do poorly on tests, get discouraged about the courses, the curriculum, and themselves, and in some cases change to other curricula or drop out of school. Students whose learning styles are compatible with the teaching style tend to retain information longer, apply it more effectively, and have more positive post-course attitudes toward the subject than do their counterparts who experience learning/teaching style mismatches.

Felder and Silverman synthesized findings from a number of studies to formulate a learning style model with dimensions. A student's learning style may be defined in part by answers to five questions:

1. What type of information does the student preferentially perceive: sensory (sights, sounds, physical sensation) or intuitive (memories, ideas, insights)?

2. Through which modality is sensory information most effectively perceived: visual (pictures, diagrams, graphs, demonstrations) or verbal (sounds, written and spoken words and formulas)?

3. With which organization of information is the student most comfortable: inductive or deductive (principles are given, consequences and applications are deduced)?

4. How does the student prefer to process information: actively (through engagement in physical activity or discussion), or reflectively (through introspection)?

5. How does the student progress toward understanding: sequentially (in a logical progression of small incremental steps), or globally (in large jumps, holistically)?

The dichotomous learning style dimensions of this model are a continua and not either/or categories. A student's preference on a given scale may be strong, moderate, or almost nonexistent, either of which may change with time or vary from one subject or learning environment to another.

According to Katsioloudis and Fantz, learning styles are personal qualities that influence the way students interact with their learning environment, peers, and teachers. They reported four learning style dimensions: sensing learners (concrete, practical, oriented towards facts and procedures) or intuitive learners (conceptual, innovative, oriented towards theories and meanings); visual learners (prefer visual representations—pictures, diagrams, flow charts) or verbal learners (prefer written and spoken explanations); active learners (learn by trying things, working with others) or reflective learners (learn by thinking things through, working alone); and sequential learners (learn in small incremental steps, linear, orderly) or global learners (learn in large leaps, holistic, systems thinkers.

Just as students have preferred learning styles, teachers have preferred teaching styles. Jain categorized teaching styles as: formal authority (teacher provides and controls flow of content, students expected to receive content); demonstrator or personal model (teacher acts as role model, demonstrating skills and processes; coaches students in developing, applying skills and knowledge); facilitator (teaching emphasizes student-centered learning); and delegator (students choice in designing, implementing learning projects; teacher in consultative role). Grasha posited that teachers actually possess each of the qualities described (including "expert" style—possessor of knowledge, expertise that students need) to varying degrees; they use some styles more often than others, and some blends of styles are dominant and others are secondary. The author further advanced that a given teaching style creates a particular mood or emotional climate in class. For example, the expert/formal authority blend may suggest "I'm in charge here" and may create a "cool" emotional climate; whereas, the expert/facilitative/delegative blend may suggest "I'm here to consult and explore with you" and may create a "warm" climate.

Katsioloudis and Fantz stated that teachers who adapt their teaching style to include both poles of each of the given learning style dimensions should come close to providing an optimal learning environment for most, if not all, students in a class. Matching teaching strategies to a student's preferred learning style is likely to promote understanding and retention of information. Complementary, through an awareness of the preferred teaching style, teachers may gain a better understanding of themselves and how their teaching style can be changed, modified, or supported to improve their interactions with students. When teachers do master differentiated teaching, ensuring that each student consistently experiences the reality that success is likely to follow hard work, the result is enhanced job satisfaction.

Section 36.2

The Inclusive Writing Classroom and Supportive Technology for Writing Problems

This section contains text excerpted from the following sources: Text beginning with the heading "Students with Learning Disabilities in an Inclusive Writing Classroom" is excerpted from "Students with Learning Disabilities in an Inclusive Writing Classroom," Education Resources Information Center (ERIC), U.S. Department of Education (ED), 2014; Text beginning with the heading "Technology to Support Writing" is excerpted from "Technology to Support Writing by Students with Learning and Academic Disabilities," Education Resources Information Center (ERIC), U.S. Department of Education (ED), 2011. Reviewed June 2016.

Students with Learning Disabilities in an Inclusive Writing Classroom

Writing is difficult for many students, and poses special challenges for students with learning disabilities. These students have historically been disadvantaged through education in classroom settings away from most peers their age. In resource rooms, teachers group students diagnosed with learning disabilities (LD), where they often work on isolated skills and do not gain a broader picture of the complexities of writing. Year by year, these students continue to fall behind their peers in regular classrooms. Teachers, researchers, and parents have challenged this kind of homogeneous grouping practice because students with LD are separated from mainstream education, limiting interaction with their mainstream peers and often receiving inferior instruction. Research has indicated that students with LD benefit from learning in an environment that engages them in peer-interaction and authentic literacy learning activities.

In order to provide students with LD equal learning opportunities and an effective learning environment, several researchers have recommended an inclusive model since the late 1990s. The inclusive model aims to educate as many students with disabilities as possible in regular classroom settings while still meeting their unique needs based on the least restrictive environment (LRE) provision of the Individuals with Disabilities Education Act (IDEA, 2004). LRE means that, to the maximum extent possible, school districts must educate students with disabilities in regular education classrooms and provide them with appropriate support such as curriculum modification, an itinerant teacher with special education training, or computer-assisted devices as examples.

IDEA requires that school districts have a continuum of placements and services available to accommodate the needs of all children with disabilities ranging from care facilities to regular classroom settings with support services. The students' needs as determined by the Individual Education Program (IEP) and each individual student's IEP team drive the degree of inclusion. It is important to point out that the inclusive model alone does not guarantee academic gains; however, students with mild LD who are educated along with their peers in an integrated educational setting have been found to benefit academically, socially, and emotionally.

Many students with LD face greater challenges than their education peers without LD when learning how to write. Writing is a complex process that requires the integration of many cognitive and social processes and comprehensive language skills. Students with learning difficulties struggle with generating topics, planning and organizing, editing, revising, monitoring the writing process, and transcribing words. They have fewer strategies with writing, less knowledge about writing, and behavior and motivational factors that impede success as school writers. Scholars who study effective techniques for teaching and learning have found considerable evidence that a process approach to writing combined with direct strategic instruction has been beneficial in improving writing skills of children with LD.

Technology to Support Writing

Among national organizations considering writing outcomes, there is widespread acceptance that writing has moved from a paper and pen activity to one that is technology-driven. Technologies are recognized as having potential both to support writing and the teaching of writing.

Technology-supported writing can advance all phases of writing — planning, transcribing, and editing and revising using tools, which include, but are not limited to, the word processor. But technology also enables writing in new ways. Technology provides new sources for and means of obtaining information (e.g., the Internet, web search engines) and enables sharing, editing, and collaboration among writers, teachers, and peers. The ability to work from remote locations permits students to gauge the quality of their writing and their level of skill against those of peers elsewhere. Finally, technology transforms writing by introducing new electronic genres and multimedia forms. In these new genres and forms, composing involves a combination of media, including print, still images, video, and sound. Digital writing is defined as "compositions created with, and oftentimes for reading or viewing on a computer or other device that is connected to the Internet." The tools used for composing are not limited to the word processor. They include many digital forms of encoding (recording) information including scanners, digital cameras, voice recorders. Networked connectivity permits writers to "draw from myriad sources, use a range of media, craft various types of communication representing a range of tools and genres, and distribute that work almost instantaneously and sometimes globally."

But, where are schools and students with disabilities in all of this? The assessment of writing in statewide high stakes testing may be both a driver and an inhibitor of writing instruction and assessments in schools. While proponents of the new forms of digital writing decry the old 'scripted genres' as being limiting to students development of 21st century writing skills, assessments such as the National Assessment of Educational Progress (NAEP) use traditional genres or purposes for writing that have defined structures and requirements for the compositions.

In addition, the use of the word processor as a tool to assess writing is not even standard among states. While empirical research suggests that digital natives perform better when using word processors, surveys indicate that non-use of word processing on statewide assessments may be influencing teachers to avoid their use and emphasize paper and pencil writing to prepare students for testing. While the new tools, media, and forms may be the now-and-future, the old media and forms continue to be the now-and-now. For students with disabilities to make advances in writing performance on measures like the NAEP, there needs to be a critical examination of the tools and technologies that may provide compensatory benefit, i.e., that assist these students to overcome barriers created by a range of persistent cognitive and physical factors.

Section 36.3

Multisensory Teaching Techniques

This section includes text excerpted from "Methods for Sight Word Recognition in Kindergarten: Traditional Flashcard Method vs. Multisensory Approach," Education Resources Information Center (ERIC), U.S. Department of Education (ED), October 2012. Reviewed June 2016.

Learning to read is a complex and often a difficult task for children and adults alike. The reading process consists of learning to decode words and learning to read words by sight. Decoding is the process of knowing and realizing that written letters have relationships to sounds. Decoding is learned through phonics instruction, where students are taught letters and their connection to letter sounds. Adults and children then are able to decode, break the words apart by sound and then blend the sounds together to read the word quickly.

Learning to read by sight is learning to recognize words and read them quickly without decoding. Retrieving and reading words quickly with meaning enables a person to read fluently. Although there is not a true definition of what fluency is, The *Eunice Kennedy Shriver* National Institute of Child Health and Human Development (NICHD) states that fluency is the ability to read quickly, accurately, and with expression. Johnston asserts that students, who can retrieve words effortlessly by sight, will be able to read text easily, with more meaning and are capable of learning many more new words. This is imperative due to the fact that a large portion of words including many of the

Dolch sight words cannot be sounded out using the rules taught within phonics instruction.

Thus, Dolch sight word training takes place in many ways using many different methods each day in schools across America. Learning Dolch sight words is a difficult process. Students struggle with committing Dolch sight words to memory, and teachers struggle with implementing best practices and strategies that will effectively impact student achievement.

A quasi-experimental action research with a pretest-posttest same subject design was implemented to determine if there is a different effect of the flash card method and the multisensory approach on kindergarteners' achievement in sight word recognition, and which method is more effective if there is any difference.

Comparative Traditional Flashcard Methods

During three baseline sessions during phase one of the study, participants read new words on flashcards for a one-minute period, while errors and words read correct were scored. There was no practice of sight words during this time. This lasted for three days. The second phase of baseline sessions lasted for two days. During this time, on day one, participants' read the flashcards from their first baseline. On day two, participants read new sight words on flashcards. These words would appear on the participants' racetracks. During the racetrack intervention phase, participants completed the racetrack for one-minute timing. There was also error drill for those words missed, which consisted of the researcher pointing to missed words and asking what word? After all words were read, all missed words were revisited and repeated until firm.

The second racetrack followed the same procedures with the exception of new words were used. When referencing a race track, this study literally used a racetrack drawn on paper with sight words placed around the track. As words were said, participants proceeded around the track. This study concluded that reading racetracks coupled with flashcards lead to gains in sight word acquisition. This could be due to intrinsic nature of the racetrack method that visually shows participants completing the "race." In addition, the speed and drill technique of traditional flashcards seem to encourage fast responses. With a small, non-representative sample in the study (three male, third-grade participants with learning disabilities), it is difficult to draw a generalized conclusion.

A replication study using racetracks was conducted by Kaufman, McLaughlin, Derby, and Waco with three special education students in a resource room. Participant one was a seven-year-old male with

ADHD and specific learning disabilities receiving services in reading and writing. Participant two was a nine-year-old male with specific learning disabilities receiving services in reading, writing, math, and social skills. The third participant was an eight-year-old male with specific learning disabilities receiving services in reading writing, and math. All three participants were in a resource room for forty-five minutes a day. Research was conducted in the resource room of an elementary school in the Pacific Northwest.

Picture Supported Methods

In other examinations of how to best teach sight words, Meaden, Stoner, and Parette investigated teaching sight words with picture supported techniques verses word only methods in a Midwestern city. The participants were age four and five years old from seven different preschool classrooms for children at-risk. The participants were randomly assigned to a control group or an intervention group. Both groups were given the same ten pre-primer Dolch words and ten primer Dolch words to learn over a four-week period. Both groups (picture supported and word only) played games such as Bingo and Shake, Drop, and Roll. The only difference was the picture supported group used the pictures for the Dolch sight words.

The outcome of the research was that the control group (written words only) learned faster (showed progress quicker). But in the end assessment, the intervention group (picture supported) read more Dolch sight words correctly. The intervention group showed their growth in the later part of the research than in the beginning as the control group did. Explanations for the control group learning words quicker but not reading correctly, demonstrates that the flashcard alone process increases speed, whereas picture supported read more correctly showing that participants used the picture (mentally) to retrieve and say the word. It is concluded from the study that flashcards can increase speed, but flashcards together with pictures can increase accuracy and speed.

Technology-Based Methods

Lewandowski, Begeny, and Rogers focused on the word recognition training with computers and tutors. The study was completed in urban central New York within an elementary school. Participants were sixty-three third graders after attrition. There were thirty-seven females and twenty-nine males, of which nineteen were Caucasian, twenty-eight African American, six Asian, four Hispanic, and nine mixed. There were fourteen students eligible for special education and fifty-nine participants were receiving free and reduced lunches. Students were randomly placed into three equal distributed groups after a pretest. The three groups were involved in one of three treatment groups receiving computer, tutor, or no treatment. Pretesting consisted of reading a training list of words, generalization list of words, and reading ten passages for one minute each. Participants were scored for words read per-minute and accuracy.

In the computer condition, the process was modeled by the experimenter. Participants focused on a textbox to see the word and hear the word. Student repeated the word silently. Participants focused on the word for five seconds. In the tutor condition, the experimenter read words to participants. Participants saw the words, heard each word, and repeated the word silently. In the control condition, the experimenter only pointed to words as participants read words, and no verbal help was given by the experimenter. Each session consisted of two practice exposures. The third session was a timed oral reading by the participants. Training lasted for three weeks. Training sessions with participants lasted for ten minutes with each participant. Posttest conditions and procedures were the same as pretest. The results indicated that the control group did not make improvements, and that the computer and tutor approaches did make significant gains. The tutor results were higher than the computer based approach; however, the two groups did not make significant gains when comparing computer and tutor results.

The results of this study show that participants had an increase in sight word recognition because of the direct instruction with error free modeling of a human tutor. Also, the human tutor was able to maintain the participants' attention while interacting with the participants. In addition, the computer offered error free sight and sound associations and the novelty of a computer to keep participants' attention. The researchers assert that computers can produce outcomes as equal if not greater than human tutors. Computer based methods can be implemented at very low cost and used as independent activities, while working with others. Nonetheless, computers integrated with human exposure were not a disadvantage to participants in acquiring sight words.

Multisensory and Explicit, Direct, and Systematic Methods

Sheehy extended her own work of morphing words and word alone strategies to include another method called The Handle technique.

This method was developed by Sheehy and Howe. The technique of teaching words involves a mnemonic approach where the understanding of a word is encoded as a non-picture cue. During the intervention, the word that a Handle is being attached to is discussed. From the participants' discussions about their personal associations and understanding of the word, a personal attribute that is the most personal and salience is attached to the word as The Handle.

Participants for Sheehy's study consisted of six students ranging from eleven and thirteen years old with severe disabilities. These students lacked a sight vocabulary. There were twelve words taught. These words were separated into three sets of four words for each condition. The conditions were: The Handle technique, the morphing method, and a word alone method. In the word only condition, participants were modeled words while being shown the word. The participants gave a contextual meaning of the words to assist in morphing words in context. The words were presented again. If the words were not read correctly, they were modeled for the participant. In the morphed words, the words were presented on a computer screen and were morphed. If the word was not named, the word was modeled and prompted to read the word again.

The Handle technique consisted of attaching a Handle that consisted of some sort of visual mnemonic cue, which in return prompts the participants to read the words. The Handle was explained during the initial stage of modeling and the explanation was written on the back of the card, and the word alone was on the front of the card. During the intervention, The Handle cuing technique was used. The word was shown alone. The participant was asked, "What is this word?" Then The Handle was shown and then the word. Results from this study revealed that words were learned through all instructional methods. However, more words were recognized with the morphing method and The Handle technique. The Handle technique and morphing procedures were found to be more effective than word alone due to the symbol accentuation and mnemonic power of visual representation of sight words. It appears that anytime the abstract is taken to concrete visual representation that participants' achievement, understanding, and learning (recall and recognition) of the sight words is increased.

The conclusions were that the generalization of the study did not show significant gains as intended. It was pointed out that this was because the interventions did not effectively promote generalization. Furthermore, the conclusion of this study did show that there were greater gains when the common stimulus was implemented. This could be related to the fact that beginning readers need stimulus to facilitate and show similarities of words to increase their ability to read words accurately. Thus, participants were visually stimulated by the color of the word's rimes showing and relating the similarity and relationships of word families. This study provides evidence that a common stimulus, color, was a factor in participants' achievement of learning to read words.

Ehri and Wilce did an analysis on the force of mnemonic power of spellings in learning non-words with first and second graders. This study was completed to see if participants' memory of non-words would be improved by seeing the spellings of the non-words and not seeing the spelling of non-words. The participants were taught a set of non-words with a number listed above the non-word. This number was then used later to evoke a response for words. For example, the number 1 would represent fav. The number would be shown and the participant would then remember the non-word associated with the number 1. Participants had study times, where words were practiced being said. In one treatment group, participants saw the words' correct spellings but no attention was given to the spellings. The other treatment group did not see the words spelled correctly.

The results were that the participants that had exposure to words spelled correctly learned the non-words faster than the group that did not see correct spellings. Conclusions were that seeing correct spellings improved the participants' memory of and for sounds and for recalling non-words. This caused students to maintain visual symbols of the sounds in memory, while seeing misspellings of non-words caused participants great difficulty in learning and recalling the non-words from memory. Therefore, the results show and establish the mnemonic power of spelling.

Other studies have been completed that actually incorporate multi-sensory teaching of phonemic awareness, alphabet activities, oral language, reading and spelling practice, reading comprehension, and vocabulary development based on the sound structure of the English language. One such study by Joshi, Dahlgren, and Boulware-Gooden was implemented with first grade students to see if their reading achievement was improved due to the implementation of a multisensory approach. The participants came from a district of approximately forty thousand students. The participants were four first grade classrooms in an inner-city school district in a southwestern city. Two of the classrooms were taught using Language Basics: Elementary, which incorporates the Orton-Gillingham Method and based Alphabetic Phonics Methods.

This is a multisensory approach that focuses on systematic and explicit instruction using auditory, visual, and kinesthetic interactions. The other two classrooms were at a different school within district and were taught using a basal reading program as prescribed. The results of the study showed statistical significance that the multisensory approach was more effective over the traditional reading basal instruction as prescribed. The conclusions for this result demonstrate that one basal reading program could not possibly meet the needs of the participants. Multisensory education involves auditory, visual, and kinesthetic interactions with direct explicit instruction in the reading content. When learning meets the diverse and multiple learning styles of participants, there is bound to be success as this study demonstrates.

Conclusion

The results of data analysis demonstrate that participants learned significantly more Dolch sight words in the multisensory approach than in the flashcard method. The multisensory approach was more effective than the traditional flash card method. In addition, participants enjoyed learning the Dolch sight words through direct, systematic, and explicit instruction with multisensory interactions more than with the flashcard method.

Another study also validates the results from the multisensory approach. Frey discovered that participants had poorly developed reading and writing skills when participants were not allowed to be involved in kinesthetic-tactile and physical movements in the classroom and engaged in conversations (auditory) sharing and demonstrating (visual) ideas coupled with direct instruction in systematic and explicit ways. Frey concludes that within their study that participants were sitting in desks for long periods of time without enough interaction with peers or teachers.

Section 36.4

Speech-Language Therapy

In a recent parent-teacher conference, maybe the teacher expressed concern that your child could have a problem with certain speech or language skills. Or perhaps while talking to your child, you noticed an occasional stutter.

Could your child have a problem? And if so, what should you do?

It's wise to intervene quickly. An evaluation by a certified speech-language pathologist can help find out if your child is having problems. Speech-language therapy is the treatment for most kids with speech and/or language disorders.

Speech Disorders, Language Disorders, and Feeding Disorders

A speech disorder refers to a problem with the actual production of sounds. A language disorder refers to a problem understanding or putting words together to communicate ideas.

Speech disorders include:

- **Articulation disorders**: difficulties producing sounds in syllables or saying words incorrectly to the point that listeners can't understand what's being said.

- **Fluency disorders:** problems such as stuttering, in which the flow of speech is interrupted by abnormal stoppages, partial-word repetitions ("b-b-boy"), or prolonging sounds and syllables (sssssnake).

- **Resonance or voice disorders:** problems with the pitch, volume, or quality of the voice that distract listeners from what's being said. These types of disorders may also cause pain or discomfort for a child when speaking.

Language disorders can be either receptive or expressive:

- **Receptive disorders:** difficulties understanding or processing language.

- **Expressive disorders:** difficulty putting words together, limited vocabulary, or inability to use language in a socially appropriate way.

- **Cognitive-communication disorders:** difficulty with communication skills that involve memory, attention, perception, organization, regulation, and problem solving.

Dysphagia/oral feeding disorders are disorders in the way someone eats or drinks, including problems with chewing, swallowing, coughing, gagging, and refusing foods.

Specialists in Speech-Language Therapy

Speech-language pathologists (SLPs), often informally known as speech therapists, are professionals educated in the study of human communication, its development, and its disorders. They hold at least a master's degree and state certification/licensure in the field, and a certificate of clinical competency from the American Speech-Language-Hearing Association (ASHA).

SLPs assess speech, language, cognitive-communication, and oral/feeding/swallowing skills to identify types of communication problems (articulation; fluency; voice; receptive and expressive language disorders, etc.) and the best way to treat them.

Remediation

In speech-language therapy, an SLP will work with a child one-on-one, in a small group, or directly in a classroom to overcome difficulties involved with a specific disorder.

Therapists use a variety of strategies, including:

- **Language intervention activities:** The SLP will interact with a child by playing and talking, using pictures, books, objects, or ongoing events to stimulate language development. The therapist may also model correct vocabulary and grammar and use repetition exercises to build language skills.

- **Articulation therapy:** Articulation, or sound production, exercises involve having the therapist model correct sounds and syllables in words and sentences for a child, often during play activities. The level of play is age-appropriate and related to the child's specific needs. The SLP will physically show the child how to make certain sounds, such as the "r" sound, and may demonstrate how to move the tongue to produce specific sounds.

- **Oral-motor/feeding and swallowing therapy:** The SLP may use a variety of oral exercises—including facial massage and various tongue, lip, and jaw exercises—to strengthen the muscles of the mouth for eating, drinking, and swallowing. The SLP may also introduce different food textures and temperatures to increase a child's oral awareness during eating and swallowing.

When Is Therapy Needed?

Kids might need speech-language therapy for a variety of reasons, including, but not limited to:

- hearing impairments
- cognitive (intellectual, thinking) or other developmental delays
- weak oral muscles
- chronic hoarseness
- birth defects such as cleft lip or cleft palate
- autism
- motor planning problems
- articulation problems
- fluency disorders
- respiratory problems (breathing disorders)
- feeding and swallowing disorders
- traumatic brain injury

Therapy should begin as soon as possible. Children enrolled in therapy early (before they're 5 years old) tend to have better outcomes than those who begin therapy later.

This does not mean that older kids can't make progress in therapy; they may progress at a slower rate because they often have learned patterns that need to be changed.

Finding a Therapist

It's important to make sure that the speech-language therapist is certified by ASHA. That certification means the SLP has at least a master's degree in the field and has passed a national examination and successfully completed an ASHA-accredited supervised clinical fellowship.

Sometimes, speech assistants (who usually have a 2-year associate's or 4-year bachelor's degree) may assist with speech-language services under the supervision of ASHA-certified SLPs. Your child's SLP should be licensed in your state and have experience working with kids and your child's specific disorder.

You might find a specialist by asking your child's doctor or teacher for a referral or by checking local directories online or in your telephone book. State associations for speech-language pathology and audiology also maintain listings of licensed and certified therapists.

Helping Your Child

Speech-language experts agree that parental involvement is crucial to the success of a child's progress in speech or language therapy.

Parents are an extremely important part of their child's therapy program and help determine whether it is a success. Kids who complete the program quickest and with the longest-lasting results are those whose parents have been involved.

Ask the therapist for suggestions on how you can help your child. For instance, it's important to help your child do the at-home stimulation activities that the SLP suggests to ensure continued progress and carry-over of newly learned skills.

The process of overcoming a speech or language disorder can take some time and effort, so it's important that all family members be patient and understanding with the child.

Chapter 37

Coping with School-Related Challenges

Chapter Contents

Section 37.1

Building a Good Relationship with Your Child's Teacher

This section contains text excerpted from the following sources:
Text under the heading "Tips for Developing a Strong Relationship
with Your Child's Teacher" is excerpted from "Tips for Developing a
Strong Relationship with Your Child's Teacher," U.S. Department of
Education (ED), 2015; Text under the heading "A Teacher's
Role in Children's Education" is excerpted from "Preparing
Special Education Teachers to Collaborate with Families,"
Education Resources Information Center (ERIC), U.S.
Department of Education (ED), 2015.

Tips for Developing a Strong Relationship with Your Child's Teacher

The start of the school year is the perfect time to build a positive relationship with your child's teacher.

It's a good idea to let your child's educator know you want to partner with him or her, and share the responsibility for your child's academic growth.

Here are some tips to bear in mind:

- Keep in touch! Make sure your child's teacher has multiple ways and times of day to contact you. Provide as many ways as possible—which might include a work, cell, and home phone number and email address if possible.

- Mark your calendar! Ask your child's teacher about the best ways and times to contact him or her. Keep in mind that most teachers are in the classroom all day, so after school may be the best time to call or to make an appointment to meet with him or her.

- Reach out! Let the teacher know that you as a parent are there to help. Volunteer to assist with school trips or functions at school that might require additional adult supervision.

- Stay informed! Within the first few weeks after school starts, find out from the teacher if you child needs any assistance in one or more subject areas. Find out what resources are available at the school and what resources the teacher would recommend to help your child keep improving.

- Team up! Remember, you and the teacher have the exact same goals. You're both working to ensure the academic development and progress of your child. So, sit down together and figure out what you can do at home to reinforce what your child's teacher is doing in the classroom. That way, your child can keep learning long after the school day ends!

A Teacher's Role in Children's Education

Teachers play a significant role in parents' decisions to become involved in their children's education. Research has shown that teachers who reach out to parents and encourage participation are more likely to motivate parents to become involved in their children's education. Teachers who encourage parent involvement and establish positive relationships with parents of children with disabilities are in a better position to provide the support needed for these parents to constructively engage in their children's education. Teacher preparation programs that have provided opportunities for teacher candidates to engage in meaningful interactions with parents of children with disabilities, while rare, have been shown to result in positive outcomes.

Given the significance of the connection between parent involvement and successful student outcomes, it is important that school employees, especially teachers, develop skills in establishing positive relationships. Cultivating supportive relationships is central to forging parent–teacher collaboration. Despite the recognition of its importance, collaboration between teachers and parents continues to be difficult to achieve. Due to the frequent complexity that parents face in raising a child with a disability, teachers may find it particularly difficult to know how to best initiate positive collaboration with these parents.

Teacher preparation programs are in a primary position to promote professional learning opportunities that prepare teacher candidates to learn how to partner with parents. All too often, graduating teacher candidates lack the skills, attitudes, knowledge, and confidence necessary for building collaborative relationships with parents. Although many teacher preparation programs acknowledge the importance of parent involvement, frequently the preparation and training that teacher candidates receive in these programs falls short of what is needed to actually foster collaboration and partnership with parents.

Federal mandates have recognized the importance of parental involvement as a strategy to improve the education of children. The No Child Left Behind (NCLB) initiative calls for the increase of parental involvement. The Individuals with Disabilities Education Act (IDEA) mandates parent participation in the education of their children with disabilities. The importance of parents as key participants in educational decisions for their children has been reinforced by the emphasis that IDEA places on collaboration between parents and teachers. Cook and Friend define collaboration as "the style professionals select to employ based on mutual goals; shared responsibility for key decisions; shared accountability for outcomes; shared resources; and the development of trust, respect, and a sense of community."

Emphasis has traditionally been placed on parent and teacher collaboration and partnership. However, increasing attention is given to communities for their role in the social, emotional, and academic achievements of students. Epstein's theory of overlapping spheres of influence reinforces the shared responsibility that schools, families, and communities have in socializing youth and ensuring students' success. School–community partnerships can be defined as connections linking schools, families, and communities in the mutual goal of promoting students' social, emotional, and academic development.

Collaboration and communication between parents and educators have been shown to be critical factors for predicting successful student outcomes. Research suggests that teachers' efforts to collaborate with parents promote parent involvement, which in turn contributes to student success. Crisman found that listening to parents and actively seeking their input makes all the difference for developing positive relationships with parents. Tolan and Woo outlined several principles for promoting educational practices that encourage school–family partnerships, including the principle that partnerships with families demand engagement across home and school, shared responsibility and decision making, and two-way communication.

Parents of children with disabilities face unique challenges. Dunst and Dempsey point out that "the role of parents with a child with a disability shows a level of complexity and intensity not generally found in the general population." Some parents who feel helpless when trying to adequately plan for their children's education can also feel hopeless and overwhelmed. For parents, learning how to provide the education and supports that their children need is an ongoing and frequently frustrating process. Given the multifaceted role that parents face, learning how to support, encourage, and empower parents of children with disabilities is a complex task for teacher candidates. Forming partnerships between educators and these parents continues to be difficult to achieve and successfully sustain.

Section 37.2

Parental Involvement in Child's Success in School and Life

This section includes text excerpted from "Intellectual Disabilities," Early Childhood Learning and Knowledge Center (ECLKC), U.S. Department of Health and Human Services (HHS), November 18, 2015.

What about School?

A child with an intellectual disability can do well in school but is likely to need individualized help. Fortunately, states are responsible for meeting the educational needs of children with disabilities.

For children up to age three, services are provided through an early intervention system. Staff work with the child's family to develop what is known as an Individualized Family Services Plan, or IFSP. The IFSP will describe the child's unique needs. It also describes the services the child will receive to address those needs. The IFSP will emphasize the unique needs of the family, so that parents and other family members will know how to help their young child with an intellectual disability. Early intervention services may be provided on a sliding-fee basis, meaning that the costs to the family will depend upon their income. In some states, early intervention services may be at no cost to parents.

For eligible school-aged children (including preschoolers), special education and related services are made available through the school system. School staff will work with the child's parents to develop an Individualized Education Program, or IEP. The IEP is similar to an IFSP. It describes the child's unique needs and the services that have been designed to meet those needs. Special education and related services are provided at no cost to parents.

Many children with an intellectual disability need help with adaptive skills, which are skills needed to live, work, and play in the community. Teachers and parents can help a child work on these skills at both school and home. Some of these skills include:

- communicating with others;
- taking care of personal needs (dressing, bathing, going to the bathroom);
- health and safety;
- home living (helping to set the table, cleaning the house, or cooking dinner);
- social skills (manners, knowing the rules of conversation, getting along in a group, playing a game);
- reading, writing, and basic math; and
- as they get older, skills that will help them in the workplace.

Supports or changes in the classroom (called adaptations) help most students with an intellectual disability. Some common changes that help students with an intellectual disability are listed below under "Tips for Teachers." The resources below also include ways to help children with an intellectual disability.

Tips for Parents

- Learn about intellectual disabilities. The more you know, the more you can help yourself and your child. See the list of resources and organizations at the end of this publication.

- Encourage independence in your child. For example, help your child learn daily care skills, such as dressing, feeding him or herself, using the bathroom, and grooming.

- Give your child chores. Keep her age, attention span, and abilities in mind. Break down jobs into smaller steps. For example, if your child's job is to set the table, first ask her to get the right number of napkins. Then have her put one at each family member's place at the table. Do the same with the utensils, going one at a time. Tell her what to do, step by step, until the job is done. Demonstrate how to do the job. Help her when she needs assistance. Give your child frequent feedback. Praise your child when he or she does well. Build your child's abilities.

- Find out what skills your child is learning at school. Find ways for your child to apply those skills at home. For example, if the teacher is going over a lesson about money, take your child to the supermarket with you. Help him count out the money to pay for your groceries. Help him count the change.

- Find opportunities in your community for social activities, such as scouts, recreation center activities, sports, and so on. These will help your child build social skills as well as to have fun.

- Talk to other parents whose children have an intellectual disability. Parents can share practical advice and emotional support. Call NICHCY (1-800-695-0285) and ask how to find a parent group near you.

- Meet with the school and develop an educational plan to address your child's needs. Keep in touch with your child's teachers. Offer support. Find out how you can support your child's school learning at home.

Tips for Teachers

- Learn as much as you can about intellectual disabilities. The organizations listed at the end of this publication will help you identify specific techniques and strategies to support the student educationally. We've also listed some strategies below.

- Recognize that you can make an enormous difference in this student's life! Find out what the student's strengths and interests are, and emphasize them. Create opportunities for success.

- If you are not part of the student's Individualized Education Program (IEP) team, ask for a copy of his or her IEP. The student's educational goals will be listed there, as well as the services and classroom accommodations he or she is to receive. Talk to specialists in your school (e.g., special educators), as necessary. They can help you identify effective methods of teaching this student, ways to adapt the curriculum, and how to address the student's IEP goals in your classroom.

- Be as concrete as possible. Demonstrate what you mean rather than just giving verbal directions. Rather than just relating new information verbally, show a picture. And rather than just showing a picture, provide the student with hands-on materials and experiences and the opportunity to try things out.

- Break longer, new tasks into small steps. Demonstrate the steps. Have the student do the steps, one at a time. Provide assistance, as necessary.

- Give the student immediate feedback.

- Teach the student life skills such as daily living, social skills, and occupational awareness and exploration, as appropriate. Involve the student in group activities or clubs.

- Work together with the student's parents and other school personnel to create and implement an educational plan tailored to meet the student's needs. Regularly share information about how the student is doing at school and at home.

Chapter 38

Alternative Educational Options

Chapter Contents

Section 38.1

Homeschooling

This section includes text excerpted from "Beyond the Brick Walls:
Homeschooling Students with Special Needs," Education
Resources Information Center (ERIC), U.S. Department
of Education (ED), March 2013.

Over the past 15 years, data from the National Center for Education Statistics (NCES) have shown an increasing trend in the numbers of children being educated within the home, including students with disabilities. During the period from 1999 to 2007, the percentage of students with disabilities who were homeschooled increased from 1.8 to 2.6% (National Center for Education Statistics). The 2007 National Household Education Surveys Program found that approximately 21% of homeschooling parents reported "other special needs" and 11% reported "physical or mental health problems" as important reasons for homeschooling (National Center for Education Statistics). According to these surveys, homeschooling has increasingly become an educational option for parents with exceptional children.

As more parents of children with disabilities consider homeschooling, this article provides information related to that decision-making process. First, an overview of homeschooling is provided, including a brief history of homeschools in the United States and a summary of laws related to homeschools and special education. Next, relevant issues for parents considering homeschooling are discussed, including characteristics of homeschool students and families, reasons that families have chosen to homeschool their children with disabilities, the benefits and challenges encountered, and the role of the public schools. Then, the current state of research on homeschools students with disabilities is explored. Finally, suggestions are made for future researchers, as well as for parents and public school educators, to consider when planning for the educational needs of children with disabilities at home.

Over the past 15 years, data from the National Center for Education Statistics have shown an increasing trend in the numbers of children being educated within the home, including students with disabilities. During the period from 1999 to 2007, the percentage of students with disabilities who were homeschooled increased from 1.8 to 2.6% (National Center for Education Statistics). The 2007 National Household Education Surveys Program found that approximately 21% of homeschooling parents reported "other special needs" and 11% reported "physical or mental health problems" as important reasons for homeschooling (National Center for Education Statistics). According to these surveys, homeschooling has increasingly become an educational option for parents with exceptional children.

As more parents of children with disabilities consider homeschooling, this article provides information related to that decision-making process. First, an overview of homeschooling is provided, including a brief history of homeschools in the United States and a summary of laws related to homeschools and special education. Next, relevant issues for parents considering homeschooling are discussed, including characteristics of homeschool students and families, reasons that families have chosen to homeschool their children with disabilities, the benefits and challenges encountered, and the role of the public schools. Then, the current state of research on homeschools students with disabilities is explored. Finally, suggestions are made for future researchers, as well as for parents and public school educators, to consider when planning for the educational needs of children with disabilities at home.

Homeschooling in the United States

Throughout history, children have been educated at home. However, the industrial revolution of the late 1800s and early 1900s resulted in compulsory U.S. public school attendance legislation, and thus, homeschooling was no longer considered an option for most U.S. families for more than a half-century. Homeschool, however, made a resurgence in the 1960s. The rise in homeschools during that time was influenced by many different social and political influences including the passage of desegregation laws; removal of prayer from schools; and John Holt's book, *How Children Fail*, which blamed public schools for failing to educate. The number of children being homeschooled steadily increased from the 1960s onward, and by 1993, homeschooling was legal in all 50 states. Today's compulsory attendance laws stipulate attendance in public or non-public schools—including homeschools— and all K-12 programs must be approved by the state. In 2007, the National Household Education Surveys Program estimated that 1.5 million U.S. children, or almost 3% of school-aged children, received homeschooling.

Laws and Regulations

The U.S. Congress first passed legislation to provide funding for the education of students with disabilities in the 1970s. This legislation has been reauthorized several times over the years and is currently known as the Individuals with Disabilities Education Act (IDEA). Although making a distinction between public and private schools in the disbursement of funds, IDEA did not define what constituted a private school nor did it specifically address funding for students in homeschools. Therefore, decisions on whether to provide funding for special education services to students in homeschools were left to individual states, and many states considered IDEA rights to be forfeited for homeschool students.

The U.S. Supreme Court has supported the power of the individual states to make decisions about support of children with disabilities in homeschools. For example, in *Hooks v. Clark County School District*, the U.S. Supreme Court upheld a Nevada school system's denial of speech therapy services for a homeschool child. The Supreme Court ruled that individual states have the power to treat a homeschool as either a private school or as a non-school; if categorized as a non-school, a student in a homeschool is not eligible for IDEA services. However, some states such as Arizona, Iowa, North Dakota, and Pennsylvania have homeschool laws that include provisions for students with disabilities. The state of Washington allows funding for special services for homeschool students who also attend public schools part time; other states or local education agencies provide special services for homeschool students on a case-by-case basis.

Several authors argued that IDEA should be amended to define homeschools as private schools so that services will be available for homeschool students with disabilities. It is notable that the U.S. Office of Special Education Programs has interpreted IDEA's Child Find provisions to be inclusive of children who are being homeschooled, even though services may not be available to eligible children who remain homeschooled. In states that do allow IDEA funds to be used for homeschool students, two additional factors are typically in play:

1. in order to receive services, the parents must also agree to submit to evaluations for their children and work with a team to develop educational plans, thereby giving up some control of their children's educational management

2. IDEA funding for all eligible students in non-public schools is not guaranteed

Whether or not a homeschool student has a disability, the homeschool must comply with its state's compulsory attendance laws. Homeschool regulations vary from state-to-state, but most states stipulate that homeschools document some or all of the following:

1. specific qualifications of the home educator

2. curriculum choices

3. required number of hours per day and days per year of instructional time

4. standardized testing

5. reports to local school systems

The burden for compliance with state homeschool laws and regulations rests on the parents. In sum, parents need to know the local homeschool regulations and the accessibility of special education services for homeschools; a good place to start searching for information is the local school board.

Homeschool Considerations

Student and Family Characteristics

The research literature on homeschooling has shown that students with many different types of disabilities and with varying levels of need have participated in homeschools. Jane Duffey *(Preventing School Failure)* conducted a national survey of parents who homeschooled their children with disabilities. The top diagnoses of homeschool children reported from 121 surveys were attention deficit hyperactivity disorder (ADHD), learning disabilities (LD), autism spectrum disorder (ASD), and speech-language impairment. However, studies have also chronicled homeschool children with epilepsy, visual impairments, intellectual disabilities, hearing impairments and deafness, and physical disabilities.

In addition, Obeng *(International Journal of Special Education)* reported qualitative interviews with two parents of pre-adolescents with severe multiple health problems. Furthermore, a study by Jane Duffey indicated that parents of students with disabilities tended to take a longer time deciding to remove their children from public school than other homeschool parents. However, once removed, the homeschool students with disabilities were also more likely to receive part time services from public schools than other homeschool students. Another attribute of some homeschool families was that only their children with disabilities were homeschooled, while the siblings continued to attend public school.

Homeschool children with disabilities come from families that are similar to all homeschool families. In a national survey of families who homeschooled children with disabilities, most families were described as white, two-parent (working father and stay-at-home mother), suburban, and with 3.5 children with 1.5 identified as having special needs. In addition, most homeschool students with disabilities received the majority of instruction from their mothers, even though fathers or other instructors have been reported. Jane Duffey also found that 12% of mothers were certified teachers, 30% of which had some training in special education. Parents reported a wide range of educational levels, from high school through master's degrees.

A very small number of homeschool parents reported having a physical or mental disability themselves. Collectively, these studies provided a picture of homeschoolers with disabilities and their families; nevertheless, there are many homeschool students and families that will not fall under these broad descriptors.

Reasons for Homeschooling

Two main philosophical perspectives for homeschooling have traditionally been described as *ideological* and *pedagogical* (Higgins, 2008). Initially categorized by Van Galen in 1988, Higgins attempted to verify whether homeschool parents could be divided into Van Galen's two discrete groups: ideologues, homeschooling because of religious reasons; or pedagogues, homeschooling to provide different methods of instruction than the schools. Higgins concluded that the philosophical position for most homeschool families indicated an overlap between the two constructs—more often, both principles played a part in the decision to homeschool. The results of studies of homeschool students with disabilities aligned with Higgins' findings: many parents expressed a desire to teach their children from religious perspectives, but more often, the main decision to homeschool was related to a desire to provide better instruction or individualization for their children.

Parents with deep philosophical differences with public education may choose to homeschool regardless of the services their children with disabilities could be offered in public school. However, other reasons for homeschooling, frequently rooted in pedagogy, include the perception that the public school has failed to meet a child's needs. That is, the main motivation for many parents to homeschool was that their children's special education needs simply were not being met. For example, a chief concern of parents of children with ASD was that schools were either unwilling or unable to provide therapies or treatments that parents considered effective. In addition, parents also attributed negative experiences with public schools as a deciding factor in choosing to homeschool.

Other reasons for homeschooling included escape from bullying and avoiding the stigma of a labeled disability. The salient point is that some parents, frustrated with their child's services, choose to homeschool and figure out how to deliver those services on their own. These findings suggest that, especially in school systems that do not have official policies and programs to support homeschool families, public schools could do a better job of outreach, connection, and communication with families to prevent much of the dissatisfaction that has led many parents to choose homeschooling over public schools.

Benefits and Challenges of Homeschooling

A majority of parents across several studies reported satisfaction with their children's progress in homeschools. Parents specified the benefits of freedom in selecting curriculum, pace of instruction, and daily routines that met their family's and individual children's needs. In this era of increased access to technology, many parents reported reliance on Internet sources for instructional support. In addition, educational consultants were often used at some point in the homeschool planning process, especially when the child had special needs. Some students were unschooled, meaning they had an unstructured schedule guided by the student's day-to-day learning interests.

However, Arora *(Journal of Research in Special Educational Need)* found that most of the interviewed families followed a structured daily routine for their children with disabilities. Furthermore, Higgins related that parents of children with disabilities were significantly more likely to use traditional teaching methods (i.e., parent directed) in homeschooling rather than more loosely structured instruction. Although there has been some indication that homeschool families shift from original values and attitudes over time, becoming more nontraditional the longer they homeschooled, it is unclear whether families whose children have special needs follow this progression. However, no matter the degree of structure or the method of instruction, parents reported enjoying much more control over their children's education when they homeschooled.

Although parents tended to give high ratings to the overall homeschool experience, many reported challenges with homeschooling students with disabilities. Some families described a lack of emotional, social, and moral support from outside sources. When support was found, it was more likely to be from other homeschool families and organized homeschool groups than from public schools. In interviews with two parents who homeschooled their children with severe multiple health problems, Obeng found that parents did not receive enough professional and social support, and as a result, the parents were feeling overwhelmed with sadness and frustration. While many other factors may influence the intensity of homeschooling challenges, certainly the severity of the child's needs and the amount of support available to the family are two major components that will affect the success of the homeschool program.

Although a commonly stated concern related to homeschooling was that students might have limited social interactions, most parents reported feeling satisfied with the socialization opportunities afforded their children from homeschool groups, sports, and religious services. However, very few researchers gathered information directly from the homeschool students with disabilities about their perspectives on socialization.

In one study that included interviews with homeschool adolescent females with LD, all three participants reported feeling uncomfortable in social situations. The first participant, an adolescent girl who also had a physical disability, reported struggling to make friends even though she had plenty of opportunities to socialize. The second adolescent reported not feeling a part of her peer group because of her learning deficits, and the third adolescent reported feelings of peer isolation because her family lived in a rural area. While it is possible that these teens would have felt the same awkwardness or isolation in a public school setting, socialization might remain an area of legitimate concern for many homeschool students and their parents.

Role of Public Schools

Unfortunately, there often seems to be disconnect between public schools and homeschools. For example, an interview of educators in Canadian schools indicated mostly negative opinions about students that had been removed from their schools for homeschooling. Administrators reported being aware that parents probably did not share their real reasons for choosing to homeschool, but also expressed frustration with parents for not working with the school to resolve problems. Conversely, parents reported not feeling genuinely welcomed to ask for support from schools, even though some administrators offered part time classes and the opportunity to re enroll students. In addition, teachers reported feeling personally offended when parents removed their children from school. Teachers' perceptions were that students tended to re enter public schools after a period of homeschooling with greater academic and social deficits. Overall, most of the educators reported negative views on homeschooling. Such negative attitudes about homeschooling seem to be pervasive across many educators and educational groups, including the National Education Association (NEA). An organization supporting public education, the National Education Association has issued resolutions over the past several years stating that homeschools with parents as instructors are inadequate educational programs.

As noted earlier, parents reported many reasons for choosing to educate children with disabilities at home, but frequently, unhappiness with the schools was a main motivation. In a personal account of her experiences homeschool her son with an ASD, Sofia *(English Journal)* described her frustrations with her son's fourth grade teachers. Sofia felt that the teachers expected all students to have normal behavior and placed inordinately high value on student compliance as a measure of success. Rather than providing differentiated instruction, teachers blamed her son's inappropriate behavior for his lack of progress. After removing her son from school, Sofia employed the services of a certified teacher for curriculum advice, based homeschool lessons on her son's areas of interest, and provided her son explicit instruction on social rules. Sofia reported that her son successfully reentered the public school system the following school year.

It is important to note that not all school systems fail to support of homeschool. One example of a school system providing homeschooling services is the Des Moines Public Schools Home Instruction Program. The Des Moines Public School System was one of the first in the United States to offer a cooperative homeschool partnership for homeschooling families. There are other homeschool partnerships in existence, and it seems that they may present a viable solution to support children with disabilities in homeschools. Funding special education services for homeschool students can offer support for families as well as special education services for students, and can potentially provide a seamless reentry for students who elect to return after a year or two of homeschooling. Even though parents of children with disabilities may have high expectations of the educational system, schools might prevent families from withdrawing due to dissatisfaction by developing a better understanding of student and family needs, and promoting stronger outreach.

Current State of Homeschooling Research

It is notable that there have not been any studies using true experimental research designs that examine the efficacy of homeschooling students with disabilities. However, two quasi-experimental exploratory studies supported the effectiveness of parents as instructors of their children with disabilities in a homeschool setting. The first exploratory study was conducted with children with learning disabilities (LD). Participating students were comprised of one middle school and three elementary level students who were paired with counterpart peers of similar ages, demographic descriptions, and abilities in public school. The duration of student engagement in academic tasks was collected over seven observations in both settings, and pretest-posttest standardized achievement tests were administered to both groups of students.

Duvall *(Education & Treatment of Children)* determined that homeschool students with LD were on task and engaged in work activities approximately two-and-a-half times more than their counterparts in a general education classroom. Pretest to posttest comparisons also indicated that homeschool students made more progress in reading and written language than their public school peers, and made equivalent progress in math. Duvall attributed the progress of the homeschool students to the higher rate of interaction with the parent-instructor and the greater degree of individualized attention provided in the homeschool setting.

Several years later, Duvall, Delquadri, and Ward replicated the earlier exploratory study with students with ADHD instead of LD. Two homeschool students with ADHD were paired with two similar students in the public school setting. Both groups of students were observed once a month for five months to collect academic engagement time data. Results indicated that the homeschool students with ADHD were academically engaged at higher rates than their counterparts, and their reading and math gains were greater or equal to their public school peers. Overall, Duvall posited that study results supported the effectiveness of untrained parents as homeschool instructors of their children with disabilities; however, the parents of children with ADHD reported doubts about their effectiveness as instructors.

Perspective of Parents who Homeschool Children with Disabilities

Many parents reported success homeschooling their children with disabilities, but others described the difficulties and the lack of support from the schools and the community. Some school systems provide part time services for students with disabilities, but many states do not support students that are in a homeschool setting. Parents need to be aware of the regulations and services available in their locales, and they need to explore the benefits and challenges of homeschooling before making the decision to homeschool a student with disabilities.

A common conclusion among studies was that a collaborative relationship between homeschools and school systems would be beneficial for students with disabilities. Other researchers concluded that public schools might prevent some loss of students to homeschools by increasing individualized instruction. Of special concern are families whose children have severe disabilities. Obeng concluded that parents who homeschool children with extensive medical needs would also benefit from psychotherapy and other supports to maintain their own health.

Kunzman and Gaither, in their review of homeschools, reported that the trend seems to be moving in favor of greater access to public schools, with 22 states reporting some accommodations for homeschoolers and only six states refusing to support homeschools. Offering part time special education services might facilitate connection with the homeschool community, and may result in the decreased exodus of students with disabilities due to parental dissatisfaction.

In conclusion, making the decision to homeschool a child with a disability requires thoughtful deliberation. Some of the many benefits of homeschooling are greater parent involvement, a strengthening of the family unit, opportunities for more natural learning experiences, increased self esteem in students with disabilities, increased individualization and student paced learning, and increased flexibility with family schedules. However, the challenges include making curriculum decisions, managing finances, accessing special education services, facilitating socialization opportunities, and finding connections with other parents for support.

In light of the increasing number of families choosing to homeschool, increased support in the form of special education services from the public schools would serve to improve the homeschooling experiences of many students with disabilities. In addition, if quality research begins to indicate that homeschooling can be done effectively, our legal and educational systems may become more willing to provide a continuum of special education support services. Furthermore, with improved relationships between public schools and families of children with disabilities, parents will choose to homeschool for the right reasons—not as an escape from the school system. The end result will be considered a win for both sides, and more importantly, for the children.

Section 38.2

Choosing a Tutor

Overview

A tutor is a teacher who offers private or small-group instruction to help students who have trouble keeping up in a regular school classroom. Tutors can teach specific skills that support learning or reinforce subjects that are taught in school. They can assist children who fall behind grade level due to motivational problems, psychiatric disorders, or learning disabilities. In many cases, tutoring leads to increased self-confidence and improved academic performance.

Signs a Tutor May Be Needed

Some of the common signs that may indicate a child would benefit from the services of a tutor include:

- receiving poor grades in school;
- struggling to master basic grade-level skills;
- falling behind in certain subjects;
- having problems with organization, time management, and study skills;
- experiencing severe test anxiety;
- exhibiting a pattern of disruptive behavior;
- showing a lack of motivation;
- making constant excuses for not doing homework;
- experiencing medical, social, emotional, or family problems; or
- having a learning disability that makes it challenging to master material and impedes progress in school.

Types of Tutors

There are several different types of tutors available to assist children with learning disabilities or attention disorders.

- Remediation tutoring is appropriate for children who need extra instruction and practice to master specific skills or subject areas, such as math or reading, in order to catch up to grade level.

- Maintenance tutoring is useful for children who work at grade level but need help with time management, organization, or study skills in order to manage their workload and meet their academic goals.

- Support tutoring includes elements of both remediation and maintenance tutoring, as needed, to help students who struggle in some areas but not others.

- Test preparation tutoring is available to teach students techniques for taking tests and help eliminate text anxiety.

- Enrichment tutoring offers activities designed to strengthen existing skills or enhance knowledge in areas of special interest.

Finding a Tutor

Tutoring is available from a wide variety of sources, including learning centers, educational therapists, private tutors, and online programs. To find a qualified tutor, parents can ask friends, acquaintances, or teachers for recommendations. The public library may also have information to help parents locate tutors and educational resources. Organizations that are dedicated to serving children with learning disabilities may also be able to provide assistance in finding a qualified tutor.

After compiling a list of possibilities, experts recommend interviewing several tutors in order to find one whose qualifications, approach, schedule, and fees provide the best fit with the family's needs. Ideally, the student should be involved in the interview process to ensure that they feel comfortable with the tutor and support the choice. Interviews with prospective tutors should cover the following main areas:

- **Experience**

Parents need to find out how much experience the tutor has in teaching the specific skills or subject areas of concern. Five or more years of experience is desirable. Parents should also ask whether the tutor has experience working with students at their child's grade level and with similar learning disabilities or attention issues.

- **Qualifications**

Parents should also inquire about prospective tutors' training and qualifications. Ideally, the tutor should be a certified teacher in the subject area being taught. If the child has learning disabilities, the tutor should be trained to use appropriate multisensory techniques to address the child's special needs. The tutor should also be willing to provide references to verify their qualifications.

- **Approach**

Parents should gather information about prospective tutors' teaching philosophy and approach. A tutor should be able to provide a clear explanation of how they will go about identifying the child's skill deficits and what strategies they plan to use in order to improve those skills.

- **Scheduling**

The next area for parents to address involves establishing a schedule for tutoring sessions. Since students with learning disabilities need practice and repetition to master skills, experts recommend scheduling a minimum of two lessons per week, with each lesson lasting one hour. It is important to schedule tutoring sessions for a time of day when the student is fresh, engaged, and ready to learn. Many tutoring programs take place immediately after school, but students tend to be tired and distracted at this time. It may take a while to see results, so parents should plan on continuing the tutoring sessions for three to four months. Finally, parents need to figure out logistical details like where the lessons will be held and how long each session will last.

- **Fees**

Tutoring can be very expensive, so parents need to ask how much each prospective tutor charges per lesson. It may also be helpful to inquire about additional fees for materials or assessments, and the tutor's policies regarding cancellations and make-up sessions. In some cases, tutoring programs may qualify as "supplemental educational services" under the federal No Child Left Behind Act. Students from low-income families who attend Title I schools that fail to meet state standards for at least three years may be eligible to receive free tutoring under this program.

- **Goals**

Parents should work closely with the tutor to establish clear goals for the tutoring sessions. The tutor should provide a written plan for accomplishing the goals. Ideally, the child's classroom teacher should participate in setting the goals so that they support school work. Experts suggest that parents avoid setting unrealistic goals or trying to accomplish too much. Instead, they should focus on specific skills or subject areas that need improvement and expect to see gradual progress rather than instant results.

- **Fit**

The personal relationship between the child and the tutor is an important factor in achieving results. Ideally, the tutor should establish a good rapport with the student, and tutoring sessions should include a mix of directed teaching, guided practice, and interactive, hands-on learning. Parents should observe some tutoring sessions to see how the relationship develops, and consider changing tutors if the child is not responding well after about eight lessons.

- **Communication**

Communication between parents and the tutor is vital in supporting the child's learning. Parents should request periodic updates from the tutor, as well as reports on academic progress from the child's teacher. Parents should also reinforce what the tutor is doing by scheduling time for the child to do homework, providing a quiet place to study, being available to help, checking homework daily, and placing a high value on education.

References

1. Shanley, Judy. "How to Choose a Tutor," LD Online, 2005.

2. Morin, Amanda. "How Different Types of Tutoring Can Help Kids with Learning and Attention Issues," Understood, 2014.

Chapter 39

Guide to Student Transition Planning

A Guide to Students for Transition

Transition planning is a process for students with disabilities that begins around middle school, and focuses on life after high school. Transition planning helps students with disabilities, as well as their parents and guardians, understand and the opportunities available to them after they graduate from high school, such as college, vocational rehabilitation, employment, and independent living. It also helps young people with disabilities develop life skills through hands-on experiences, so they can become successful, independent members of society.

What Is Transition Planning?

The National Collaborative on Workforce and Development (NCWD) for Youth defines transition planning as:

"...a coordinated set of activities for a student with a disability that:

1. Is designed within an outcome-oriented process, that promotes movement from school-to-post-school activities, including post-secondary education, vocational training, integrated employment (including supported employment), continuing

---

This chapter includes text excerpted from "Guide to Student Transition Planning," Disability.gov, April 8, 2014.

and adult education, adult services, independent living or community participation

2. Is based upon the individual student's needs, taking into account the student's preferences and interests

3. Includes instruction, related services, special education, community experiences, the development of employment and other post-school adult living objectives, and when appropriate, the acquisition of daily living skills and functional vocational evaluation."

The transition planning process should begin around middle school and continue throughout high school. The student, his or her parents or guardians, teachers, and school counselors should work together to develop a plan for life after high school. This plan should take into account the student's strengths, preferences and interests, as well as any accommodations needs and other key factors. The types of questions to think about are similar to what any student would need to address, with a few additional considerations:

• What types of things interest this student? Is he or she creative and thinking about going into the arts? Is there an interest in a particular field, such as journalism or mathematics?

• Is the student thinking about going to college? If so, which type of school would be a good fit (community college, in-state four-year university, out-of-state university, etc.)?

• Is the student thinking about training for a trade? If so, what schools or programs are available? Which would be a good fit for him/her?

• Which standardized tests does the student need to take to apply for colleges or technical/trade schools? Will the student need any accommodations while taking these tests?

• What types of accommodations would the student need in college or at technical/trade school?

• What are the student's financial needs? Does he or she want to apply for student aid? Which types of aid would be best (e.g., loans, grants, scholarships)? When are the applications due? What information needs to be provided?

• Which type of living situation is the student interested in (e.g., at home, college dorm, on his/her own) and what types of accommodations will the student need?

- Is the student interested in going directly into the workforce? What job training, internship or apprenticeship opportunities are available?

Where Can I Learn about Options for Life after High School?

After graduating from high school, there are a wide range of options for your future; choosing your path is a big decision. Some options include:

- Going to college

- Attending a trade or technical school

- Participating in a job training or internship program

- Volunteering

- Getting a job

The resources below can help young people with disabilities decide what option or options are right for them:

- The PACER Center's "College or Training Programs: How to Decide" offers ideas to consider before graduation to help youth with disabilities decide the right path for them. The Center's "Mapping Your Dreams" fact sheet provides additional information to help transition-age students figure out what they want to do after high school.

- The HEATH Resource Center's "Awareness of Post-secondary Options" provides an overview of the different choices available after high school so young people with disabilities can make an informed decision about their future. "What Do I Want To Be When I Grow up?" helps young people identify their interests, values, and preferences related to work and use that information to consider possible careers. The Center's "Opportunities in Career and Technical Education at the Post-Secondary Level" helps explain the career training options that are available for students, including high school and post-secondary certificates, two and four-year college degrees and technical and trade schools. The Center also offers a fact sheet on "Non-Degree Post-Secondary Options for Individuals with Disabilities" (there is also a follow up to the fact sheet).

- The National Youth Transitions Center offers information, programs and events to help young people with disabilities, including Veterans, make the transition from high school to higher education or the workforce. Programs include career counseling, school-to-work readiness training, work-based learning experiences, leadership training and family education and support. The Center also houses the Youth Transitions Collaborative and the National Veterans Center.

- TransCen Online Learning Tools are free online training courses students and parents can do at their own pace to learn more about options after high school.

- NCSET's "Person-Centered Planning: A Tool for Transition" has information about creating a transition planning process that focuses on the needs and interests of students with disabilities. It includes information on transition planning as part of IEPs and how young people can play a leading role in making decisions about their future.

- The Youthhood (www.youthhood.org) website helps young people plan for the future, figure out what they want to do after high school, and think about issues such as employment, housing and health care.

- Youth.gov has information for transition-age youth, including students with disabilities. Learn about youth employment, mental health and substance abuse issues and mentoring.

- The I'm Determined! (www.imdetermined.org) website offers information and resources for students, parents and teachers about the transition process and post-secondary options. It includes information about educational rights, employment, living independently and self-determination. It also has fact sheets, videos and a transition planning guide.

- The Learn How to Become (www.learnhowtobecome.org) website has information and resources on careers and education and training options so young adults can find the right career and determine a plan for success.

- The Autism Society's "Transition Planning for Students with Autism" guide has information to help students prepare for life after high school, including to search for a job and a place to live.

- Think College's Transition Checklist provides a list of topics that should be taken into consideration when discussing transition from high school to college for students with intellectual disabilities.

- The GetMyFuture (www.careeronestop.org/getmyfuture/index.aspx) website has information to help young people move from school to work and find careers that fit their interests and skills. Learn about finishing high school, writing a resume, training for a job and starting your own business. You can also use the website to find scholarship opportunities, look for a job in your area and get contact information for state job programs and agencies.

What Laws Protect Students' Educational Rights during the Transition Process?

- The Individuals with Disabilities Education Act's (IDEA) definition of transition services is, "a coordinated set of activities for a student with a disability that:
  - Are focused on improving the academic and functional achievement of the student to facilitate movement from school to post-school activities;
  - Are based on the individual student's needs, taking into account his/her strengths, preferences, and interests; and
  - Include instruction, related services, community experiences, the development of employment and other post-school adult living objectives, and, if appropriate, acquisition of daily living skills and functional vocational evaluation."

- Transition planning should be included as a part of a student's Individualized Education Program (IEP) or Individualized Learning Plan once the student has turned 16, or at a younger age if determined appropriate by the IEP Team. The IEP should include "measurable post-secondary goals based upon age-appropriate transition assessments related to training, education, employment and, where appropriate, independent living skills," as well as transition services needed to assist the student in reaching those goals. Some schools also work with local businesses to offer work-based learning opportunities, such as youth apprenticeships, paid and unpaid work experience, job shadowing, mentoring, and community service. Check with your guidance counselors or teachers to find out which work-based learning opportunities are available through your high school.

- Legal protections after high school (including accommodations): It's important to understand that the IDEA **does not** apply to students after they graduate from high school. Protections for post-high school students are provided by the Americans with Disabilities Act (ADA) and Section 504 of the Rehabilitation Act, and students must meet certain criteria to be eligible for accommodations. A college, university or trade/technical school may not provide the same accommodations a student received in high school. Students should discuss their accommodations needs with the disability student service office or a student adviser at the college, university or trade school they are interested in attending. For more information, read the U.S. Department of Education's (ED) guide "Students with Disabilities Preparing for Post-Secondary Education: Know Your Rights and Responsibilities" and the HEATH Resource Center's "Transitioning from High School to College: A Spotlight on Section 504."

- Testing: ADA Title III regulations prohibit discrimination by "any private entity that offers examinations or courses related to applications, licensing, certification or credentialing for secondary or post-secondary education, professional or trade purposes." These regulations require that any request for documentation must be reasonable and limited to the need for the modification, accommodation, or auxiliary aid or service requested. Entities must give considerable weight to documentation of past modifications, accommodations or auxiliary aids, or services received in similar testing situations, or those provided in response to an IEP or under Section 504 of the Rehabilitation Act. Learn about accommodations available for people with disabilities taking the General Educational Development (GED) test.

- Employment rights: The ADA also provides protections for employees who need assistive technology as a "reasonable accommodation." Section 508 of the Rehabilitation Act protects federal employees' access to information and electronic technology. Learn more about the laws and regulations that protect employees and job seekers with disabilities by reading Disability.gov's "What Are My Legal Rights on the Job as a Person with a Disability?" The U.S. Equal Employment Opportunity Commission's (EEOC) fact sheet "Job Applicants and the Americans with Disabilities Act" provides information about what questions employers can and cannot ask about your disability on job applications and during the interview process and what types of accommodations employers must provide to job applicants with disabilities.

How Do I Plan for the Transition to College or a Trade or Technical School?

Many high school graduates with disabilities choose to continue their education by attending college. There are several things to consider about going to college, including what is the right school, what sort of living situation is best (e.g., at home, in a dorm), whether or not to apply for student aid, which type of aid (grants, loans, scholarships) to apply for, etc. The following resources can help begin the college planning process:

Planning for College or Trade School:

- "A Practical Guide for People with Disabilities Who Want to Go to College" offers tips and ideas to help students with disabilities plan for college. The guide addresses topics such as finding the right school, applying for financial aid and determining what accommodations are needed.

- The U.S. Department of Education's (ED) College Navigator tool helps students choose the right school based on location, programs, and tuition.

- The HEATH Resource Center's College Application Process online training provides information to help students with disabilities understand the college admissions process and outlines some of the differences between high school and college. The Center also offers free online trainings about preparing to take the SAT or ACT and how to write a college application essay.

- "College Planning for Students with Disabilities" is a handbook that guides students with disabilities through the important steps and considerations necessary to prepare for college. It covers issues such as self-advocacy and a student's legal rights and responsibilities.

- ISEEK's Tips to Prepare for College webpage offers practical advice for students from middle school through adult learners on steps to take to prepare for college.

- The KnowHow2Go website offers information and resources for middle and high school students and Veterans and military members about planning for college, including making a plan, exploring your interests and how to pay for college. It includes the Four Steps to College online tool.

401

- The Education Quest Foundation's Students Transitioning to College webpage offers information on managing money, selecting a major and what to expect from the first year of college.

- The U.S. Department of Education's "Funding Your Education: The Guide to Student Financial Aid" provides information for students and families about federal student aid to pay for college, technical or training school or other post-secondary education. The guide explains the application process; the various federal loans, grants, and work-study programs available; and how to apply for federal student aid. Find in-depth information about financial aid by reading Disability.gov's "Guide to Student Financial Aid." Financial Aid for Students with Disabilities" offers additional information for paying for college or trade school.

- Affordable Colleges Online offers information about post-secondary education options for every budget. Use the website's search tool to find affordable options. The "Guide to Online Learning for Students with Disabilities" provides information about distance learning for students with disabilities. Learn how to work with student disability services to get accommodations and assistive technology for students with hearing, vision, cognitive or physical disabilities.

- Some colleges and universities offer programs specifically designed for students with intellectual and developmental disabilities. Examples of these types of programs include the George Mason University LIFE program, Temple University's Academy for Adult Learning and Virginia Commonwealth University's ACE-IT in College program. There are also college programs specifically for students with autism spectrum disorders, including Asperger Syndrome.

- Think College offers additional college planning resources for people with intellectual disabilities and their parents. Use the site's college search tool to find college programs for students with intellectual disabilities. The student section offers advice from college students about how college is different from high school, tips for success and information about financial aid options, including scholarships, grants, and loans.

- The Guide for College Students Living with a Chronic Condition has information and resources about topics like balancing school work while managing a chronic illness, financial aid options and returning to school after treatment.

- The University of Minnesota Institute on Community Integration offers Student Stories with advice from students with intellectual disabilities on how to successfully make the transition to college.

- "Navigating College–A Handbook on Self Advocacy for Students with Autism" is a handbook from the Autistic Self Advocacy Network for current and future college students with autism. It discusses getting accommodations in college, disability disclosure and advocating for yourself. Also includes information on living independently, staying healthy while in college and dealing with social issues. Read the Navigating College blog to learn more. The Autism Society of America also has the "Preparing to Experience College Living" guide for students with autism moving from high school to higher education.

- Learning Disabilities (LD) Online offers resources for students with learning disabilities who want to go to college. The website includes information about taking standardized tests and entrance exams, such as the SATs. The National Center for Learning Disabilities offers additional information about post-high school options for students with LD. The College Programs for Students with Learning Disabilities webpage offers a list of colleges that offer programs specially designed for students with LD.

- The PACER Center's "Off to College: Tips for Students with Visual Impairments" offers tips and helpful hints for students with visual impairments getting ready to go to college, as does the Texas School for the Blind and Visually Impaired.

- PepNet 2 provides information on equality for students who are deaf or hard of hearing during college entrance exams and other tests.

- Use the Career OneStop online tool to learn about education and training programs that offer certificates or diplomas in a variety of fields, or browse programs by occupation.

Making the Transition to College or Trade School:

The college experience is very different from high school, and there are steps students with disabilities can take to make the transition easier. Be sure to meet with your college or university's disabled student services office to discuss your accommodations needs and ways they can help students with disabilities get the most out of their time at school. The resources below can also help make the transition from high school to college smoother.

- The Going to College website offers high school students with disabilities tools and resources to help identify their strengths and learning styles, discover what to expect at college and learn how to prepare for higher education. The site's Getting Accommodations section has information to help students get the accommodations they need while in college.

- The U.S. Department of Education's publication "Students with Disabilities Preparing for Post-Secondary Education: Know Your Rights and Responsibilities" offers information on how legal rights and protections for students with disabilities change after high school. It includes information on accommodations, including for those needed for test taking.

- The National Collaborative on Workforce and Disability (NCWD) for youth's "Making My Way through College" helps students with disabilities prepare for and succeed in college. Also has information on moving from college to the workforce.

- The HEATH Resource offers an online training about accommodations for college students.

- Graduates in Science, Technology, Engineering, and Math (STEM) fields are in high demand. The need for qualified workers in STEM fields is growing, and jobs in these fields are also often high paying. In fact, the top ten bachelor degree majors with the highest median earnings are all in STEM fields. Efforts are being made to make sure students with disabilities have opportunities in STEM fields. Examples include the U.S. Department of Labor High School/High Tech program, the American Association for the Advancement of Science Entry Point Internship Program, and the University of Washington Disabilities, Opportunities, Internetworking and Technology (DO-IT) Center.

Part Five

Living with Learning Disabilities

Chapter 40

Coping with a Learning Disability

Coping with a Learning Disability

Parents are always important influences in the lives of their children, but their influence is particularly important in the lives of children with learning disabilities or attention deficit hyperactivity disorder (ADHD). Parental support, encouragement, and positive reinforcement can instill children with the confidence, determination, and self-esteem they need to cope with the special challenges they face. Although parents cannot cure their children's learning difficulties, they can provide valuable social and emotional tools to help the children become strong and resilient and view their deficits as surmountable obstacles that can be overcome with hard work and optimism. Experts recommend the following parenting approaches to help give children with learning disabilities or ADHD the best chance at success:

Provide structure and routines.

Children with learning disabilities often struggle with organization skills, so providing clear guidelines for structuring time and space and developing understandable routines can be very helpful. Visual aids—such as labels, lists, and pictures—can help children organize their belongings and remember how to put things away. Routines are important to help children manage time. Since many children with learning disabilities have trouble listening to and following instructions, it can be helpful to break tasks down into simple steps and communicate directions using short phrases. Parents can help children practice organization and time management skills by including them in planning activities, such as a birthday party, special meals, vacation, or planting a garden. Charting the tasks to be done, making lists, shopping for supplies, and checking off items are fun ways to develop organizational skills and promote independence.

Set reasonable expectations.

Parents can help children with learning disabilities expand their skills by breaking complex tasks down into simple steps that the child can accomplish. After the child can perform one step without assistance, the next step can be introduced. Learning how to set the table for dinner, for instance, might begin by having the child count out the appropriate number of spoons. Next, the child can put one spoon at each place. The parent should provide initial assistance and then gradually reduce their support as the child masters the task.

Maintain consistent discipline.

Parents should establish rules and expectations and explain them in clear, simple language. Children with learning disabilities may struggle to understand lengthy instructions and complex sentences. Reinforcement of the rules should be firm and consistent, with corrections applied in a warm and patient manner.

Practice social skills.

Parents can help children address difficulties with personal relationships by anticipating what might happen in various social situations and practicing appropriate responses ahead of time. They can act out scenarios—such as the child wanting to join in a game on the playground—and encourage the child to come up with different approaches for solving the problem. It may be helpful for the parent to demonstrate the wrong way of handling a situation and allow the child to offer suggestions for improvement.

Focus on strengths rather than weaknesses.

Children with learning disabilities are usually well aware of their areas of weakness. It is important for parents to reassure children that they are not defined by their learning disabilities. In addition to offering coping skills, parents should focus on the child's strengths, nurture their talents, and encourage them to pursue activities in which they excel, such as art, science, photography, computers, or sports.

Promote self-esteem.

Low self-esteem is common among children with learning disabilities. As they compare themselves to peers or siblings, they notice that they struggle to perform some tasks that come easily to others, and they begin to view themselves in a negative way. Parents can help by offering frequent and specific praise for things the child does well. Concrete comments help children understand expectations, feel confident about their progress and accomplishments, and gain self-esteem. Visual evidence such as certificates, charts, checklists, stars, and stickers can be used to reward the child for hard work on household tasks, such as making the bed, picking up toys, setting the table, or taking out the garbage.

Offer role models.

Parents can help children maintain a positive outlook by showing them that many successful people have had to overcome similar difficulties. Many books and videos are available that feature individuals who struggled to achieve their goals in the face of disability, illness, discrimination, or other challenges. Children may also gain inspiration from meeting highly effective members of society with learning disabilities or ADHD, such as firemen, business executives, politicians, park rangers, athletes, or celebrities.

Become an advocate for education.

Parents of children with learning disabilities or ADHD must take an active role in ensuring that their children receive the tools and accommodations they need in order to learn. Although schools are required to develop an Individualized Education Plan (IEP) for children with disabilities, the IEP may not maximize student achievement. Parents must understand special education laws in order to be effective advocates for their children at school and ensure they get the support services to which they are entitled. Yet parents also need to recognize that formal schooling will only be one part of the solution for their children's learning disabilities and avoid becoming excessively frustrated by dealing with the limitations of school systems.

Identify and reinforce the child's primary learning style.

Every child has a learning style that works best for them. Visual learners respond best to information they are able to see or read, for instance, while auditory learners respond best to material they can hear, and kinesthetic learners respond best to an active, hands-on approach. For parents of children with learning disabilities, it is particularly important to identify and reinforce the child's unique learning style, both at home and at school. Visual learners will benefit from using materials like books, videos, computers, flashcards, and visual aids like diagrams, drawings, lists, and color coded or highlighted notes. Auditory learners will find it helpful if parents read notes or study materials aloud to them, provide a tape recorder for them to record lessons, give them access to books on tape or CD, and encourage them to use verbal repetition or word associations to memorize information. Kinesthetic learners will perform best if parents reinforce lessons with hands-on experiments, field trips, role-playing activities, model building, and memory games.

Foster intellectual curiosity.

All children benefit from being excited and engaged in the learning process. Parents who convey a love of learning to their children can help them develop their natural curiosity and sense of wonder about the world. This spirit of inquiry can help make learning a fun, positive experience for children with ADHD or learning disabilities.

Emphasize classifying and categorizing objects.

Noticing similarities and differences, or picking out the relevant attributes of objects, can be difficult for children with learning disabilities. Parents can help them develop these skills by introducing simple categorization and classification of objects by color, shape, or use from an early age.

Encourage language usage and math activities.

Talking with children is the most important way for parents to help them develop language skills. Children with learning disabilities sometimes experience language delays, but parents still need to keep up informal, unstructured conversation to guide their language development. Simple math skills can also be introduced from an early age in the form of counting games and number songs, as well as activities that involve estimating distances, measuring amounts, or comparing quantities.

Teach children how to play.

To help children with learning disabilities interact with their peers in social situations, parents can help them learn to play. Children with visual-spatial difficulties may need help to develop the skills needed to stack blocks, for instance, while children who struggle with symbolic skills may need help learning to pretend. Preparing in advance for group activities, and giving the child a safe environment in which to learn from their mistakes, can be enjoyable for parents as well.

Build skills for life success.

Children with learning disabilities need to be aware that success in school is not the only means of achieving success in life. Parents should emphasize that children can still achieve their dreams and lead a happy, fulfilling life if they struggle in school. The key is to build the skills and characteristics that help people achieve life success, including self-confidence, perseverance, setting goals, being proactive, asking for help when needed, and handling stress.

Emphasize healthy habits.

To perform at the peak of their abilities and be able to work hard and concentrate on the task at hand, it is vital that children with learning disabilities develop healthy eating, sleeping, and exercise habits. The overall health of the body has a direct impact on the brain's ability to process information. Parents should also encourage children with learning disabilities or ADHD to develop healthy emotional habits to help them express feelings of anger, frustration, or discouragement in an appropriate way and learn how to calm themselves and regulate their emotions.

References

1. Johnson, Doris J. "Helping Young Children with Learning Disabilities at Home," LD Online, 2000.

2. Kemp, Gina. "Helping Children with Learning Disabilities," HelpGuide.org, May 2016.

3. Smith, Sally L. "Parenting Children with Learning Disabilities, ADHD, and Related Disorders," Learning Disabilities Association of America, 2002.

Chapter 41

Family and Relationship Issues

Chapter Contents

Section 41.1

Caring for Siblings of Kids with Learning Disabilities

As a parent, you want to give equal attention to all of your children. But when parenting a child with special needs, that can be hard. Your child with a disability needs you. But so do his or her siblings. It may feel like there's never enough of your attention to go around—and your other kids might begin to feel left out.

It can help to understand what your typically developing child or teen might be thinking and feeling. Kids love their siblings. They want to understand why there are some things that a sibling with a disability cannot do, and how they can help.

By answering questions in an age-appropriate way and being open and honest, you can help ease worries, clear up any confusion, and maybe even give your other kids a chance to help out. Kids who feel understood, loved, and secure about their place in the family can thrive—and the bond between siblings can grow.

Here's what might come up with kids at different ages and stages of development.

Preschoolers (Ages 3 to 5)

By nature, preschoolers feel that everything is about them and what they want—from the game they want to play to the toy they ask for at the store. So helping them understand why a sibling might need more of your more time or attention can be hard.

It can help to set aside one-on-one time with your child. This can be a challenge, but even a few minutes spent playing ball or allowing your little one to "help" you in the kitchen at mealtime can provide the mommy or daddy time that your child needs.

When kids ask about their sibling's abilities, explain the condition using simple language in a way they can understand. Use real words, like "cerebral palsy" instead of "boo boo." This prevents confusion in kids who get their own cuts and scrapes—you don't want them to be overly concerned about a bump on the head.

Say something like, "Your brother has trouble walking because he has cerebral palsy." If your child asks, "What is cerebral palsy?" state in simple terms that it's a condition that makes it harder for a child to do the same things other kids do.

Kids this age are also "magical thinkers"—so, the drink poured at the tea party is very hot and the monsters under the bed are very real. When kids have a sibling with special needs, this type of thinking can mean that they worry that the disability is an illness, like the common cold. Reassure your child that he or she cannot "catch" a condition like cerebral palsy, and that nothing either child did created the condition—it is no one's "fault."

Big Kids (Ages 6 to 12)

By elementary school, kids start to better understand the "why" of a diagnosis. Expect that you will get more complicated questions, and don't be afraid to answer them.

For example, for questions about a sibling with limited mobility, your explanation might expand to "His legs don't work because he was born with a health problem." The next question might be "Will he ever walk?" to which you need to answer honestly: "I don't know if he will, but we're going to try to help him do that. That's why he has therapy."

Your child might be sad or worried about his or her sibling's health. But playing together and enjoying each other's company can help. Encourage your typically developing child to read books to his or her sibling, build block towers together, and do craft activities with fingerpaint or clay.

This is also the age when kids start having to explain their sibling's condition to their friends. Some friends might ask rude questions or even participate in bullying behavior such as name-calling, which can leave your child feeling embarrassed, angry, or guilty.

You can help your child whether these encounters by rehearsing some conversations. If someone asks, "What's wrong with your sister?" for example, your child can simply say: "She has cerebral palsy." Or if a classmate uses an unkind term to describe the sibling with special needs, let your other kids know that as hard as it is, they must not act out in anger. Instead, help them explain the situation: "It's harder for my sister to learn new things than it is for you or me, but that doesn't make it OK to say mean things about her."

Sibling rivalry also builds at this age, so don't be surprised if kids act jealous of their brother or sister with special needs. After all, they see their sibling getting extra attention, or being allowed to stay up later or excused from doing chores.

Comparisons are normal, but explain that while it seems unfair, this is simply the way it has to be. Just as a child might feel that the sibling is getting extra attention, there are many opportunities that the sibling with special needs cannot have. Fair does not always mean equal.

Teens (Ages 13 and up)

During the teen years, siblings often feel increased pressure to care for their siblings with special needs. You might rely on your teen to babysit or help more with chores around the house. Teens might feel pressure to take on more responsibility than they should at this age.

As a parent, make sure you are not asking too much of your teen. Make certain responsibilities, such as babysitting, a choice. This will help teens feel that they have control over how much they help out. For example: "It would be great if you could watch your sister, but if you want to go out with your friends, that's OK."

Also, be sure that you don't expect too much when it comes to chores, school work, or extracurricular activities. Typically developing children sometimes feel extra pressure to be perfect so that their parents don't have to worry about them.

Teens are struggling with their independence from parents. And a teen who has a sibling with special needs also may struggle with the idea of life apart from that sibling. Let your teen know that wanting more independence and experiencing more of the world is normal, healthy, and encouraged, within safe limits.

As teens near adulthood, they might start to worry about the future, and wonder who is going to help care for the sibling once they've moved out—or if something happens to you. Reassure your teen that whatever the future holds, help with caring for his or her sibling will depend on how much your teen is comfortable taking on. Then, have a plan ready for when changes come that will benefit all members of the family.

Handling Strong Emotions

Just as parenting a child with special needs can be joyful and frustrating, kids, and teens who have a brother or sister with special needs will have ups and downs.

Some siblings roll with the punches and don't let much bother them, while others are more sensitive and take things to heart. These kids need healthy ways to work through their emotions. Writing in a journal, being physically active, or participating in creative arts like dance or music are good ways to handle strong emotions.

But if you notice changes in your child's sleep routine, appetite, mood, or behavior, it could be a sign of anxiety, depression, or another problem. If this happens, seek help from a mental health professional for your child.

Section 41.2

Dealing with Learning Disabilities in Relationships

This section includes text excerpted from "Marriage Advice for Parents of Children with Special Needs," © 1995–2016. The Nemours Foundation/KidsHealth®. Reprinted with permission

Marriage Advice for Parents of Children with Special Needs

If you're raising a child with special needs, you probably devote much of your time and energy to his or her care. And then you might have other children who need you, too. But there's someone else who you shouldn't forget: your spouse or partner.

Working on your relationship might seem like another task on an already long to-do list. But when your marriage is strong, you work better as a team. You communicate better. You fight less. And this can make life easier and better not just for you, but for your children, too.

Here are 10 ways that even overwhelmed parents can strengthen their marriages:

1. **Keep talking.** Silence says a lot about your relationship, because it begs the question: What are you not talking about? Parents of kids with special needs often hold in their emotions.

One parent might feel guilty while another feels angry. One parent might feel overwhelmed while the other feels neglected. Talk about these emotions, but don't judge each other for them. Two people in the same situation can have completely different emotional reactions, and neither is right or wrong. In fact, hearing about why your partner feels or acts a certain way can be helpful and give you a new perspective. Keep talking about the big stuff and you'll be able to keep talking about anything.

2. **Work together.** Resentment over an imbalance of childcare duties and other responsibilities can hurt your relationship. If you feel like you're doing most of the work, talk about it and see if there are better ways to split duties. Have the conversation when you're both well-rested and getting along, not in the heat of an argument or when tempers flare. Then, identify each other's strengths together—maybe one person is better at handling the doctor's appointments, while the other can better handle bathing and feeding. Once these roles are decided, allow your partner to "step up" and resist the urge to take over.

3. **Avoid "boss–employee" roles.** One parent often assumes most of the responsibilities for childcare and health care decisions. Over time, he or she might start making all the decisions, without first asking a spouse, "What do you think?" Suddenly one parent is the boss and the other feels like the hired help. This leads to resentment. If you're the primary caregiver, don't forget to keep your spouse informed on issues related to medical care, schooling, and other aspects of parenting. This helps to share the sometimes overwhelming demands of caring for a child with special needs. And when this happens, primary caregivers can feel less overwhelmed and partners can feel less like assistants and more like equals.

4. **Keep the spark.** When you're exhausted and overwhelmed, you might think there's no time or energy left for physical intimacy. But romance is what binds you together as a couple, and the healthiest marriages prioritize alone time. Intimacy allows you to take care of yourself and your partner in a way that also strengthens the relationship.

5. **Keep alone time as a couple.** Make a commitment to have 20 minutes of alone time daily. Share a meal or a favorite

beverage and talk about your day. If possible, you might even arrange for a babysitter or respite care and have a regular date night. When you're alone together, try to discuss topics other than your children. Doing this strengthens your bond as a couple and makes you more likely to work together as a team when issues come up.

6. **Argue (sometimes).** Disagreements are normal in any relationship. Don't ignore your differences of opinion; instead, embrace them. Talk them through and truly listen to one another. But make sure your arguments are focused on solutions that take into consideration both partners' feelings. Having small disagreements here and there can prevent big, emotionally draining arguments down the line.

7. **Tackle your exhaustion.** Raising a child with special needs requires a lot of energy. You are "on" from morning to night, and sometimes after that. How can you find time for your marriage when you are physically or emotionally drained? Figure out what on your to-do list can be ignored. Maybe the house isn't perfectly organized; maybe you don't host the next holiday dinner; maybe you eat on paper plates just to make cleanup easier. It's OK to cut corners to create time you can devote to yourself and your partner.

8. **Take time for yourself.** Let's face it: a spouse can feel like just another person who needs or wants your attention. And if you are emotionally exhausted, no matter how much you love that person, you might have nothing left to give. Nourish your spirit and you'll be able to give more to your entire family. Maybe you wake up a few minutes early and enjoy a long shower, or you arrange for respite care so you can get to the gym or go for a walk a few times a week. Figure out what would work for your lifestyle and do it—without guilt. The better you feel, the better you'll be able to care for others.

9. **Learn to listen.** When your partner has had a tough day, fight the urge to one-up his or her frustrations with your own struggles. Instead, listen. Sympathize with the situation, acknowledge that he or she needs a break, and express appreciation for how hard your partner works. By listening and acknowledging, you help avoid resentment, which is toxic to a marriage.

419

10. **Say "thank you."** Did your partner get up early so you could sleep in? Did your spouse take a day off of work to finally address that "honey-do" list? Did you get some time out of the house to yourself? Appreciation is a powerful emotion. When you say thanks, you acknowledge your spouse's efforts and are reminded of where they came from—the love he or she has for you.

When the Going Gets Tough

Every relationship has its ups and downs now and then. But if you feel like yours has had more "downs" than "ups" lately, perhaps it's time to get help from a professional

Many good resources are available to help spouses and families. You might start by asking a member of your child's care team or your family doctor for references of health professionals who specialize in this type of work. Couples counseling, couples retreats or seminars, books, and other resources help many couples overcome obstacles and get back on track.

Section 41.3

Parenting Issues for Adults with Learning Disabilities

This section includes text excerpted from "Chapter 12: The Impact of Disability on Parenting," National Council on Disability (NCD), September 27, 2012. Reviewed June 2016.

People with disabilities face significant barriers to creating and maintaining families. These obstacles—created by the child welfare system, the family law system, adoption agencies, assisted reproductive technology providers, and society as a whole—are the result of perceptions concerning the child-rearing abilities of people with disabilities. But are these views informed? Does disability affect one's ability to parent?

Social science research examining the effect of disability on parenting is scarce. Historically, the absence of data has encouraged the bias against parents with disabilities. Ora Prilleltensky, professor at the University of Miami and a person with a disability, says, "Despite the growing numbers of disabled adults who are having children, parents with disabilities continue to be primarily ignored by research and social policy. The sparse literature that can be found on the topic typically focuses on the relationship between parental disability and children's well-being. In some cases, a negative impact is hypothesized, studied and 'verified'; in other cases, the correlation between indices of dysfunction in children and parental disability is explored; and in others yet, the negative impact on children and the need to counsel them is taken as a given."

Parents with Intellectual or Developmental Disabilities

Parents with intellectual or developmental disabilities face similarly significant and detrimental discrimination, which raises the question, do intellectual and developmental disabilities affect parenting ability? According to Preston, research has historically been focused on the pathological bias against parents with intellectual and developmental disabilities, "pointing out that much of the literature on parents with intellectual disabilities has failed to distinguish between characteristics that facilitate and those that inhibit parenting abilities. Most of these studies have focused only on identifying parents with intellectual disabilities who provide inadequate childcare, rather than identifying predictors of adequate childcare such as coping and skill acquisition—despite the fact that a substantial number of parents with intellectual disabilities have provided adequate care."

According to professors at the University of Minnesota School of Social Work, "Despite disproportionately greater involvement in the child welfare system, a growing body of research on the outcomes for children of parents with disabilities does not necessarily support the assumption that parents with disabilities are more likely to abuse or neglect their children. Studies have found that children of parents with intellectual and developmental disabilities can have successful outcomes."

Chris Watkins notes, "Almost all studies have found a sizeable percentage of parents with developmental disabilities to be functioning within or near normal limits. In addition, many studies have found that parents labeled mentally retarded can and do benefit from training and support. Even researchers and commentators who have reached the most negative conclusions about cognitively disabled parents caution that such parents must be evaluated as individuals before reaching conclusions about their parental adequacy, or their ability to benefit from training and support."

Several researchers have used qualitative methods to investigate life experiences and outcomes of children of parents with intellectual disabilities. In Denmark, J. Faureholm interviewed 20 young adult children of mothers with intellectual disabilities. Despite the difficult circumstances of their growing up, including being bullied and ostracized by their peers, most of the children discovered an underlying personal strength that enabled them to overcome these experiences, and all but one maintained a close and warm relationship with their parents. Similarly, in England, internationally recognized researchers Tim Booth and Wendy Booth also interviewed adult children of parents with "learning difficulties." They said, "The majority recalled happy, if not necessarily carefree, childhoods. Only three regarded their childhoods as wholly unhappy." Significantly, most of the interviewees expressed positive feelings of love and affection toward their parents, and all maintained close contact with their parents. Tellingly, those who had been removed by the child welfare system had subsequently reestablished and maintained contact with their birth parents. "In both studies, family bonds endured despite time and circumstance intervening."

Recent research further demonstrates the absence of a clear correlation between low IQ and parental unfitness. In fact, studies have indicated that it is impossible to predict parenting outcomes on the basis of the results of intelligence testing. Thus, Chris Watkins says, "The available research suggests that factors unrelated to disability often have a more significant impact on parental fitness than does disability itself. The research also suggests a tremendous variance in the impact that disability has on parental fitness. Importantly, parenting services have been shown to make a difference for many parents with insufficient parenting skills. While few conclusions can be drawn about the parenting abilities of developmentally disabled parents as a group, it is clear that individual inquiry is required before decisions are made to remove children from parents."

Conclusion

Current research, limited though it is, demonstrates that disability does not necessarily have a negative effect on parenting. Certainly, much more research in this area is needed; specifically, research that does not pathologize parental disability in a negative way. Moreover, research should focus on the effect of supports for parents with disabilities.

Chapter 42

Educating Others about Your Child with a Learning Disability

Overview

One of the many vexing questions facing parents of children with learning disabilities is deciding whether and how to explain their child's diagnosis and difficulties to other people. On the one hand, parenting a child with learning disabilities may seem challenging enough without dealing with other people's reactions and opinions. On the other hand, not discussing the child's unique challenges—and explaining how they affect the child's behavior and needs—may create an uncomfortable situation or make it seem as if the parents are embarrassed or hiding something. The decision about whether to disclose also affects the child. When other people are properly informed and educated about the child's learning disabilities, they may be better equipped to offer understanding and support. In this way, the child may feel increased comfort, trust, and confidence in seeking accommodations.

Making the Child Aware of a Learning Disability

The first step in the process of disclosure is to make the child aware of their learning difficulties. The timing of this step can be tricky, and

"Educating Others about Your Child with a Learning Disability," © 2016 Omnigraphics. Reviewed June 2016.

it must be handled in a sensitive, age-appropriate manner. In the absence of an explanation, the child will still notice that they struggle with classroom activities or need more assistance than other students. They may start to believe that they are stupid or inferior, rather than merely different in the way they process information. Yet it is also important to avoid detailing all of the potential difficulties that could arise from the diagnosis, because too much negative information could convince the child that there is no point in trying to learn. The following steps can help guide parents through the process of making a child aware of a learning disability:

- Before talking to the child, the parents should first educate themselves about the diagnosis and the full range of the child's strengths and weaknesses.

- When opening the discussion, the parents should reassure the child that they are healthy.

- Then the parents should explain that the child's brain works differently in some ways, which will make certain tasks more difficult and other tasks easier.

- Next, the parents should reinforce the fact that they will provide all the help the child needs to be successful. The parents should be active advocates for the child at school to ensure that all available supports and accommodations are used.

- The parents must communicate clearly and make sure the child understands and feels free to ask questions.

- The parents should also discuss their expectations, as well as the child's hopes and dreams for the future. They should take a positive outlook and emphasize the power of perseverance and hard work to overcome difficulties and frustration.

- Finally, the parents should offer sincere praise and compliments to the child for hard work and positive accomplishments, and make sure the child knows that they are loved and valued.

Informing Others about a Child's Learning Disability

Although a child's diagnosis and unique learning style is personal, the details must be shared with many people who are involved with the child's life, education, and welfare.

Some of the people who require a full understanding of the child's learning disability include:

- Healthcare providers

Doctors, nurses, social workers, psychologists, therapists, and other medical professionals who work with the child should be made aware of the child's learning disability and how it may affect the provision of healthcare services. A dentist, for instance, should be told that short appointments work better for a child with attention deficit hyperactivity disorder (ADHD), or that certain types of lights or sounds might trigger reactive behavior in a child with sensory processing disorders.

- Education providers

Teachers, paraprofessionals, tutors, coaches, scout leaders, camp counselors, and religious leaders who guide the child's educational and recreational experiences should also be made aware of the child's learning disability. Parents should describe the child's strengths and talents, as well as weaknesses and challenges. They should also provide examples of approaches that might aid learning and eliminate confusion or frustration for the child.

- Strangers in the community

Store clerks, restaurant servers, bus drivers, and other people the child might encounter in social situations do not need as much information as medical and educational providers. But parents can help smooth their interactions with the child by anticipating problems and intervening in advance. Experts suggest using a firm, positive tone to explain the child's needs, preferences, and behaviors.

- Social acquaintances

People who are likely to see the child regularly—including classmates, friends, and parents of friends—should be provided with some explanation about the child's learning difficulties. They at least need to know what activities might create challenges or engender disruptive behaviors.

Educating Family Members about a Child's Learning Disability

Perhaps surprisingly, immediate and extended family members can be among the most challenging people to inform about a child's learning disability. Although some family members will accept the news and immediately offer support, others may deny a problem exists or even blame the parents or the child. The closeness of family relationships—along with the fact that learning disabilities are often inherited—increases the potential for strong feelings of pain, grief, anger, and guilt. Siblings of the child with learning disabilities may feel jealous of the extra attention they receive or resentful that they may be held to different expectations. Despite the potential difficulties, however, informing and educating family members is important for both the parents and the child in order to break down barriers of communication and understanding, reduce feelings of isolation, help set realistic expectations, and expand the support system.

Experts recommend using simple, easy-to-understand language and avoiding clinical terminology. They suggest emphasizing the child's talents and positive qualities as well as explaining their areas of difficulty. After sharing the basic information, parents should help family members come up with strategies to interact positively with the child. They should also allow the family members to ask questions and make an effort to provide thoughtful, sensitive answers. Since some people will want additional information, it may be helpful to come prepared with articles, reports, or organizations to contact for further information. Education of family members usually cannot be accomplished in one sitting, so multiple discussions may be needed. The child may be included in some of the later discussions.

When sharing information with a large family group, it may be best to begin by talking to those family members who are most likely to be supportive. These allies can help reinforce the message with others who may be more resistant. If a family member reacts with denial or blame, it may be helpful to ask a teacher, therapist, or supportive family member to intervene. It is also important to remember that some people may need time and space to process their feelings. While some family members may never fully understand the learning disability, they may still be able to find a comfortable role in the child's life and provide the child with love, attention, and support.

References

1. "Educating Others about Your Child's Learning Disability," SmartKids, January 18, 2016.

2. "Talking with Family about Your Child's Learning Disability," GreatSchools, March 18, 2016.

Chapter 43

Bullying and Learning Disabilities: What Parents Need to Know

What Is Bullying?

Bullying is unwanted, aggressive behavior among school aged children. It involves a real or perceived power imbalance and the behavior is repeated, or has the potential to be repeated, over time.

Both kids who are bullied and kids who bully others may have serious, lasting problems.

Bullying and Children and Youth with Disabilities and Special Health Needs

Children with physical, developmental, intellectual, emotional, and sensory disabilities are more likely to be bullied than their peers. Any number of factors—physical vulnerability, social skill challenges, or intolerant environments may increase their risk. Research suggests that some children with disabilities may bully others as well.

Kids with special health needs, such as epilepsy or food allergies, may also be at higher risk of being bullied. For kids with special health

This chapter includes text excerpted from "Bullying and Children and Youth with Disabilities and Special Health Needs," StopBullying.gov, U.S. Department of Health and Human Services (HHS), July 13, 2012. Reviewed June 2016.

needs, bullying can include making fun of kids because of their allergies or exposing them to the things they are allergic to. In these cases, bullying is not just serious; it can mean life or death.

A small but growing amount of research shows that:

- Children with attention deficit or hyperactivity disorder (ADHD) are more likely than other children to be bullied. They also are somewhat more likely than others to bully their peers.

- Children with autism spectrum disorder (ASD) are at increased risk of being bullied and left out by peers. In a study of 8-17-year-olds, researchers found that children with ASD were more than three times as likely to be bullied as their peers.

- Children with epilepsy are more likely to be bullied by peers, as are children with medical conditions that affect their appearance, such as cerebral palsy, muscular dystrophy, and spina bifida. These children frequently report being called names related to their disability.

- Children with hemiplegia (paralysis of one side of their body) are more likely than other children their age to be bullied and have fewer friends.

- Children who have diabetes and are dependent on insulin may be especially vulnerable to peer bullying.

- Children who stutter may be more likely to be bullied. In one study, 83 percent of adults who stammered as children said that they were teased or bullied; 71 percent of those who had been bullied said it happened at least once a week.

Children with learning disabilities (LD) are at a greater risk of being bullied. At least one study also has found that children with LD may also be more likely than other children to bullying their peers.

Effects of Bullying

Kids who are bullied are more likely to have:

- Depression and anxiety. Signs of these include increased feelings of sadness and loneliness, changes in sleep and eating patterns, and loss of interest in activities they used to enjoy. These issues may persist into adulthood.

- Health complaints

- Decreased academic achievement—GPA and standardized test scores—and school participation. They are more likely to miss, skip, or drop out of school.

Bullying, Disability Harassment, and the Law

Bullying behavior can become "disability harassment," which is prohibited under Section 504 of the Rehabilitation Act of 1973 and Title II of the Americans with Disabilities Act of 1990. According to the U.S. Department of Education (ED), disability harassment is "intimidation or abusive behavior toward a student based on disability that creates a hostile environment by interfering with or denying a student's participation in or receipt of benefits, services, or opportunities in the institution's program."

Disability harassment can take different forms including verbal harassment, physical threats, or threatening written statements. When a school learns that disability harassment may have occurred, the school must investigate the incident(s) promptly and respond appropriately. Disability harassment can occur in any location that is connected with school—classrooms, the cafeteria, hallways, the playground, athletic fields, or school buses. It also can occur during school-sponsored events.

What Parents Can Do

If you believe a child with special needs is being bullied:

- Be supportive of the child and encourage him or her to describe who was involved and how and where the bullying happened. Be sure to tell the child that it is not his or her fault and that nobody deserves to be bullied or harassed. Do not encourage the child to fight back. This may make the problem worse.

- Ask the child specific questions about his or her friendships. Be aware of signs of bullying, even if the child doesn't call it that. Children with disabilities do not always realize they are being bullied. They may, for example, believe that they have a new friend although this "friend" is making fun of them.

- Talk with the child's teacher immediately to see whether he or she can help to resolve the problem.

- Put your concerns in writing and contact the principal if the bullying or harassment is severe or the teacher doesn't fix the problem. Explain what happened in detail and ask for a prompt response. Keep a written record of all conversations and communications with the school.

- Ask the school district to convene a meeting of the Individualized Education Program (IEP) or the Section 504 teams. These groups ensure that the school district is meeting the needs of its students with disabilities. This meeting will allow parents to explain what has been happening and will let the team review the child's IEP or 504 plans and make sure that the school is taking steps to stop the harassment. Parents, if your child needs counseling or other supportive services because of the harassment, discuss this with the team. Work with the school to help establish a system-wide bullying prevention program that includes support systems for bullied children. As the U.S. Department of Education (ED) recognizes, "creating a supportive school climate is the most important step in preventing harassment."

- Explore whether the child may also be bullying other younger, weaker students at school. If so, his or her IEP may need to be modified to include help to change the aggressive behavior.

- Be persistent. Talk regularly with the child and with school staff to see whether the behavior has stopped.

Getting Additional Support

If a school district does not take reasonable, appropriate steps to end the bullying or harassment of a child with special needs, the district may be violating federal, state, and local laws. For more information, contact:

1. The U.S. Department of Education Office for Civil Rights

    Phone: 800-421-3481

    Website: www2.ed.gov/about/offices/list/ocr/ complaintintro.html

2. The U.S. Department of Education Office of Special Education Programs

    Phone: 202-245-7468

    Website: www2.ed.gov/about/offices/list/osers/osep/index.html

3. The U.S. Department of Justice Civil Rights Division

    Phone: 1-877-292-3804

    Website: www.justice.gov/crt/complaint/#three

Chapter 44

Social Skills: A Difficult Area for Many with Learning Disabilities

Scope of the Problem

Estimates of the prevalence of social problems in students with learning disabilities (LD) in the United States range from 38% to 75%. About 2,800,000 children have been identified as having LD; hence a sizable population of students has LD as social problems. Moreover, social problems have been reported across ages (preschool-elementary-junior-senior high schools-college-adulthood), race and ethnicity (some inconsistencies), settings (rural-urban), raters (parents, teachers, peers, and self-assessments), methods and measures (surveys, observations, and laboratory studies), countries (United States, Canada, Israel, Australia, and South Africa), and time (30+ years).

The results of studies on social problems have been replicated many times in many places, and appear to be resistant to the vagaries of time, place, and methodologies.

This chapter includes text excerpted from "Disability Inclusion," Centers for Disease Control and Prevention (CDC), March 17, 2016.

Characteristics of Students with LD: The Social-Emotional Domain

Self-Concept

Self-concept is one of the most widely researched topics in LD. One of the most frequently cited findings is that students with LD have lower academic self-concepts than peers. Although students with LD consistently and accurately rate themselves lower than achieving classmates on academic achievement, their self-concept for social status appears to be inconsistent. For example, Bursuck and Kistner, Haskett, White, and Robbins found students with LD accurate in evaluating themselves more negatively on social skills than comparison students insofar as they received lower peer ratings. But Bear and Minke (1996) and Clever, Bear, and Juvonen (1992) found inflated ratings on their self-esteem on social factors. If the sample included students with LD who did not have social problems, inflated scores may have reflected accurate social perceptions.

On the other hand, inflated self-perceptions of social skills ratings may represent a deficit in social perception. It is also possible that if the child has one friend, the child could perceive him/herself socially skilled in spite of receiving lower sociometric ratings from peers. Moreover, in the absence of teasing or bullying, social status may be more amorphous than academic status.

While an accurate perception of social rejection is likely to produce sad, depressed feelings, deficits in social perception may help the child maintain positive feelings about the self. In sum, although students with LD are likely to perceive themselves more negatively on measures of academic self-concepts throughout their school years, their social self-concepts may vary depending on a variety of personal and situational factors.

Affect / Emotions

A relatively ignored area in education is the impact of affect/emotions on social relationships and learning. Yet, research in psychology, medicine, and nursing has demonstrated strong relationships between positive and negative affect and most human functions, including learning, social relationships, and health. Negative affect (i.e., anger, fear, anxiety, disgust, depression) depresses memory and produces inefficient information processing. It affects the performance of complex cognitive functions that require flexibility, integration, and utilization of cognitive material. In contrast, positive affect increases access to information stored in memory, boosts positive feelings about self, generosity and goodwill toward others, and facilitates conflict resolution. Moreover, affect is contagious. That is, we can "catch" elation, euphoria, sadness, anger, and depression from the people around us. As a result, people seek the company of those who exhibit positive affect, while avoiding people who are depressed, sad, or angry.

Several studies have compared students with and without LD on their negative feelings; namely, depression, anxiety, and loneliness. The results of these studies consistently have found that students with LD are more likely than comparison students to experience these negative emotions. Feelings of loneliness have been found to range from 10% to 18% in children without disabilities but to range as high as 25% or more among children with developmental disabilities. Feelings of loneliness appear to be rooted in reality. For example, Pavri and Luftig found that students with LD were also less popular and more controversial than their peers.

However, we should not assume that negative affect is the result of poor academic achievement and difficulty making friends. Data suggest that negative affect may well be the precursor of both. For example, Margalit and Al-Yagon reported that preschool students who were identified as learning disabled a year later were more depressed and lonelier than higher achieving classmates. Because preschool children's loneliness pre-dates the experience of school difficulties and being identified as learning disabled, negative affect is not the result of academic difficulties. Furthermore, data showing that peer rejection predates identification as having LD suggest that peers are reacting to social skill deficits and that young peers may avoid preschoolers who are sad in order to avoid the social contagion of negative affect.

Studying emotionality is another way to examine the impact of affect on social status. Hypothesized that high emotionality and poor emotional regulatory skills interfere with coding social cues and assessing situations from different cognitive and affective perspectives, thus preventing a flexible approach to goal selection. Highly emotional children, or children upset by others' emotionality, may experience difficulty focusing on a variety of responses and evaluating them. Elementary school students with high emotionality and poor emotion regulation skills have been found at risk for behavior problems, but the research has not yet been extended to students with LD. Some of the behavior problems exhibited by students with LD may be traceable to poor emotional regulatory skills.

In sum, affect and emotions, which are regulated by the nervous system, have been implicated as a cause and/or correlate in LD because

(a) negative affect has negative effects on learning and social relations and (b) problems in emotional regulation influence responses in social situations. Negative affect and/or poor emotional regulation are likely to "color" children's perceptions and interpretations of others' behaviors toward them as well as others' responses to them.

Social Information Processing

Social perception. Social perception is defined as the recognition and labeling of prosody, facial expressions, gestures, and body language. Accurate judgments of emotions and feelings can be made without verbal cues, but require attention to often subtle, fleeting cues. Negative interactions with others have been related to neglect of subtle social cues or a lack of ability to perceive and accurately read social cues. A variety of methods have been used to study the social perception of students with LD, including their accuracy in perceiving others' attitudes or behaviors toward them.

Nonverbal perception. Studies of nonverbal perception have been based on children's accuracy in labeling photographs or silent-film scenarios, and auditory and visual recordings of everyday emotions (anger, disgust, surprise, sadness, fear, and happiness). Students with LD consistently perform worse than comparison students. The auditory-only input is more difficult than the combined auditory-visual input. Of note, teachers' ratings of children's social skills are significantly correlated with students' accuracy in labeling emotions. Furthermore, students with LD appear to be aware of their deficiencies in nonverbal communication and social problem solving.

Social Cognition

When asked to generate solutions to social dilemmas, students with LD perform less ably than average-achieving and low-achieving peers in encoding the dilemmas and in generating competent solutions. Although students with LD are able to generate a diversity of potential competent solutions, they indicate a preference for significantly more incompetent solutions than average-achieving students.

Children's "reading" of their social environment may be the dominant factor that shapes their selection of responses. Donahue, Szymanski, and Flores suggest that what looks like an incompetent response may actually serve an important, adaptive, and strategic social purpose given a history of social difficulties and consequent social environments. That is, the incompetent response may reflect the role the child plays in his or her social milieu.

Communicative Competence

Communicative competence (i.e., pragmatics) refers to the functional use of language to express social intentions that are consistent with cultural norms. Acquisition of pragmatic skills requires learning the elements of the language system (i.e., vocabulary, syntax, semantics) and the rules for language use in social transactions (e.g., turn taking).

A meta-analysis of pragmatic language skills found that students with language and/or learning disabilities demonstrated consistent and pervasive pragmatic deficits in conversation across settings, conversational partners, age groups, and types of pragmatic skills measured. Specifically, children and adolescents with LD display problems in topic selection, initiation and maintenance, conversational turn taking, requesting and producing clarification, narrative production, presenting logical opinions and different points of view, gaze and eye contact, being tactful in formulating and delivering messages, and comprehension of humor and slang.

Lapadat attributed the deficits to underlying language deficits rather than insufficient social knowledge. Considering that decades of research have linked language and reading skills, it is notable that Most, Al-Yagon, Tur-Kaspa, and Margalit found that preschool children differed from comparison children on measures of phonological awareness, loneliness, and social acceptance. This study suggests a connection between language skills, academic performance, and social status.

Social Behavior

A host of negative or inappropriate behaviors have been attributed to students with LD, including a lack of skills in initiating and sustaining positive social relationships, acting more aggressively, and exhibiting more negative verbal and nonverbal behaviors than classmates. Some tend to be withdrawn whereas others behave disruptively. Teachers report that children with LD are more disruptive, less cooperative, insensitive, less tactful, and engage in more attention-seeking behavior than classmates. Parents rate them as less attentive, more active, not following directions or completing tasks. Peers rate them as more aggressive or disruptive. Finally, a meta-analysis indicated children with LD are more likely than others to suffer personality or immaturity problems.

Interventions

Several studies have attempted to teach the social skills that have been identified in the research as being problematic among students with LD. Although positive effects have been reported in some research, meta-analytic analyses have found limited positive effects on social behavior. These intervention studies were based on group designs and classroom-based interventions.

Researchers have been testing the impact on children's academic and social status of various classroom-based interventions. For example, Charles Greenwood and colleagues at Juniper Gardens have demonstrated, time and again, the positive effects of peer tutoring on academic learning and social relationships. Another promising method is cooperative goal structures. For a time, having teams of children work on thematic units was a popular way to integrate children's learning across subjects, and to provide opportunities for children to work collaboratively in ways that promote friendships and collegiality.

More recently, Vaughn, Elbaum, Schumm, and Hughes found a moderate increase in the friendship quality and peer acceptance of students with LD in classrooms using a consultation/collaborative teaching model. The Circle of Friends model, bibliotherapy or writing groups are other methods that could integrate social skills training into language arts curricula. Bryan and Bryan developed Amazing Discoveries, a program that integrated social skills training into science.

Although teachers are more likely to find classroom-based interventions acceptable than individualized social skills training, interventions that are individualized are more likely to be effective. That is, group designs may teach important social skills but not address the actual social deficits of the students in a particular sample. A mismatch between the needs of the student and the instruction may explain the relatively weak results of these studies. Positive results have been found when interventions are matched to student problems. See, for example, the attribution retraining studies by Borkowski, Weyhing, and Carr and Schunk and Cox. These studies demonstrated that academic achievement and self-perceptions could be systematically improved. Indeed, students receiving attribution retraining plus academic instruction did better academically than students who received only academic instruction.

Affect interventions have also been demonstrated to be effective in laboratory and classroom settings. A series of studies found that 45-second affect inductions using self-induced positive thoughts, happy music, room freshener, or teacher pep talks had positive effects on social problem solving, math, spelling, learning to read unfamiliar words and students' willingness to help out at a school event. Although these effects have been estimated to be effective only for about 20 minutes, generating positive moods in the classroom is likely to have a positive impact not only on learning but on cooperative behaviors and conflict resolution.

In general, the skills taught as part of classroom instruction are unlikely to generalize to other settings. However, Elksnin described procedures that facilitate generalization of social skills. Extending special education's basic principles to teaching social skills, Elksnin suggests focusing on sequential modification, introduction of contingencies, training with several examples, training across settings, and mediating training generalizations. Further, Deshler and Schumaker established models for individualizing instruction and teaching generalization in learning many complex skills.

The scientific database delineating the social problems of students with LD is in place and foundations have been established for classroom-based interventions and individualized instruction. We can argue that the research has limitations and that more research is needed, but the fact is that the social difficulties of students with LD have been systematically demonstrated over and over again. We know what has to be done. We know how to do it. But if we are to effectively help children with LD improve their social status and social skills, a number of major issues must be addressed.

First, classroom-based interventions may reduce the factors that create negative academic and social self-perceptions and poor social relationships by reducing the visibility of individual performance and increasing the opportunity for legitimate, prosocial interactions. And it may be possible to weave individualized social skills training into academic curricula. Classroom-based interventions hold the promise of establishing positive social environments for all students; they are feasible and promote academic learning. But for students who have problems in affect/emotions, perception, cognition, and language, it is critical that interventions address the needs of individual students. Thus, class-wide interventions are likely to provide the supports that must be in place to facilitate peer group acceptance, but are unlikely to provide the individualized instruction that children with learning/ social disabilities need. Students with social LD require individualized instruction (i.e., special education that addresses their social needs).

Full inclusion is another common intervention for improving the social skills of children with disabilities. Part of the rationale for integrating children with special needs into general education classrooms was the opinion that the resource room pullout service delivery system contributed to low social status. It was believed that placing students with disabilities into general education classrooms would increase their opportunities to interact with typical children, learn social skills by observing good role models, gain peer acceptance, and feel better about themselves.

Several research studies have examined whether full inclusion has improved the self-perception and social status of students with LD. Based on meta-analyses, self-concepts are not influenced by class placement. Regardless of whether students with LD are in general education classes, resource rooms, self-contained classes, or special schools, they have lower academic self-concepts than typically achieving students. In other words, there is no systematic association between self-concept of students with LD and their educational placement.

Similarly, the social competence of students with LD does not seem to be higher in inclusive than in non inclusive settings based on teachers' ratings. Students with LD were found to be less well liked and more frequently rejected than average-/high-achieving students, and the number of students with LD who were not liked by classmates in the fall increased in the spring despite placement in classes of teachers who were highly accepting of students with LD. In sum, merely placing students in inclusive classrooms is not sufficient to create social inclusion and acceptance.

Chapter 45

Self-Esteem Issues and Children with Learning Disabilities.

Overview

Self-esteem refers to positive feelings of worth, acceptance, and value that people hold with regard to themselves. Children who have high self-esteem feel proud, confident, secure, and capable. These feelings enable them to act independently, take responsibility for their actions, stand up for themselves, and face challenges. They are more likely to be resilient and keep trying if they make a mistake, and to have the courage to make good decisions in the face of peer pressure. Children with low self-esteem, on the other hand, lack confidence and do not believe they have value and are worthy of respect. They are less likely to stand up for themselves or ask for help, and they are more likely to give in to peer pressure.

How Self-Esteem Develops

Self-esteem begins to develop in infancy. In childhood, when the primary influences are loving parents, most people have very positive self-esteem. Toddlers, for instance, often respond with enthusiasm when asked if they are smart or able to do something. Young children try new things, experience repeated successes, and receive praise for their efforts. This pattern gives them confidence to face additional challenges and makes them feel good about themselves. Over time, they develop the positive characteristics associated with high self-esteem.

As children reach school age, however, they gradually begin incorporating more negative feedback from the classroom and other parts of the outside world. They experience failures, and their efforts are not always rewarded. Around the age of seven, children begin comparing themselves to their peers and realizing that others may possess stronger skills in some areas. As a result, their confidence and self-esteem may begin to wane.

Learning Disabilities and Self-Esteem

This process affects children with learning disabilities to a greater degree than most other children. Children with learning disabilities tend to experience more failure and receive more negative feedback. They also compare themselves unfavorably to their peers in terms of academic skills and performance. Schoolwork comes less easily to them and can sometimes seem impossible. Although many children with learning disabilities or attention issues are accepted by their peers, some become targets of teasing or bullying.

As a result, research suggests that children with learning disabilities tend to have lower self-esteem than their peers. After years of academic struggles and frustration, they often view themselves as being "stupid" or "slow" in comparison with other children. They tend to generalize these feelings and perceive themselves negatively in other areas of life as well. Due to low self-esteem, children with learning disabilities may lose interest in learning, develop self-defeating ways of dealing with challenges, and perform poorly, which only reinforces their low self-worth.

Ways Parents Can Impact Self-Esteem

Fortunately, parents, siblings, friends, teachers, and other influential people can help bolster children's self-esteem. Experts stress that it is possible for children to learn to improve the way they view themselves and their abilities. For parents of children with learning disabilities, being supportive yet realistic is the key to helping children build their self-esteem. While praise and positive feedback is important, it becomes meaningless if it is offered insincerely. When parents lavish praise on everything a child does, the child may begin to distrust it or overreact to negative feedback. Parents can incorporate the following suggestions to help children with learning disabilities develop higher self-esteem:

- Emphasize that the child is bright and healthy, and that they just have a deficit in a certain area of learning.

- Encourage the child's non-academic interests—such as art, music, or sports—and highlight their areas of strength—such as kindness or a sense of humor.

- Provide an example of how to value personal strengths while also acknowledging and working to improve upon weaknesses.

- Offer examples of successful people who have overcome learning disabilities and achieved their dreams.

- Express clear, realistic expectations instead of criticisms. For instance, instead of complaining that the child's room is always messy, ask the child to put away their toys and make their bed.

- Ensure that the child has plenty of opportunities to be successful.

- Help the child view mistakes as learning experiences for next time.

- Avoid comparing the child to other people—such as siblings or classmates—and only evaluate their performance in relation to previous efforts.

- Help the child develop positive strategies for learning and coping with challenges.

- Help the child build effective problem-solving and decision-making skills. Rather than providing solutions, help them brainstorm creative approaches and consider the possible consequences of each one.

- Teach the child to reframe negative statements.

- Help the child find friends who accept them and make them feel valued.

- Encourage the child to help others by volunteering in the community. Having something valuable to offer to other people bolsters self-esteem.

- Provide a safe haven where the child feels loved, appreciated, and supported. Studies show that children who are made to feel special by an adult develop increased hopefulness and resilience.

Self-esteem is a tremendous asset to help children manage learning disabilities successfully. Parents can play an important role in building self-confidence and empowering children with learning disabilities to overcome the challenges they face.

References

1. Cunningham, Bob. "The Importance of Self-Esteem for Kids with Learning and Attention Issues," Understood, 2016.

2. Lyons, Aoife. "Self-Esteem and Learning Disabilities," Learning Disabilities Association of Illinois, 2012.

3. Tracey, Danielle. "Self-Esteem and Children's Learning Problems," Learning Links, November 2012.

Chapter 46

Life Skills for Teens and Young Adults with Learning Disabilities

Overview

Although young people with learning disabilities or attention deficit hyperactivity disorder (ADHD) often face academic challenges, research indicates that problem-solving abilities and life skills may provide better indicators of future happiness and success than school grades. The key attributes, according to researchers, are social, emotional, and ethical literacy. These characteristics enable people to be creative problem solvers, flexible learners, and good decision makers in their adult lives. Parents can teach these skills and competencies through their words and actions. For instance, parents who engage in positive self-talk and model creative problem-solving strategies can help promote those capabilities in their teenagers. Young people with learning disabilities or ADHD can also benefit from training in specific life skills such as cooking, managing finances, and driving in order to increase their ability to function independently.

"Life Skills for Teens and Young Adults with Learning Disabilities," © 2016 Omnigraphics. Reviewed June 2016.

Cooking Skills

Cooking is a basic functional skill that is required for young people to become independent adults and enjoy a good quality of life. For teenagers with learning disabilities or ADHD, the process of determining what they need for a recipe, making a shopping list, obtaining ingredients, following directions, and preparing meals provides valuable real-life practice in math and reading skills.

In teaching young people with learning disabilities how to cook, it is important to choose recipes that offer the opportunity to touch on various educational goals. Cooking can allow students to work on such challenges as prioritizing tasks and performing them in sequence, reading charts, measuring, and keeping track of time. All of these skills can be generalized to other life tasks. To maintain student motivation, it may be helpful to allow them to choose a food item that they like to eat and are likely to want to prepare at home.

The first step in the process of cooking is making a shopping list and purchasing the ingredients. Students might type the list of ingredients into a computer or use an app that generates a shopping list and includes photos of the various items. At the grocery store, students can be made familiar with the general layout of the store and assisted in identifying the aisles where different items can be found. Students should take responsibility for collecting the items, crossing them off the list, and purchasing the items.

The most important part of teaching cooking skills to young people with learning disabilities is providing directions in a way that they can understand. Depending on the student's disabilities, the recipe may need to be in large print or include photo instructions. Once the student masters the basic steps in cooking, such as using the oven and other kitchen tools, measuring ingredients, chopping, and mixing, they will be able to apply these skills to future recipes.

Managing Finances

Managing money and banking can be difficult for young adults with learning disabilities or ADHD. Teens who tend to behave impulsively, for instance, may have trouble sticking to a budget due to repeated spur-of-the-moment purchases. Similarly, young people who struggle with organization may experience problems in keeping bills and bank statements straight or balancing their checkbook. People with visual processing issues may invert or misalign numbers in check registers, leading to errors in computing the balance.

Parents can help teens with learning disabilities or ADHD avoid some of these problems by teaching and practicing money management skills. Some tips for helping young people gain competence in handling financial matters include the following:

- During the early teen years, parents should help the young person create a basic weekly budget. List sources of income—such as an allowance or earnings from chores or jobs—and anticipated expenses, including clothing, entertainment, snacks, and miscellaneous expenses. Use separate envelopes for each budget category and place enough cash in each envelope at the beginning of the week to cover the anticipated expenses.

- Parents should set up a desk or table where the young person can keep all the tools needed to manage financial matters successfully, such as pencils, paper, calculator, stapler, tape, paper clips, envelopes, and stamps. Also equip the space with an accordion file or file drawer to organize papers under different headings and a calendar to record the due dates of bills.

- By the end of high school, teens should learn the skills of using a checkbook and paying bills. Carbon checks may be helpful to provide a sample of a properly completed check and to ensure that all transactions are recorded. Some teens may prefer to manage money by using software such as Quicken or online banking services.

- When a young person reaches the age of eighteen, they should learn about the benefits and drawbacks of credit cards. Starting with a card with a low limit from a reputable bank, the teenager should be taught to pay monthly bills in full to avoid interest charges and establish a good credit history.

- Parents should also take teens with them to a variety of retail stores to help them gain consumer skills, such as locating items they commonly use, asking for assistance, and making purchases.

- Parents should also teach young people about the general workings of contracts, such as apartment leases, cell phone agreements, and gym memberships.

- Finally, parents should discuss the etiquette surrounding tipping for good service from restaurant servers, hotel bellhops, cab drivers, hair stylists, and other providers. Explain how to determine the amount of the tip and have the young person help calculate it.

Using Public Transportation and Driving

People with learning disabilities and ADHD can become socially isolated without access to transportation options. Public transportation, where available, enables people with learning disabilities to gain independence and control over their lives. It may also increase opportunities for socialization and participation in the community. Yet people with learning disabilities face some barriers to using public transportation. Travel information, such as route maps and timetables, is often presented in a way that is hard for people with learning disabilities to understand. In addition, many people with learning disabilities lack confidence or fear for their safety while using public transportation. Transport services offered by government agencies may inspire greater confidence, but they often are not flexible enough to facilitate independent living. Proposals to resolve these problems include improving maps and timetables and assigning "travel buddies" to help increase young people's confidence as they grow accustomed to using public transportation.

Learning to drive a personal automobile can provide a great deal of independence for teenagers. For those with learning and attention issues, however, driving may create unique challenges. Young people with ADHD, for instance, may struggle to tune out distractions and focus on the road. Those with impulsivity may overestimate their driving abilities or drive too fast, which puts them at risk for accidents. Dyslexia and other reading issues can create problems for teens behind the wheel, as well. They may find it difficult to read road signs, scan the dashboard for information, or use a map or GPS device to plan a route. Other learning issues can affect a teenager's ability to see where objects are positioned in space, whether in relation to themselves or to other objects. They may experience challenges in judging distances, reading maps, or telling left from right. Recognizing these challenges enables parents to put strategies and supports in place to help teens with learning disabilities to become safe and successful drivers.

References

1. Cohen, Jonathan, and Eve Kessler. "Life Skills That Make a Difference," Smart Kids, n.d.

2. Debenham, Lucy. "Transport for People with Learning Disabilities," About Learning Disabilities, February 14, 2014.

3. "Dollars and Sense: Financial Skills for Teens with Learning Disabilities," GreatSchools, June 22, 2015.

4. Pulsifer, Lisa. "Teaching Cooking Skills to Students with Intellectual Disabilities," Bright Hub Education, January 7, 2012.

5. Rosen, Peg. "How Learning and Attention Issues Can Impact Driving," Understood, October 22, 2015.

Chapter 47

Transition to Adulthood

Chapter Contents

Section 47.1

Adult Transition Services

This section contains text excerpted from the following sources:
Text beginning with the heading "A Quick Summary of Transition"
is excerpted from "Transition to Adulthood," Center for Parent
Information and Resources (CPIR), October 2014; Text beginning
with the heading "Adult Services: What Are They? Where Are They?"
is excerpted from "Adult Services: What Are They? Where Are They?"
Center for Parent Information and Resources (CPIR), October 2014.

A Quick Summary of Transition Services

- Transition services are intended to prepare students to move from the world of school to the world of adulthood.

- Transition planning begins during high school at the latest.

- Individuals with Disabilities Education Act (IDEA) requires that transition planning start by the time the student reaches age 16.

- Transition planning may start earlier (when the student is younger than 16) if the Individualized Education Program (IEP) team decides it would be appropriate to do so.

- Transition planning takes place as part of developing the student's IEP.

- The IEP team (which includes the student and the parents) develops the transition plan.

- The student must be invited to any IEP meeting where postsecondary goals and transition services needed to reach those goals will be considered.

- In transition planning, the IEP team considers areas such as postsecondary education or vocational training, employment, independent living, and community participation.

- Transition services must be a coordinated set of activities oriented toward producing results.

- Transition services are based on the student's needs and must take into account his or her preferences and interests.

IDEA's Definition of Transition Services

Any discussion of transition services must begin with its definition in law.

Transition services means a coordinated set of activities for a child with a disability that—

- Is designed to be within a results-oriented process, that is focused on improving the academic and functional achievement of the child with a disability to facilitate the child's movement from school to post-school activities, including postsecondary education, vocational education, integrated employment (including supported employment), continuing and adult education, adult services, independent living, or community participation;

- Is based on the individual child's needs, taking into account the child's strengths, preferences, and interests; and includes—

  - Instruction;

  - Related services;

  - Community experiences;

  - The development of employment and other post-school adult living objectives; and

  - If appropriate, acquisition of daily living skills and provision of a functional vocational evaluation.

Transition services for children with disabilities may be special education, if provided as specially designed instruction, or a related service, if required to assist a child with a disability to benefit from special education.

Considering the Definition

A number of keywords in the definition above capture important concepts about transition services:

- Activities need to be **coordinated** with each other.

- The process focuses on **results**.

- Activities must address the child's **academic and functional achievement.**

- Activities are intended to smooth the young person's movement into the post-school world.

You can also see that the definition mentions the domains of independent and adult living. The community employment adult services daily living skills vocational postsecondary education. This clearly acknowledges that adulthood involves a wide range of skills areas and activities. It also makes clear that preparing a child with a disability to perform functionally across this spectrum of areas and activities may involve considerable planning, attention, and focused, coordinated services.

Transition activities should not be haphazard or scattershot. Services are to be planned as in sync with one another in order to drive toward a result.

What result might that be? From a federal perspective, the result being sought can be found in the very first finding of Congress in IDEA, which refers to "our national policy of ensuring equality of opportunity, full participation, independent living, and economic self-sufficiency for individuals with disabilities." Preparing children with disabilities to "lead productive and independent adult lives, to the maximum extent possible" is one of IDEA's stated objectives.

Students at the Heart of Planning Their Transition

For the students themselves, transition activities are **personally defined**. This means that the postsecondary goals that are developed for a student must take into account his or her interests, preferences, needs, and strengths. To make sure of this, the school:

- must invite the youth with a disability to attend Individualized Education Program (IEP) team meeting "if a purpose of the meeting will be the consideration of the postsecondary goals for the child and the transition services needed to assist the child in reaching those goals under," and

- "must take other steps to ensure that the child's preferences and interests are considered" if the child is not able to attend.

As you keep reading below, keep the importance of student involvement in mind, because there are many excellent materials and guides available to help students become involved in their own transition planning...and many good reasons to do so.

When Must Transition Services Be Included in the IEP?

What's not apparent in IDEA's definition of transition services but nonetheless critical to mention is the timing of transition-related planning and services: When must transition planning begin?

The answer lies in a different provision related to the content of the IEP:

- **Transition services**. Beginning not later than the first IEP to be in effect when the child turns 16, or younger if determined appropriate by the IEP Team, and updated annually, thereafter, the IEP must include—

  - Appropriate measurable postsecondary goals based upon age appropriate transition assessments related to training, education, employment, and, where appropriate, independent living skills; and

  - The transition services (including courses of study) needed to assist the child in reaching those goals.

So, the IEP must include transition goals by the time the student is 16. That age frame, though, is not cast in concrete. Note that, in keeping with the individualized nature of the IEP, the IEP team has the authority to begin transition-related considerations earlier in a student's life, if team members (which include the parent and the student with a disability) think it is appropriate, given the student's needs and preferences.

A Closer Look at What to Include in the IEP

Breaking the provisions into their component parts is a useful way to see what needs to be included, transition-wise, in the student's IEP. This is also where the rubber meets the road, so to speak, because what's included in the IEP must:

- state the student's postsecondary goals (what he or she hopes to achieve after leaving high school);

- be broken down into IEP goals that represent the steps along the way that the student needs to take while still in high school to get ready for achieving the postsecondary goals after high school; and

- detail the transition services that the student will receive to support his or her achieving the IEP goals.

Writing goal statements can be a challenging business, because it's not always obvious what needs to be included in a goal statement. Goal-writing is a topic worthy of an entire discussion on its own.

The Domains of Adulthood to Consider

The definition of transition services mentions specific domains of adulthood to be addressed during transition planning. These are:

- postsecondary education,
- vocational education,
- integrated employment (including supported employment),
- continuing and adult education,
- adult services,
- independent living, or
- community participation.

These are the areas to be explored by the IEP team to determine what types of transition-related support and services a student with a disability needs. It's easy to see how planning ahead in each of these areas, and developing goal statements and corresponding services for the student, can greatly assist that student in preparing for life after high school.

Types of Activities to Consider

- Instruction;
- Related services;
- Community experiences;
- The development of employment and other post-school adult living objectives; and
- If appropriate, acquisition of daily living skills and provision of a functional vocational evaluation.

The IEP team must discuss and decide whether the student needs transition services and activities (e.g., instruction, related services, community experiences, etc.) to prepare for the different domains of adulthood (postsecondary education, vocational education, employment, adult services, independent living, etc.) That's a lot of ground to cover!

But it's essential ground, if the student's transition to the adult world is to be facilitated. A spectrum of adult activities is evident here, from community to employment, from being able to take care of oneself (e.g., daily living skills) to considering other adult objectives and undertakings.

Adult Services: What Are They? Where Are They?

Many different individuals come together to help the student plan for transition. Typically, transition planning is handled by members of the IEP team, with other individuals becoming involved as needed. It's important to involve a variety of people, for they will bring their unique perspectives to the planning table. The team draws upon the expertise of the different members and pools their information to make decisions or recommendations for the student.

In addition to the regular players at the IEP table (parents, student, special education and general education teachers, related service providers, administrators, others), when transition is going to be discussed, representatives of outside agencies may be invited, especially those who are well informed about resources and adult services in the community. Here's a list of four different agencies to consider, plus the ever-useful "Other" category. Each is discussed in some detail further below.

1. Vocational Rehabilitation Agency (VR)

2. Service agencies operating programs and services for individuals with intellectual disabilities or mental health concerns

3. Independent living centers (ILCs)

4. Social Security Administration (SSA)

5. Others to consider involving

The Vocational Rehabilitation (VR) Agency

The Vocational Rehabilitation (VR) agency has traditionally been a primary player in determining the way transition services are delivered. Typically, VR helps persons with cognitive, sensory, physical, or emotional disabilities to find employment and achieve increased independence. Funded by Federal and state money, VR agencies typically operate regional and local offices. VR services usually last for a limited period of time and are based on an individual's rehabilitation plan. If needed, an individual with disabilities can request services at a later time, and a new rehabilitation plan will be developed.

VR has its own eligibility requirements. Therefore, not all students receiving special education services can receive VR services. You will need to check with the VR agency in your own area to learn what eligibility requirements apply.

Examples of **employment services** that may be available through VR include:

- vocational guidance and counseling

- medical, psychological, vocational, and other types of assessments to determine vocational potential

- job development, placement, and follow-up services

- rehabilitation, technological services and adaptive devices, tools, equipment, and supplies

Examples of *postsecondary education services* that may be available through VR include:

- apprenticeship programs, usually in conjunction with Department of Labor (DOL)

- vocational training

- college training towards a vocational goal as part of an eligible student's financial aid package

Examples of **independent living and adult services** that may be available through VR include:

- housing or transportation supports needed to maintain employment

- interpreter services

- orientation and mobility services

Service Agencies for Individuals with Intellectual Disabilities or Mental Health Concerns

Depending on the student's individual needs, it may be important for the transition team to include representatives from service agencies addressing intellectual disabilities or mental health. These agencies provide a comprehensive system of services responsive to the needs of individuals with mental health concerns or intellectual disabilities.

Federal, state, and local funding are used to operate regional offices; local funding is often the primary source. Services are provided on a sliding payment scale.

Examples of employment-related services often available through these service agency include supported and sheltered employment, and competitive employment support for those who need minimal assistance.

Examples of independent living and adult services you may find available include:

- case management services to access and obtain local services
- therapeutic recreation, including day activities, clubs, and programs
- respite care
- residential services (group homes and supervised apartments)

The services provided by these agencies, however, vary greatly from community to community due to differences in local funding and priorities. Again, you will need to check with your state's agencies that offer such services.

Independent Living Centers (ILCs)

Independent Living Centers (ILCs) are nonresidential, community-based agencies that are run by people with various disabilities. ILCs help people with disabilities achieve and maintain self-sufficient lives within the community. Operated locally, ILCs serve a particular region, which means that their services vary from place to place. ILCs may charge for classes, but advocacy services are typically available at no cost.

Social Security Administration (SSA)

The Social Security Administration (SSA) operates the federally funded program that provides benefits for people of any age who are unable to do substantial work and have a severe mental or physical disability. Several programs are offered for people with disabilities, including:

- Social Security Disability Insurance (SSDI)
- Supplemental Security Income (SSI)
- Plans to Achieve Self-Support (PASS)

- Medicaid

- Medicare

Examples of employment services that may be available through SSA work incentive programs may include

- cash benefits while working (e.g., student-earned income)

- Medicare or Medicaid while working

- help with any extra work expenses the individual has as a result of the disability

- assistance to start a new line of work

With respect to adult and independent living services, SSA programs may support medical benefits, as well as allow the individual to use income as basis for purchase or rental of housing.

SSA can be a great source of support and assistance to youth with disabilities as they leave high school and move into adulthood. It's very important for a student's transition team to investigate whether or not the student is eligible for any of SSA's programs and, if so, to involve SSA as part of transition planning.

Others to Consider Involving in Transition Planning

Other individuals or agencies may serve as one-time or ongoing consultants to the team, sharing a particular expertise or insight, while others may be valuable sources of specific information that helps the team plan and make decisions. Consider the useful information to be gained from any of the following:

Postsecondary education and training providers such as representatives from colleges, or trade schools, who can help the student explore types of training available as well as remind the group that lifelong learning for all individuals is important.

Department of Labor job services agencies, which offer transition services and employment programs, many of which are meant for individuals with disabilities (although others may not have a disability focus).

One-Stop program representatives, who can tell the team about job training available under the Workforce Investment Act (WIA) to help students prepare for their first job or further education and training.

Community leaders such as religious leaders, directors of recreation programs, and county extension agents, who may help the team address a particular need that a student has;

Community recreation centers such as Boys Clubs, YMCA, or 4-H Clubs, which may provide job counseling and youth development activities.

Employers, who can provide training and job opportunities and who can explain the expectations that the business community has for future workers.

Team members do not necessarily have to come from social service agencies. Students and their families may also invite a relative, friend, or advocate who can provide emotional support, access to their personal networks, or other unique expertise. If possible, it is also helpful to have team members from similar language and cultural backgrounds as the student. These members can help the team understand how cultural or language issues impact the transition process. Some typical transition outcomes, such as going away to college, getting a paying job, moving out of the family home, and making decisions independently of the family are valued differently by different cultures.

It is very important to invite service representatives and other individuals identified as transition consultants to IEP meetings that will be focused on only transition. They do not need to be at every IEP meeting of the student. If they cannot attend the meetings focusing on transition, talk to them about the IEP and bring their ideas or comments to the meeting.

Section 47.2

Employment Services

This section includes text excerpted from "Employment Connections," Center for Parent Information and Resources (CPIR), February 2016.

Employment Connections

For many youth with disabilities looking ahead to life after high school, employment will be an immediate and serious consideration. And the time to consider it well and thoroughly is during the high school years, during transition planning, and through transition services that are carefully matched to the goal of employment.

Getting Started

First, is employment a goal the student has for himself or herself? In what area or domain might he or she be interested? There are so many possibilities when you think about having a job, it's important for students to identify what types of jobs are suited to their interests, needs, and preferences. This alone can involve quite an inquiry, but it's a very important beginning link in the chain of planning.

Understanding the Network That's Out There to Help

There's nothing like knowing the players in the field. They are excellent sources of help, info, tools, and connections.

Reasonable Accommodations in the Workplace

Many individuals with disabilities need accommodations and support in the workplace. Here are two premier resources that can help you learn what's considered "reasonable," what types of accommodations can be made, and where employers can tap into specialized free guidance about accommodations.

What about a Job Coach?

Job coaches play an important role in the workplace for many people with disabilities, especially those whose disabilities are severe. These professionals help the new employee learn the job and how to navigate the world of work. Support may be for a limited period of time or provided on an ongoing basis, depending on the needs of the individual. Connectability (mentioned above) gives the following suggestions to parents: "Here's how you can help determine whether a job coach may be appropriate for your son or daughter:

- As you work with your son or daughter's IEP Team to develop work opportunities and career exploration opportunities, be sure to ask if job coaching is appropriate and how your school can provide it.

- When your son or daughter starts volunteering (or working after school, or in the summer), look for natural supports (someone already working at the site, or willing to provide some of the activities listed for a job coach).

- If your son or daughter has trouble keeping a job or being successful on-the-job, consider whether a job coach might be helpful, and talk with your son or daughter about exploring this option."

Supported Employment (SE)

You may hear the term "supported employment" used to describe a range of supports that an individual with disabilities may receive at work, but the term actually is most closely associated with its use in the Rehabilitation Act of 1973, as amended. In that context, supported employment is an approach to addressing the employment needs of individuals with the most significant disabilities, those–

- for whom competitive employment has not traditionally occurred; or

- for whom competitive employment has been interrupted or intermittent as a result of a significant disability; and

- who, because of the nature and severity of their disability, need intensive supported employment services in order to perform designated work.

For many youth, especially those with significant disabilities, supported employment may be important to consider and pursue. Such services are typically available through vocational rehabilitation programs, but Vocational Rehabilitation (VR) is not the only place you'll find supported employment in operation. SE is considered a "place and train" model: the individual receives job-specific training after placement, rather than prevocational training before placement.

Section 47.3

Independent Living

This section includes text excerpted from "Independent Living Connections," Center for Parent Information and Resources (CPIR), February 2016.

Independent Living Connections

Independent living is about life, isn't it? It's about choice, seeing to your own affairs, and pursuing your talents, interests, passions, and selfhood as independently as possible. We all would like to see our young people grow to adulthood and find their place in the world, doing for themselves to the best of their ability.

Disability can complicate independence, to be sure, which is why independent living can be an important part of helping a young person with a disability get ready for life after high school. The more involved the disability, the more likely it is that independent living will be a subject of serious discussion—and preparation.

This resource page is designed to help you and yours take apart the concept of independent living, examine its many elements, and put the concept back together again with concrete plans and insight into what it takes to turn the concept into reality.

Philosophical Underpinnings

One search of the web using the term "independent living" and it's clear to see that a great deal of passion and commitment exists in the independent living movement and community. It's rather breath-taking, in fact. You'll see phrases like: all people achieving their maximum potential, barrier-free society, self-determination, self-respect, dignity, and equal opportunities, consumer-driven, empowerment. At its heart, the passion in the independent living community is fueled by individuals with disabilities themselves. And it's worldwide, this passion for selfhood. Consider this statement found on the website of the Independent Living Institute in Sweden.

Independent Living does not mean that we want to do everything by ourselves and do not need anybody or that we want to live in isolation. Independent Living means that we demand the same choices and control in our every-day lives that our non-disabled brothers and sisters, neighbors and friends take for granted. We want to grow up in our families, go to the neighborhood school, use the same bus as our neighbors, work in jobs that are in line with our education and interests, and start families of our own. We are profoundly ordinary people sharing the same need to feel included, recognized, and loved.

Defining Independent Living

The National Secondary Transition and Technical Assistance Center (NSTTAC) posts the following definition of independent living.

Independent Living or life skills are defined as "those skills or tasks that contribute to the successful independent functioning of an individual in adulthood" (Cronin, 1996) in the following domains: leisure/recreation, home maintenance and personal care, and community participation.

So now we have yet more domains of adulthood, all these related to independent living:

- leisure/recreation

- home maintenance and personal care

- community participation

Each of these, of course, has its own aspects and concerns that the Individualized Education Program (IEP) team will want to consider and plan ahead for, as appropriate for the student's needs and plans. We'll talk in a moment about what any one of these areas might involve, in terms of learning concrete skills.

463

Does the Student Need Transition Planning and Services in the Domain of Independent Living?

It's important to understand that not all students with disabilities will need an in depth investigation of, and preparation for, independent living after high school. As the Department of Education stated in its Analysis of Comments and Changes:

The only area in which postsecondary goals are not required in the IEP is in the area of independent living skills. Goals in the area of independent living are required only if appropriate. It is up to the child's IEP Team to determine whether IEP goals related to the development of independent living skills are appropriate and necessary for the child to receive FAPE.

Whether or not will very much depend on the nature and severity of the student's disability. As the Department notes, it's up to each student's IEP team to decide if planning for independent living is needed. If the team feels that the student can benefit from transition planning and services in this domain, then independent living will be an area of discussion during IEP meetings where transition is discussed.

If the student with whom you are involved is going to need transition planning and services in the domain of independent living, then keep reading.

What's Involved in Independent Living?

Independent living clearly involves quite a range of activities, skills, and learning needs. Consider just the three mentioned in the definition posted at NSTTAC: leisure/recreation, home maintenance and personal care, and community participation. Each of these can be broken down in its own turn to include yet more skills, activities, and learning needs. Just think about what's involved in "home maintenance and personal care" alone. Everything from brushing teeth to shopping for food to cooking it to cleaning up afterwards, to getting ready for bed, locking the front door, and setting the alarm clock for the next day. It's enough to boggle the mind, all the little facets and skills of taking care of ourselves as best we can, with support or solo.

So how is an IEP team to take on the task of planning for a student's independent living in the future? Much will depend on the nature and severity of the student's disability. Some students will not need transition planning or services to prepare for independent living. Others will need a limited amount, targeted at specific areas of need or interest. And still others, especially those with significant support needs, will need to give independent living their focused attention.

Fortunately, a great deal has been written about the skills of independent living, and we won't reinvent that wheel. Have a look at some of these resources. They'll more than give you food for thought about what to consider for yourself or yours, as will any local or state policy at work in your area.

Independent Living Centers (ILCs)

One of the most useful resources in the independent living area are the nationwide network of independent living centers (ILCs). ILCs are nonresidential, community-based agencies that are run by people with various disabilities. ILCs help people with disabilities achieve and maintain self-sufficient lives within the community. Operated locally, ILCs serve a particular region, which means that their services vary from place to place. ILCs may charge for classes, but advocacy services are typically available at no cost.

Other Resources to Explore

There really are too many organizations and associations to be fair about listing any. The ones we've identified below, listed in alphabetical order, will lead you into specific lines of investigation, such as the need for transportation, a personal assistant, a service animal, or other support for living independently. Pursue the resources that seem relevant to your student's needs and interests. There, you'll find links to many other organizations also interested in independent living, the participation of individuals with disabilities in community life, and the the self-determination to live life as fully and inclusively as possible.

Chapter 48

Employment Issues for People with Learning Disabilities

Chapter Contents

Section 48.1

Youth with Learning Disabilities: The Challenges

This section includes text excerpted from "Literacy, Employment and Youth with Learning Disabilities," Literacy Information and Communication System (LINCS), U.S. Department of Education (ED), September 2010. Reviewed June 2016.

Overview

Youth with learning disabilities (LD) face multiple challenges that complicate their training and learning trajectories. This section provides an overview of how learning disabilities impact employment and literacy development for youth.

Characteristics

Learning disabilities are a group of disorders that can impact many areas of learning, including reading, reading comprehension, writing, spelling, math, listening, oral expression, information processing, and organization, with reading difficulties being the most common. Youth with LD demonstrate different types and degrees of difficulties and strengths. Learning disabilities are lifelong; they are not outgrown and often impact individuals in the workplace. It is important to note that many youth with LD lack a clear understanding of their disability and its potential impact on their ability to perform a job. As a result, many make poor career choices.

Employment Challenges

Being an employee is just one valued adult role, but it is a significant indicator of adult success and autonomy in the United States. Working is how people contribute to their communities and to the economy. The National Longitudinal Transition Study 2 (NLTS-2) (2003) findings indicate between 57 and 69 percent of youth with LD have the goal to attain competitive employment in their individualized education program (IEP), and 43 percent would like to attend a vocational training program. While they value and strive for employment success, youth with LD often experience difficulties and require interventions in the workplace. The NLTS-2 found that only 46 percent of youth with LD actually had regular paid employment within two years of leaving high school. Studies by Kaye and Reder suggest that youth with LD experience high rates of unemployment and underemployment, fewer work hours, lower wages, and lower annual incomes as adults than their nondisabled peers.

According to the National Center for Learning Disabilities (NCLD), there are five common reasons why youth with LD experience challenges at work:

1. **Efficiency**: Slow pace of work, difficulties with organization

2. **Accuracy**: High error rate associated with reading tasks and/or written correspondence

3. **Sequencing of tasks**: Problems following instructions or completing projects with multiple steps

4. **Time management**: Trouble with planning, being on time or meeting deadlines

5. **Social skills**: Problems with meeting new people, with professional interactions and with discussing the impact of LD on tasks to be completed

These are some of the predominant issues that limit the success of workers with LD, many of whom also struggle with "soft" skills and self-determination or empowerment skills.

Soft Skills. According to the 2006 report "Are They Really Ready to Work?" while the "three R's" (reading, writing, and arithmetic) are still fundamental to every employee's ability to do the job, employers view "soft" skills as even more important to work readiness. Youth frequently lack these skills, which include collaboration skills, critical thinking, problem solving, and oral and written communication skills. This report supports the previous findings of Gerber and Gerber and Brown that unemployment and underemployment for individuals with LD is often tied to their deficits in social competency. According to Gerber (n.d.), social skills are an important underpinning for success in any employment setting. What youth "need to know" has been gathered from employers and industry into the Secretary's Commission on Achieving Necessary Skills (SCANS) report from the U.S. Department of Labor (DOL) and widely circulated among education and workforce programs. These nonacademic limitations may have a greater adverse impact on achieving and maintaining employment than those associated with poor academic performance.

Self-Determination. The employment cycle characteristic of youth with LD is in part due to a lack of a focus on self-determination and empowerment by teachers, transition specialists, workplace programs and the youth themselves. Most youth and adults with LD do not receive needed accommodations on the job because they have chosen not to disclose their disability to their employer, reflecting a lack of self-awareness, self-determination, and self-advocacy. Self-disclosure to employers by working youth occurs only approximately four percent of the time. Many more youth do not accept that they have a learning disability or understand how it may impact their workplace performance, and therefore do not disclose their disability or request accommodations, leading to an unproductive working situation.

Section 48.2

Meeting the Needs of Youth with LD in Workplace Programs

This section includes text excerpted from "Literacy, Employment and Youth with Learning Disabilities," Literacy Information and Communication System (LINCS), U.S. Department of Education (ED), September 2010. Reviewed June 2016.

In response to the numerous challenges that systems and professionals face in their efforts to transition youth with learning disabilities (LD) to the workplace, the literature identifies four specific program elements that can assist in this effort: professional development; literacy development; technology supports; and youth self-determination and empowerment. By contextualizing and reinforcing these elements, we can help youth with LD gain the skills and confidence they need to become 21st-century workers.

Professional Development Collaboratives

High-quality professional development of existing staff can lead to better practice with youth, improve program quality and increase the positive outcomes of youth. But for professional development to be considered high quality and have the impact the planners envision, it must be much more than the typical decontextualized one-time workshops without follow-up. High-quality professional development that leads to sustained change in practitioners' habits and practice must be content focused, incorporate active learning for participants, be consistent with participants' goals and other program initiatives, and be part of an ongoing learning initiative.

Throughout the field of workforce development, there seems to be little professional training available for youth service practitioners and no formal system for accessing the training that is available. Research shows that most youth service practitioners do not have access to coherent education, training and professional development opportunities that can prepare them for this work. Similarly, despite the availability of national standards for preparation of transition specialists, there are too few professionals trained to fill transition specialist positions and too few training programs. The result is that too many transition specialists are serving without proper credentials and training.

Effective professional development can be accomplished through local or regional cooperatives that represent strengths and expertise in workplace training, adolescent literacy, technology integration, disability services, and professional development delivery. An established, strategic team approach to professional development that builds ownership and provides ongoing support has proved much more effective than purchased workshops by outside experts and consultants. A team approach can develop when an active partnership and joint planning among programs and providers are in place to create shared practices.

The Next Generation Youth Work Coalition recently conducted a scan of more than 70 federal programs and 15 state systems' programs and funding priorities to identify potential areas of support for workforce development and youth-serving professionals. While overall they found funding and system-spanning infrastructure support sorely lacking for youth-serving organizations, they did find communities with successful cross-agency networks. The report, which details a variety of state examples, shows how professional development cooperatives can be established and funded.

Professional Development to Reinforce Literacy Learning

A handful of big ideas in adolescent literacy research can inform how workforce development programs approach this topic to design programs for youth, build strategic partnerships and plan professional development. Research suggests that programs and instructors should pay particular attention to the interrelated big ideas of background knowledge and vocabulary, comprehension strategies, the synergies of reading and writing, and interest and motivation.

Although workforce development professionals are not expected to become reading specialists, through their work, they should reinforce, extend and contextualize the literacy instruction youth are receiving elsewhere. This section provides an overview of these areas of literacy instruction and how workforce professionals might provide reinforcement.

Background knowledge and vocabulary. Youth who struggle with academics, including those with LD, will likely benefit from focused attention on their background knowledge and vocabulary as part of literacy instruction. As youth move from general survey courses in secondary school to more in-depth disciplines and career training topics, specific background knowledge and vocabulary assumed in reading materials and preparation tasks become even more important. Pre Teaching and making explicit the background knowledge and vocabulary assumptions needed for success in a training program are keys to helping youth engage the material thoughtfully. This is especially true for students who are English language learners; even if their oral English is quite proficient, the content areas and specific job-related vocabularies are often completely unfamiliar. Learners with LD need explicit, multisensory instruction that helps them connect new vocabulary with the sounds and spelling patterns, and need many opportunities to use and hear new words in context.

Workforce development providers can coordinate with literacy providers to share lists of expectations for background knowledge and vocabulary related to specific programs and courses. Programs can also make vocabulary learning a program wide, strategic effort to give learners the context and reinforcement they need to learn.

Comprehension strategies. All students benefit from ongoing comprehension strategy instruction throughout their academic careers as the texts and expectations continue to change dramatically across content areas (a biology lab report is constructed and written quite differently than a history text, for example). The same is true for vocational preparation and workplace literacies. How texts are constructed, the key structural phrases and words, and the unique vocabularies of specific disciplines contribute to the unique "academic literacies" of each discipline.

A variety of comprehension strategies are appropriate for all readers, but struggling readers often have a very limited repertoire. They need explicit modeling and guided practice to learn new strategies or to apply different strategies appropriate for specific texts (Torgesen et al., 2007). Supporting and reinforcing comprehension instruction youth receive in academic settings requires a deliberate increase in the amount and quality of time devoted to open, sustained discussion of reading content. Far from watering down expectations, this recommendation calls on instructors of all types of courses to increase the intellectual intensity with which they engage their learners in discussions of text and modeling of comprehension. This discussion time can be used to model and role-play thoughtful, respectful workplace conversations and critical thinking skills—soft skills that struggling students often lack and that workforce development programs are keen to impart.

Learners with LD have difficulty in comprehension for a variety of reasons. They may struggle to decode the text, stay focused, monitor their comprehension, make inferences or generalize to the larger reading purpose. They need many opportunities to experience guided practice, hear strategies modeled and be prompted to employ appropriate strategies. Workforce development providers can coordinate planning with partnering literacy providers to reinforce a shared set of comprehension strategies and teaching vocabulary.

Synergy of reading and writing. Just as academic literacies challenge reading comprehension, they also challenge learners' writing proficiencies. While students may be able to write a personal narrative or creative story, they may struggle to construct an acceptable technical report or daily event log. Explicit writing instruction and guided practice reinforce vocabulary and comprehension strategies to help learners generalize and internalize the academic literacies and gain confidence with them. And while reading and writing are complementary processes, struggling writers, especially those with LD, need explicit strategy instruction and guided practice to become proficient and flexible writers. The underdeveloped writing skills of many adult education students and even GED graduates are considered a major barrier to workplace and postsecondary success.

In addition, skills youth need for the workplace include the ability to write for multiple audiences and purposes, alone or collaboratively, and to use a variety of tools and platforms to do so. Learners with LD commonly continue to struggle with many of the components of writing, including spelling, handwriting, planning, revising and editing. As with reading comprehension, workforce development providers can coordinate planning with partnering literacy providers to reinforce a shared set of writing strategies and approaches, including the use of similar technologies.

Interest and motivation. Interest and motivation are absolutely key to learning, and youth with LD who have experienced years of school failure may be reluctant to re-engage with any academic system. Yet youth with LD are as driven by their personal interests as their peers. Although they may need specific skill development, they also need strategy development and interesting, authentic contexts and content. Tapping into their interests, uncovered through informal conversations, assessments and observations, energizes their motivation to do the extra work required to succeed. In several studies of youth and adults, Fink found that even severely dyslexic students reported reading a significant amount of text and actively engaging in inquiry for extended periods when driven by their interests.

Contextualized workplace education programs draw on youths' interest in authentic learning because youth can see the value and direct applicability of the training to their jobs. In-house and on-the-job literacy development benefits both employers and employees, as its "applicability to real-world situations is immediate and highly effective", and it improves workplace productivity. Many youth with LD have difficulty generalizing reading skills to specific tasks, especially in the workplace. The use of contextual learning in the workplace, specific to the job tasks, can help them compensate.

Resources and technical assistance centers. Below are sources of additional information on adolescent literacy and learning disabilities, training materials and links to further professional learning opportunities:

Adolescent Literacy, www.AdLit.org, provides online articles and links to research-based information on instruction and supports for youth literacy development.

Carnegie Corporation of New York, www.carnegie. org, sponsors the Carnegie Council for Advancing Adolescent Literacy, which produces reports on how to advance literacy and learning for all students, including such topics as the cost of implementing adolescent literacy programs and reading in the disciplines.

The **International Reading Association,** www.reading.org, maintains a focus area for adolescent literacy and professional development resources and research.

LD OnLine, www.LDOnLine.org, offers hundreds of resources and articles specific to addressing the academic and life success of individuals with LD. The technology section hosts articles on how to integrate technology into teaching, learning, and independent living.

Literacy Matters, www.LiteracyMatters.org, hosts an online collection of professional development modules, archived workshops and resources addressing the instruction of adolescent literacy, and a section for activities for learners.

The Role of Technology to Support Youth With LD Digital literacy is crucial in the 21st-century workplace as businesses automate tasks and equipment; using digital means to communicate and collaborate is rapidly becoming an expected skill of workers and citizens in general. Ensuring that learners have the skills to use mainstream technologies productively is an important component of their preparation. For workers with LD, technology is essential. Youth in workforce development programs should be given explicit instruction and guided practice to become proficient with these technologies.

Technology can be used to differentiate instruction and services and to reinforce literacy learning. Through strategic program design, purchases and use, programs can create a more universally designed and flexible learning environment in which learners can gain familiarity with the types of mainstream technology tools that are available in the workplace and those that are available as specific accommodations. Options for online or computer-based courses in foundational skills and practice, high school credit recovery toward a diploma or specialized training can extend a program's menu of services. Below are suggestions for how programs might incorporate the use of various technologies that assist literacy acquisition and performance for learners with LD.

Equip a computer lab with a variety of mainstream and assistive technologies. Make these technologies available to all learners to use on assignments and for independent study. Provide orientation and ongoing guidance on their use through dedicated technology staff, volunteers, and peer tutors. Use the lab for professional development trainings on the equipment and to offer distance training for staff. Install keyboarding tutorials and challenge learners to improve their skills. Offer a variety of common adaptive input devices such as alternative keyboards and mouse types so that learners can "test drive" them. Ask vendors for demo copies of software and hardware, and encourage an atmosphere of exploration.

Customize learner profiles. Many users would benefit from learning how to customize software to meet their personal learning needs. Have technology staff work with learners to create unique profiles that take advantage of the accessibility features and settings of mainstream operating systems and software. For example, users who have visual impairments, dyslexia or who tire easily when reading will find that the following, simple adjustments may improve their ability to stay focused: enlarging or changing text fonts, changing contrasting colors of background to text, customizing a toolbar to remove distractions; increasing the size of the cursor or decreasing the speed at which it responds. Another simple customization is sequentially designed "hot keys" that decrease the number of keystrokes or sequences to be remembered or executed and help users navigate the computer. Other simple adjustments can be found at www.microsoft.com/enable/default.aspx and www.apple.com/accessibility/ma-cosx/vision.html.

Text-to-speech (TTS) software with electronic references. Literacy software with TTS and study skill features can help learners read and comprehend. Many learners with dyslexia have better listening comprehension than reading comprehension; providing TTS supports comprehension and vocabulary. Robust literacy software programs have study features such as highlighting, bookmarking, note-taking systems, dictionaries and pronunciation supports, and word processors. Using TTS with highlighting as the text is read provides a model of fluent reading, supports vocabulary development and frees attention for annotation and active comprehension.

Voice recognition software. For students who have severe dysgraphia or spelling disabilities that inhibit their writing, voice recognition software offers an alternative way to express their thoughts. Training times have been greatly reduced and accuracy increased in the latest generation of this technology. Although training the user on the software is still important and represents a time commitment, for some users, it is well worth it. Customize and create macros and templates for content-related tasks that will pre-fill information for common tasks and assignments.

Spell-checkers. Despite the ubiquity of spell-checkers in mainstream word processors, strategies to use them efficiently are rarely taught.

Install the program on all computers in the program. Teach how to use it and expect learners to access it. They should know how to attempt a spelling in order to generate a list of suggestions, how to skim the list of suggested words and how to check whether the correct word has been chosen. Teach learners how to use spell-checkers in conjunction with dictionaries, thesauruses, glossaries, and other reference sources and to listen to their writing through a text-to-speech program as a means of proofreading. Consider purchasing a program specifically designed to catch the common mistakes made by dyslexic writers. **Word prediction software** is built on common patterns of English writing and misspellings and has the ability to "learn" from a user's mistakes. These programs predict, offer a suggested next word or phrase and assist writers with poor spelling, poor motor control and difficulty with word recall.

Presentation and diagramming software. Encourage learners to represent what they know by offering them presentation software such as PowerPoint, simple Web pages or graphic organizers. Students who struggle with language can excel with visual representations when trained to use the programs. **Graphic organizer software with outlining and drafting capabilities** is a type of visual representation that makes relationships and concepts visible and can be used before or during reading to aid comprehension. By mapping relationships visually, abstract connections and sequences can be made explicit. Software programs that convert visual presentations to outline or draft views help learners convert their thinking into writing.

Electronic references such as dictionaries, thesauruses, encyclopedias, translation dictionaries, and reading pens. Definitions and explanations are now portable and immediate. Identify dictionaries and other online reference tools to use in the program, teach and model their use and expect learners to use them to develop vocabulary skills. Look for tools with TTS that read the word and the definitions and support word study. If the number of computers is limited, consider purchasing handheld devices with many of the same features. Encourage learners to acquire and use their own devices.

Resources to assist in technology planning. Below are sources of online technical assistance to guide programs in making wise technology purchases and implementation decisions:

- *Consumer Guide,* www.techmatrix.org/con- sumerGuides.aspx, is a decision support tool for administrators and purchasers of educational technology

- *Differentiating Instruction* Through Technology, www.airlearning.org, is a free, online professional development course that pairs technology tools and resources to concepts and principles of differentiating instruction to meet student needs

- *Disability Network,* www.disnetwork.org, provides a guide to incorporate accessible computer technology into One-Stop Career Centers

- *EdTech Locator,* www.EdTech Locator.org, provides a roadmap of technology integration that begins with an assessment of how programs currently use technology and suggests steps for deeper utilization

- *Tech Matrix,* www.TechMatrix.org, is a database of products reviewed for universal design and accessibility features with links to manufacturers' Web sites and a collection of research on the use of technology for instruction

- *Total Cost of Ownership toolkit,* www. classroomtco.org, provides a planner that assists purchasers to project maintenance, technical support and upgrade costs when considering various technology initiatives

Self-Determination with a Focus on Youth Empowerment

A youth-centered approach to workplace learning and literacy is a holistic way to serve youth that addresses their unique and often multiple needs while empowering them to make informed decisions about learning and work. An "empowerment approach" to literacy learning in the workplace recognizes that youth may have lost power and control over their lives owing to their disability or low literacy skills. They must develop an internal locus of control that places the responsibility for their actions with their own decisions and behaviors rather than outside forces or even their disability. Empowering youth with LD connotes a process of literally restoring their power by helping them to recognize and develop the skills and capacities for exercising some reasonable control over their lives and their decisions. To enable this process, professionals working with youth with LD need to create opportunities that challenge and guide youth to make decisions, experience the consequences and reflect on the results.

Self-determination training for youth with disabilities has become an important focus in special education and transition programs on the basis of research showing that self-determination skills are essential to the successful transition from school to work for individuals with disabilities. The concept of self-determination for students with disabilities includes several facets, such as self-awareness (awareness of strengths and weaknesses); self-advocacy (the ability to speak up and represent one's own needs and rights); self-efficacy or self-confidence; decision making; independent performance or self-management; self-evaluation or reflection; and adjustment. Two literature reviews on self-determination research found that self-determination is a predictor of successful transition to adult life and positive adult outcomes; that it is teachable through integrated curriculum and instruction; and that it is valued by teachers, students, and family members, who all see the benefits in independence, self-efficacy and self-management. Teaching these skills in the context of workforce training and guided employment promotes generalization of these skills.

As mentioned above, many youth with disabilities do not fully understand their legal rights to request accommodations in the workplace or postsecondary training environment. The shift in legal standing from entitlement under IDEA to eligibility under the ADA shifts the responsibility to the individual. Self-awareness and self- advocacy depend on knowledge. Youth with LD are often unclear about their own profiles of strengths and weaknesses and cannot articulate what accommodations may assist them. Those who are undiagnosed or misdiagnosed are at a greater disadvantage. Furthermore, youth may fear discrimination if they disclose a disability to an employer. It is important for workplace preparation professionals to offer clear and unambiguous training in this area.

Whether or not to self-disclose a disability and request accommodations at a training or employment site is an individual's decision, but youth need to consider the consequences. Disabilities need not be disclosed at the time of an interview unless they are required for a productive interview (e.g., an interpreter or accessible space). Programs can help youth explore the consequences of disclosing upon hire and can role-play the conversations for multiple situations. Youth need to understand that employers and training programs cannot provide accommodations unless they are requested within a reasonable time frame. Accommodations are negotiated between the employer and employee and must be requested in advance; the term "reasonable" in the ADA regulations means that an accommodation may not have to be provided exactly as requested or provided immediately. Training on how to ask for and negotiate an accommodation in a positive manner is critical for generalization to future training environments.

Awareness of assistive technology should be part of any empowerment approach to helping youth with LD succeed in the workplace and other adult settings. While accommodations are specific to situations and people, there is no doubt that assistive technology can promote success in the workplace for many youth with LD. Assistive technologies can provide critical supports that increase learning independence and empower youth to access and master workplace learning and tasks. For the maximum boost to personal productivity and independence, however, users need to be matched to the appropriate technologies and be proficient and comfortable with their use, which require awareness and evaluation followed by guided practice and modeling.

Vocational rehabilitation offices, federally funded Assistive Technology Access Programs or local community college resources for disabled students are sources of evaluation expertise and trial equipment or labs. Each state has an office or agency devoted to disability rights and policies.

Section 48.3

Helping Your Child Choose a Career and Find a Job

This section includes text excerpted from "Tips on How Parents Can Put Their Children with Disabilities on the Path to Future Employment," Office of Disability Employment Policy (ODEP), U.S. Department of Labor (DOL), December 12, 2007. Reviewed June 2016.

Tips on How Parents Can Put Their Children with Disabilities on the Path to Future Employment

Start Early

Starting early is a key component to your child's future success. Start by exploring the work world together and conveying your expectations that he/she can and will work when he/she grows up. Provide opportunities for your child to gain early work experience through volunteer work in your community.

Promote Education

Keep your child engaged in classroom activities. When parents expect their children with disabilities to continue their education beyond high school, the children tend to receive better grades than their peers whose parents do not have these expectations. In addition to the basic skills your child learns in the classroom, it is important that the child also learns how and when to tell others about any accommodations he or she may need.

Encourage Work-Based Learning Experiences

Schools and community-based organizations may offer internships, job-shadowing, and mentoring opportunities that focus on employment. While postsecondary education is important, it is also important to remember that it is not the only gateway to well-paying jobs. Vocational education classes can provide an alternate route for exposing young people with disabilities to careers and preparing them for work.

Create Leadership Opportunities

Encourage your child to connect with mentoring activities designed to establish strong relationships with other adults and peers. Encourage your child to become a mentor to younger youth. Participating in sports, student government, chorus, or volunteer groups can also build leaderships skills. There are also a few leadership organizations specifically focused on youth with disabilities:

- Kids as Self-Advocates
- The National Youth Leadership Network
- The National Consortium on Leadership and Disability for Youth

Set Goals

Teach your child how to set goals and work towards achieving them. Start small and work toward larger goals. With an older child, goal setting might relate to entering a chosen field.

Develop Social Skills

Friendships play a key part in youth development. Through the day-to-day activities that accompany making and maintaining friendships, you will be assisting your child in developing the ability to interact and get along with others, another essential skill employers look for and value in an employee.

Be Open to New Ideas

Listen to the ideas of experts—teachers, medical staff or community providers. Know in the end, however, that you are the one who knows your child best. Share expert's' input with your child, and, particularly as your child gets older, involve your child in any decision-making that affects him or her.

Additional Resources for Parents of Children with Disabilities:

- Office of Disability Employment Policy (www.dol.gov/odep)
- Office of Disability Employment Policy Guideposts to Success: (www.dol.gov/odep/categories/youth)
- Disability.gov (www.Disability.gov)
- The Job Accommodations Network (JAN) (AskJAN.org)
- PACER Center: (www.pacer.org)

Section 48.4

Tips for Disabled Job Seekers

This section includes text excerpted from "10 Things Job Seekers Should Know," Disability.gov, January 29, 2016.

Ten Things Job Seekers Should Know

1. **Your Employment Rights.** The Americans with Disabilities Act (ADA) guarantees that job applicants and employees

with disabilities have certain rights. The ADA covers things like what questions employers can ask about your disability or medical condition during an interview and what pre-employment medical tests they can require you to take. The ADA also requires employers to provide reasonable accommodations for employees with disabilities. Job accommodations are tools or modifications that help people with disabilities do their job. They can include assistive technology, such as screen readers for employees who are blind, or changes to work schedules, duties or locations. Teleworking can also be used as an accommodation for certain types of jobs. The Job Accommodation Network offers accommodation ideas by type of disability or limitation. If you feel you have been discriminated against on the job or during the interview or application process, you can file an employment discrimination complaint with the Equal Employment Opportunity Commission (EEOC) field office closest to where you live. Learn about other laws that protect the rights of people with disabilities in the workplace and the agencies that enforce them.

2. **Job Placement Programs.** Looking for assistance training for and finding a job? Your state Vocational Rehabilitation (VR) agency can help! VR agencies provide career counseling, job training and job placement services for people with disabilities. They also offer job accommodations and other supports, such as job coaching, to help workers with disabilities stay on the job. The Workforce Recruitment Program (WRP) connects college students and recent graduates with disabilities with federal government employers nationwide for internships or permanent employment. People who receive Social Security disability benefits and are interested in entering or returning to the workforce should check out the Social Security Administration's Ticket to Work (TTW) program. Anyone ages 18 to 64 who receives SSDI or SSI benefits because of a disability is eligible to participate.

3. **Writing Resumes and Cover Letters That Get Noticed.** When you're looking to get into the job market, a good first step is to create or update your resume and cover letter. Think of these documents as your marketing tools to help an employer understand why you're the best fit for the job. The Harvard Business Review has great advice on how to write a strong cover letter, including tips like researching the employer and the specific job you're applying for and

referencing that information. CareerOneStop has a very useful fact sheet on different types of cover letters and how to write them. Also from CareerOneStop is a resume guide that gives you a step-by-step plan for how to create a resume that will catch the eye of employers. More help can be found in the Department of Labor's Return-to-Work Toolkit. Find information on resume design, tips, tricks, and trends in Learn How to Become Resume Revolution section.

4. **A Social Angle.** Social media sites such as Facebook, LinkedIn, and Twitter can provide many leads and opportunities when searching for a job. Using social media to look for work has numerous benefits, including increasing networking opportunities. Having a strong presence on social media websites, or creating a "personal brand," is a great way to connect with employers and others in your chosen field. Job recruiters use social media to spread the word about job openings, as well as to learn more about potential employees. This means it's important that any "digital footprints" on social media be appropriate and professional in order to make a good impression on recruiters. There are many smart strategies job seekers can use to make the most out of social media accounts, such as participating in industry-related Twitter chats and joining relevant Facebook groups. Jump start successful use of social media for job searching through this free email course. Different social media platforms can serve different functions in searching for work, so it's helpful to learn how to use and maintain social media profiles on popular networking sites.

5. **A Deeper Look at LinkedIn.** If you're looking for a job and you want to know where the recruiters are, look no further than LinkedIn. Ninety-five percent of recruiters say they use the site to search for and contact job candidates. Not only is it a great place to showcase what you have to offer, but LinkedIn is also a useful tool for networking with contacts, connecting with new people, conducting research, and more. You'll want to begin by making sure your profile is up to date. Build a winning profile with a professional-looking photo, include details about your past work experiences and use common keywords for your profession. The Society for Human Resources Management offers advice for networking and job searching on LinkedIn and other social media sites. Don't overlook LinkedIn Groups as a job-seeking tool. Groups allow you to connect

with others in a similar field of interest and make yourself known by the information and articles you share in those groups. What's Next lists the ten best LinkedIn groups for job seekers. Temple University has a fact sheet on how to network on LinkedIn, which includes ten helpful tips on how to connect with others while job searching.

6. **Finding a Job.** Your resume is in hand and you're ready to look for that new job opportunity. But where do you start? Get help with your job hunt through organizations that specialize in helping people find employment, such as your local American Job Center, state Vocational Rehabilitation agency or state job bank. Since much of the job search process takes place online these days, you may also wish to look for job postings on a variety of websites, particularly CareerOneStop. The site allows you to explore career options and search for jobs. If you're looking for federal government employment, all open federal jobs are posted on USAJobs.gov. There are four basic steps to using the site:

1. Create an account, which includes your profile and resume.

2. Search for jobs and carefully review the "Qualifications and Evaluation" section to make sure you meet the criteria.

3. Apply for jobs by following the instructions in the "How to Apply" section of each listing. Keep in mind that job openings on USAJOBS.gov expire at 11:59 p.m. Eastern Time on the published closing date, meaning that the agency will no longer accept applications after that time.

4. To check the status of your application or get answers to specific questions about the job posting, contact the agency directly.

You may also want to read these six tips about finding a job with the federal government and how to avoid government job scams. You should never pay to find information on government employment—this information is available for free.

1. **Ace That Interview**. One of the keys to acing a job interview is to take steps beforehand to prepare. Recruiters are searching for candidates who not only have the necessary skills and experience for a position, but also demonstrate strong knowledge of a company or organization's culture. Start preparation for an interview by following this 7-Step Interview Prep Plan.

Use this helpful Interview Checklist to stay on track with preparation efforts. Be sure to research the organization and read the job description carefully, taking note of facts that may be useful during the interview. Study commonly-asked interview questions and plan out the main points you'll use to respond to them. Also, take some time to plan questions to ask the interviewer. Before the interview, plan an appropriate outfit and gather things such as a notebook and a pen, copies of your resume and work samples and anything else the interviewer would likely request to see. Follow these interview tips, which include reminders to arrive early and to be confident, to help ensure a successful interview. Remember to always follow up an interview by sending a thank you note, either by email or hand written, to the person or people who interviewed you.

2. **Moving from School to Work**. As young people reach the age at which they are ready to enter the workforce, it's important to know what resources are available to aid in a smooth transition from school to work. The National Collaborative on Workforce and Disability for Youth has a website that provides guidance on all aspects of the school-to-work transition process. First, it's helpful to have an understanding of the laws that protect people with disabilities in the workforce and well as job assistance services that are available, such as One Stop Centers and state Vocational Rehabilitation Agencies. To determine a career plan, youth can use the Guiding Your Success Tool on their own or in collaboration with peers, parents or guidance counselors. Families and caregivers can play key roles in mentoring and preparing young adults to move into the workforce by guiding the development of soft skills and other work-related skills. Parents, teachers and guidance counselors who work with youth with disabilities should always remember to encourage self-advocacy throughout the school-to-work transition process. Young people can take charge of their future by learning about options including employment supports and being self-employed.

3. **There's No Workplace Like Home**. Working from home, sometimes called teleworking or telecommuting, is a popular option for many people with disabilities. It allows for more flexibility and eliminates the need for transportation, which can be a barrier to employment. TeleworkTools.org has information for people interested in teleworking. It includes

information about jobs with telework potential and a self-assessment you can take to see if you're ready for home-based employment. Learn about the traits of successful teleworkers and what it takes to work professionally from home. Telework can also be considered a reasonable accommodation under the ADA. Looking for telework jobs? The National Telecommuting Institute (NTI) is a nonprofit organization that helps place people with disabilities in telework jobs. Learn about the types of work-at-home positions NTI offers. Employment Options is a certified Social Security Administration Employment Network in the Ticket to Work Program that helps people who receive Social Security disability benefits find work from home jobs. Unfortunately, some work-from-home jobs you see advertised may not be legitimate.

4. **Job Help for Veterans**. There are many resources to help Veterans with disabilities find jobs and transition from military to civilian life. The U.S. Department of Veterans Affairs (VA) Veterans Employment Center has a job bank, resume builder, and military skills translator. The National Resource Directory has a section with employment information for wounded warriors, transitioning ServiceMembers and Veterans about choosing a career, finding a job, starting a business and getting workplace accommodations. You can find additional assistance through the VA's Veteran Employment Service Office, including contact information for Veterans Employment Specialists in your area. Your State Veterans Affairs Office can also connect you to job training and placement programs near you. Use CareerOneStop's Veterans website to search for civilian jobs based on your military experience. Learn about the Gold Card Initiative for Post-9/11 Veterans and how to get Veteran's employment services from your local American Job Center. Paralyzed Veterans of America's Operation PAVE also offers one-on-one vocational assistance to Veterans and their families. Want to work for the federal government? FedsHireVets has information about federal employment, including what Veterans' preference is and how it can be used.

Section 48.5

Learning Disabilities and Federal Government Employment

This section includes text excerpted from "10 Things You Want to Know about Federal Government Employment," Disability.gov, January 2015.

Federal Government Employment

1. The Best Places to Work in the Federal Government for People with Disabilities. Two new reports now make it easier for people with disabilities to assess various agencies in the federal government as possible employers. Last month, the Partnership for Public Service released its 2014 Best Places to Work in the Federal Government report, which ranks federal agencies across ten workplace categories, such as support for diversity, and demographics, including age, gender, race and ethnicity. Rankings and scores were based on the U.S. Office of Personnel Management's (OPM) annual Federal Employee Viewpoint Survey and other agency data. Among some of the highest ranked agencies are the National Aeronautics and Space Administration, Federal Deposit Insurance Corporation (FDIC), and the Surface Transportation Board.

OPM also released a revised report detailing agency improvements in recruiting, hiring and retaining people with disabilities in the federal workforce. Due in part to Executive Order 13548, the federal government has set a goal to become a model employer of individuals with disabilities. The report shows that in Fiscal Year 2013, more people with disabilities were hired by the federal government than at any other point in the past 33 years. Additionally, more people with targeted disabilities were hired than at any time in the past 18 years.

2. Getting Your Foot in the Door at a Federal Agency. Several internship programs can help people with disabilities get their "foot in the door" in federal employment. One example is the Workforce Recruitment Program (WRP), a recruitment and referral program that connects federal and private sector employers to motivated college students and recent graduates with disabilities. Candidates who apply to WRP are pre-screened through interviews by federal recruiters. Qualified candidates are then added to the WRP database, which includes information about each applicant's skills and notes from recruiter interviews. Federal and private sector employers can also search the database for capabilities tailored to specific job requirements. The program works, too. Check out these two success stories featuring employees with disabilities who were hired after completing their internships, one at the Pentagon and the other at the FDIC.

Another valuable program is Project SEARCH, which helps students with significant intellectual and developmental disabilities secure competitive employment, including in federal agencies. Project SEARCH is a one-year school-to-work internship program that takes place entirely in the workplace setting and includes a combination of classroom instruction, career exploration, hands-on work experiences, and on-the-job training. To get started, use the interactive map to find a program in your area.

3. Where Do I Apply? All federal government jobs are posted on USAJOBS.gov. There are four basic steps to using the site:

- Create an account, which includes your profile and resume.

- Search for jobs and carefully review the "Qualifications and Evaluation" section to make sure you meet the criteria.

- Apply for jobs by following the instructions in the "How to Apply" section of each listing. Keep in mind that job openings on USAJOBS.gov expire at 11:59 p.m., Eastern Time on the published closing date, meaning that the agency will no longer accept applications.

- Check the status of your application or contact agencies for specific follow-up questions.

USAJOBS.gov offers a number of tutorials and tips on writing your federal resume, applying for federal jobs if you are someone with a disability and communicating your worth. You may also want to read these six tips about finding a job with the federal government and how to avoid government job scams.

4. Resumes and Cover Letters. Like any other opportunity, your federal resume and cover letter should showcase your skills and employment experience, as well as prove to the hiring manager that you are the best candidate for the job. For some helpful advice, read the U.S. Bureau of Labor Statistics' guide on applications, cover letters and resumes. Since resumes for government jobs are structured differently. Look closely at the job description and use its keywords and phrases in your resume, as long as they are consistent with your past experience. It's normal for jobseekers to feel like their resumes are in a "black hole," but Job-Hunt.org suggests avoiding small mistakes that may impede your success.

5. Federal General Schedule and Pay Grades. The federal government has different classifications and pay systems that determine an employee's position and compensation in federal jobs. Having an understanding of them will help you decide before you apply whether you are qualified for a particular position. The General Schedule or "GS" classification and pay system covers most professional, technical, administrative, and clerical positions for civilian federal employees. The GS system has 15 grades, starting from GS-1 (the lowest) to GS-15 (the highest), each with 10 salary steps. Federal agencies classify the grade of each job based on its level of difficulty, responsibility, and required qualifications. Individuals with a high school diploma and no additional experience typically qualify for GS-2 positions; those with a Bachelor's degree qualify for GS-5 positions; and those with a Master's degree qualify for GS-9 positions. According to the U.S. Department of Labor (DOL), jobs at a GS-7 level or higher typically require an advanced degree that is directly related to the work of the job opening.

6. Schedule A. Job applicants with intellectual disabilities, psychiatric disabilities or severe physical disabilities, who are interested in federal employment, can use the Schedule A Hiring Authority, often referred to as "Schedule A." To be considered for employment through Schedule A, you must provide documentation of your disability in a Schedule A Letter, which is prepared by your licensed medical provider, licensed vocational rehabilitation specialist or a state or federal agency that provides disability benefits. Keep in mind that Schedule A does not guarantee that you will be hired for the job; you must meet the qualifications and be able to do the work. A guide from the U.S. Equal Employment Opportunity Commission, The ABCs of Schedule A, provides tips for applicants with disabilities on getting federal jobs. Young adults with disabilities who are seeking employment in the federal government should take note of this fact sheet on Schedule A hiring for youth. Finally, watch the bite-sized training on applying for federal jobs using Schedule A to make sure you are familiar with the whole process.

7. Hiring America's Heroes. A key piece of the federal government hiring strategy is recruiting and employing veterans, including those with disabilities. In 2009, President Barack Obama signed Executive Order 13518 to help the men and women of the armed forces find jobs; In addition to Schedule A, learn about special hiring authorities for veterans, such as Veterans' Recruitment Appointment (VRA). You can also review the Federal Employment training module and test your knowledge. The VA, in partnership with DoD, manages a Veterans Employment Center and offers support for transitioning service members with disabilities.

8. Job Accommodations. Congratulations, you got the job! Now you have to do it. For many people with disabilities this means working with your employer to create workplace supports and accommodations, so you can be as productive as possible. There are many resources that guide employees on how to ask for accommodations and what to ask for based on particular disabilities. One such resource is the Job Accommodation Network (JAN), which is a full service employment accommodation resource center for people with disabilities and employers. JAN offers information by disability, as well as comprehensive resources on topics affecting the entire employment life cycle. Another great resource is the DoD's Computer/Electronic Accommodations Program (CAP). CAP specializes in technology accommodations, including assistive technology, for people with disabilities and wounded Service members throughout the federal government. The fastest way to request an accommodation is online. Visitors can browse possible technology accommodation solutions for various disabilities, as well as get answers to frequently asked questions. CAP also has an onsite demonstration and assessment facility at the Pentagon called CAPTEC, where employees with disabilities can receive a personalized needs assessment and compare different solutions.

9. Other resources. For those seeking employment with the federal government, there are a multitude of resources that can help you get on your way. DOL's Office of Disability Employment Policy (ODEP) is your first stop for information on federal government programs and other employment issues that affect people with disabilities, including transitioning youth. This past year, a large emphasis has been placed on the employment and career advancement of people with disabilities through accessible technology—a key tenet of the ODEP-funded Partnership on Employment & Accessible Technology (PEAT), which is a consortium of leaders who are working with employers and technology providers to encourage the widespread adoption of accessible workplace technology practices. People with disabilities who want to learn how to return to work while receiving disability benefits should register for Work Incentive Seminar Events (WISE) or watch the archived versions to learn about the Social Security Administration's Ticket to Work program.

10. Disability as Part of Diversity. Employers, including federal agencies, increasingly view disability as a part of their diversity and inclusion efforts. Fostering a culture that values individuals' different attributes and experiences can help an employer benefit from varied perspectives. The 2011 Government-Wide Diversity and Inclusion Strategic Plan outlines how the federal government will promote diversity and inclusion in the federal workforce. Federal employers can review the Guidance for Agency-Specific Diversity and Inclusion Strategic Plans, as well as the Toolkit for Federal Agencies on Implementing Executive Order 13548, which outlines a five-step process for hiring people with disabilities. Another helpful resource is the Employer Assistance and Resource Network's (EARN) Disability Is Diversity: Effective Hiring Practices for Federal Employers research-to-practice brief. Federal hiring managers also can create an account on eFedLink to access resources, promising practices and information on federal initiatives.

Chapter 49

Coaching for Adults with Learning Disabilities

Overview

With regard to people with learning disabilities or attention deficit hyperactivity disorder (ADHD), coaching refers to a type of intervention that provides individuals with strategies, tools, and support to help them overcome difficulties and accomplish goals. Coaches can be an important part of the treatment team, serving as teachers, mentors, counselors, and role models who guide individuals with learning disabilities on a path toward rewarding self-discovery. Coaches are not medical professionals, however, and are not trained to diagnose learning or attention issues or treat psychological disorders. Instead, they help people deal with the life problems associated with learning disabilities or ADHD, such as issues involving self-control, decision making, and social skills.

Several different types of coaches are available to help individuals with learning disabilities develop and practice strategies for coping with the challenges they face. Academic coaches, for instance, can help teenagers build the skills they need to become independent learners and succeed within a school environment. In addition, parents can be trained to apply a coaching program to assess the child's skills and behavior and work together with the child as a team to

"Coaching for Adults with Learning Disabilities," © 2016 Omnigraphics. Reviewed June 2016.

practice strategies for overcoming the hurdles of learning disabilities and ADHD. Applying a coaching program can help parents reduce conflict at home. Whereas the traditional reward-and-punishment approach to behavior management places the parent in an adversarial role with the child, the coaching technique establishes a supportive, team environment.

One of the main goals of coaching for people with learning disabilities or ADHD is helping them avoid labels and develop ways to describe their challenges and advocate for themselves. Rather than simply saying that they have ADHD, for example, clients might be encouraged to explain that they sometimes have trouble managing unscheduled time or seeing tasks through to completion. Ideally, the coaching process enables individuals to understand their strengths and limitations and find ways to manage daily demands. Coaches focus on listening to their clients, encouraging honest and open communication, teaching them to apply tools and strategies, and helping them develop self-confidence and independence.

Coaching for ADHD

Coaches can provide valuable support and strategies to help teenagers and adults with ADHD. ADHD creates challenges with many executive functions, including paying attention, avoiding distractions, managing time, prioritizing tasks, staying organized, following through on projects, and accomplishing goals. A coach who specializes in ADHD can help clients clarify the specific issues they face and break down problems into manageable steps. ADHD coaches are able to adjust problem-solving strategies as needed to deal with the specific issues the client may face, such as impulsiveness or distractibility.

Coaches have a complete understanding of the difficulties ADHD presents. Tasks that appear effortless to some people, such as getting to work or school on time, may be extremely challenging for someone with ADHD. Coaches can serve as cheerleaders to offer praise and encouragement when clients accomplish such goals. It is important to note, however, that coaching programs may not be appropriate for people who struggle with other disorders in addition to ADHD, such as depression or substance abuse. Psychotherapy is generally needed to treat these issues, although coaching can provide valuable support during recovery.

Finding a Coach

Choosing a qualified coach to assist adults with learning disabilities or ADHD involves multiple steps, including the following:

- Research possible coaches through reputable organizations. Several organizations dedicated to helping people with learning disabilities or ADHD offer national directories of service providers or lists of accredited coaches within a state or local area.

- Inquire about potential coaches' background and qualifications. Ideal candidates will have a degree in education, special education, or psychology and keep their training current by attending conferences. It is also important to ask how many years they have been coaching, how many clients they have served, and whether they hold certifications from professional organizations.

- Obtain referrals from other professionals, such as a psychiatrist or therapist, in addition to testimonials from former clients.

- Conduct an interview with each potential coach to delve deeper into their experience, specialties, and approach. An ideal candidate will have experience providing the specific kind of help the client needs, whether it involves helping a teenager with ADHD submit college applications or helping a small business owner get organized and stick to a schedule. For the client, it may be helpful to come up with a clear idea of what you hope to achieve through coaching and then ask each potential coach how they would approach the problem.

- Remember that the coach's role is to facilitate change and provide support, but the client is responsible for actually doing the work. In addition, sustainable behavioral changes take time to accomplish. Clients who expect an immediate solution to all of their problems are certain to be disappointed by any coach.

- Avoid coaches who suggest concrete solutions rather than helping the client find the most useful strategies for solving the problem.

- Take time to make an informed decision, and let potential coaches know that you plan to interview multiple candidates to find the best fit.

- Trust your instincts and choose someone with whom you feel comfortable and develop a good rapport. For the coaching relationship to be effective, it is vital that you are able to work closely together as a team.

References

1. Miles, Lisa A. "ADHD Coaching: Look to the Willow Tree," Psych Central, 2016.

2. Tartakovsky, Margarita. "ADHD Coaching—Nine Tips to Find the Right Coach," Psych Central, 2016.

Chapter 50

Special Needs Trusts

Overview

A trust is a financial arrangement in which a third party holds property or assets on behalf of a beneficiary. A special needs trust (SNT)—also known as a supplemental needs trust—is a particular type of trust that is established on behalf of a person with special needs to provide them with financial support after their parents or other caregivers die. Some people with disabilities are unable to work to support themselves, so extra financial assistance may be necessary to ensure their future security, welfare, and quality of life. But leaving money directly to a loved one with special needs often jeopardizes their ability to qualify for government benefits, such as Supplemental Security Income (SSI) and Medicaid.

These federal programs were established to provide a safety net of healthcare coverage and money to cover basic needs for elderly people and people with disabilities. However, the income threshold to qualify for these programs is very low. Although the value of a home, furnishings, a car, clothing, and other personal items does not count toward income for the purposes of receiving Medicaid and other government benefits, cash and investments can affect eligibility. People with disabilities who have financial resources above the threshold—even if the money comes from an inheritance or gift—are likely to lose their benefits. Special needs trusts are designed to let beneficiaries retain their

"Special Needs Trusts," © 2016 Omnigraphics. Reviewed June 2016.

eligibility for benefits while also giving them access to additional funds to cover needs and services that the government does not provide.

Setting up a Special Needs Trust

The first step in setting up a special needs trust is to create a trust document. Although a number of books and websites offer do-it-yourself instructions and forms to create a basic trust, many families seek assistance from an attorney to create a personalized trust. Knowledgeable legal advice can ensure that the trust is valid, complies with state laws, and meets the evolving needs of the beneficiary.

The trust document establishes the terms of the trust. Basically, the person who creates the trust, known as the grantor, places funds or property in the hands of another person, known as the trustee. The trustee has full control and discretion over the assets held in the trust, and they are legally obligated to manage the trust for the benefit of the person with disabilities, known as the beneficiary. Once the trust document has been finalized, it must be signed by all parties and notarized in order to take effect.

Funding the Trust

The trust will then receive a tax identification number from the Internal Revenue Service (IRS), which is required to open a bank account in the name of the trust. At this point the trust can be funded. Anyone who wants to help support the beneficiary can contribute property to a special needs trust. Most trusts are established by parents to support children with disabilities, but grandparents, siblings, friends, and others can contribute as well.

Trusts receive funds in a variety of ways. Relatives may leave property to the trust in a will, for instance, or designate the trust as a beneficiary to receive the value of stocks and bonds, a retirement plan, or a life insurance policy. Other types of property can be held in a special needs trust as well, such as jewelry, collections, cars, patents, business interests, and real estate. The key for estate-planning purposes is to leave property to the special needs trust instead of gifting it directly to the person with special needs.

Choosing a Trustee

Choosing a trustee is an important step in establishing a special needs trust. The trustee has complete control over the funds in the trust. Rather than giving money to the beneficiary directly, the trustee provides funds to purchase goods and services in accordance with the terms of the trust document. To perform this role effectively, the trustee must be familiar with the beneficiary's needs. They must also know the law in order to avoid making purchases that affect the beneficiary's eligibility for government benefits. In addition, the trustee is responsible for keeping records, paying taxes, managing trust investments, and selling tangible property in order to get cash to spend on the beneficiary.

Many families choose to hire a professional to serve as trustee. Although professionals charge an annual fee for administering the trust, this option ensures that the funds will be managed properly. In some cases, a family member who is familiar with the beneficiary's needs and has their best interests at heart will serve as co-trustee. The trust document should spell out how decisions will be made in case conflicts arise between co-trustees.

Using Trust Assets

The trustee is charged with using the trust funds to support the beneficiary. The trustee cannot give cash to the person with disabilities directly without jeopardizing their eligibility for government benefits. Instead, the trustee must use the funds to pay for goods and services that are not covered by Medicaid or SSI and that improve the beneficiary's quality of life. Some of the items that can be paid for with trust assets include:

- personal care attendants, therapies, and physical rehabilitation

- out-of-pocket medical and dental expenses

- educational expenses

- recreational activities and experiences, such as vacations or concerts

- items such as clothing, home furnishings, or a computer

- services such as Internet, cell phone, housekeeping, or maintenance

- pet food or veterinary care

A special needs trust continues to exist until the funds are depleted, the beneficiary no longer needs or is no longer eligible for government benefits, or the beneficiary dies.

Advantages and Disadvantages

The main advantage of having a SNT is that it enables the beneficiary to remain eligible for government programs and services, while also providing funds to pay for additional goods and services to enhance the beneficiary's quality of life. If the person with disabilities is unable to manage their own finances, the SNT provides a trustee to handle this function and ensure that the funds are used for their care. Finally, the funds used to create a SNT are tax-deductible.

One disadvantage of special needs trusts is the high cost involved in setting up the trust and managing the funds. In addition, some people with disabilities feel frustrated by the lack of control and independence the arrangement provides them. Finally, the passage of the Affordable Care Act in 2010 prohibited health insurance companies from denying coverage to people with preexisting health conditions. This provision enabled many people with disabilities to obtain healthcare coverage from sources other than Medicaid. As a result, special needs trusts may no longer be necessary for the purpose of preserving eligibility for Medicaid benefits.

References

1. Elias, Stephen. "Special Needs Trusts: The Basics," Nolo, 2016.

2. Fleming, Robert. "What Are Special Needs Trusts?" Learning Disabilities Association of America, 2016.

3. Hannibal, Betsy Simmons. "How Special Needs Trusts Work," Nolo, 2016.

4. Stuart, Melissa. "The Pros and Cons of a Special Needs Trust: Ensuring Your Child's Future," September 6, 2012.

Part Six

Additional Help and Information

Chapter 51

Glossary of Terms Related to Learning Disabilities

accommodations: Techniques and materials that allow individuals with various disabilities to complete school or work tasks with greater ease and effectiveness. Examples include spellcheckers, tape recorders, and expanded time for completing assignments.

assistive technology: Equipment that enhances the ability of students and employees to be more efficient and successful. For individuals with disabilities, computer grammar checkers, an overhead projector used by a teacher, or the audio/visual information delivered through a CD-ROM (compact disk read-only memory) would be typical examples.

attention deficit disorder (ADD): A severe difficulty in focusing and maintaining attention. Often leads to learning and behavior problems at home, school, and work. Also called attention deficit hyperactivity disorder (ADHD).

axon: The fiber-like extension of a neuron through which the cell carries information to target cells.

basal ganglia: Deeply placed masses of gray matter within each cerebral hemisphere that assist in voluntary motor functioning.

brain injury: The physical damage to brain tissue or structure that occurs before, during, or after birth that is verified by

---

This glossary contains terms excerpted from documents produced by several sources deemed reliable.

electroencephalography (EEG), MRI, CAT, or a similar examination, rather than by observation of performance. When caused by an accident, the damage may be called traumatic brain injury (TBI).

brainstem: The structure at the base of the brain through which the forebrain sends information to, and receives information from, the spinal cord and peripheral nerves.

cerebellum: A portion of the brain that helps regulate posture, balance, and coordination.

cerebral cortex: The intricately folded surface layer of gray matter of the brain that functions chiefly in coordination of sensory and motor information. It is divided into four lobes: frontal, parietal, temporal, and occipital.

collaboration: A program model in which the learning disabilities (LD) teacher demonstrates for or team-teaches with the general classroom teacher to help a student with LD be successful in a regular classroom.

developmental aphasia: A severe language disorder that is presumed to be due to brain injury rather than because of a developmental delay in the normal acquisition of language.

direct instruction: An instructional approach to academic subjects that emphasizes the use of carefully sequenced steps that include demonstration, modeling, guided practice, and independent application.

dyscalculia: A severe difficulty in understanding and using symbols or functions needed for success in mathematics.

dysgraphia: A severe difficulty in producing handwriting that is legible and written at an age-appropriate speed.

dyslexia: A severe difficulty in understanding or using one or more areas of language, including listening, speaking, reading, writing, and spelling.

dyspraxia: A severe difficulty in performing drawing, writing, buttoning, and other tasks requiring fine motor skill, or in sequencing the necessary movements.

executive functioning: A group of skills that help people focus on multiple streams of information at the same time and revise plans as necessary.

free appropriate public education (FAPE): A term used in the elementary and secondary school context; for purposes of Section 504, refers to the provision of regular or special education and related aids and services that are designed to meet individual educational needs of students with disabilities as adequately as the needs of students without disabilities are met and is based upon adherence to procedures that satisfy the Section 504 requirements pertaining to educational setting, evaluation and placement, and procedural safeguards.

frontal lobe: One of the four divisions of each cerebral hemisphere. The frontal lobe is important for controlling movement, thinking, and judgment.

gray matter: Neural tissue, especially of the brain and spinal cord, that contains cell bodies as well as some nerve fibers, has a brownish gray color, and forms most of the cortex and nuclei of the brain, the columns of the spinal cord, and the bodies of ganglia.

hippocampus: A component of the limbic system that is involved in learning and memory.

learning styles: Approaches to assessment or instruction emphasizing the variations in temperament, attitude, and preferred manner of tackling a task. Typically considered are styles along the active/ passive, reflective/impulsive, or verbal/spatial dimensions.

limbic system: A set of brain structures that regulates our feelings, emotions, and motivations and that is also important in learning and memory. Includes the thalamus, hypothalamus, amygdala, and hippocampus.

locus of control: The tendency to attribute success and difficulties either to internal factors such as effort or to external factors such as chance. Individuals with learning disabilities tend to blame failure on themselves and achievement on luck, leading to frustration and passivity.

midbrain: The upper part of the brainstem, which controls some reflexes and eye movements.

minimal brain dysfunction (MBD): A medical and psychological term originally used to refer to the learning difficulties that seemed to result from identified or presumed damage to the brain. Reflects a medical rather than educational or vocational orientation.

myelin: Fatty material that surrounds and insulates axons of some neurons.

neuron: A unique type of cell found in the brain and body that is specialized to process and transmit information.

neurotransmitter: A chemical produced by neurons to carry messages to other neurons.

perceptual handicap: Difficulty in accurately processing, organizing, and discriminating among visual, auditory, or tactile information. A person with a perceptual handicap may say that "cap/cup" sound the same or that "b" and "d" look the same. However, glasses or hearing aids do not necessarily indicate a perceptual handicap.

placement: A term used in the elementary and secondary school context; refers to regular and/or special educational program in which a student receives educational and/or related services.

plasticity: The capacity of the brain to change its structure and function within certain limits. Plasticity underlies brain functions, such as learning, and allows the brain to generate normal, healthy responses to long-lasting environmental changes.

prefrontal cortex: A highly developed area at the front of the brain that plays a role in executive functions such as judgment, decision-making, and problem-solving, as well as emotional control and memory.

receptor: A protein that recognizes specific chemicals (e.g., neurotransmitters, hormones) and transmits the message carried by the chemical into the cell on which the receptor resides.

related services: A term used in the elementary and secondary school context to refer to developmental, corrective, and other supportive services, including psychological, counseling and medical diagnostic services and transportation.

self-advocacy: The development of specific skills and understandings that enable children and adults to explain their specific learning disabilities to others and cope positively with the attitudes of peers, parents, teachers, and employers.

sensitive period: Windows of time in the developmental process when certain parts of the brain may be most susceptible to particular experiences.

specific learning disability (SLD): The official term used in federal legislation to refer to difficulty in certain areas of learning, rather than in all areas of learning. Synonymous with learning disabilities.

synapse: The site where presynaptic and postsynaptic neurons communicate with each other.

temporal lobe: One of the four major subdivisions of each hemisphere of the cerebral cortex that assists in auditory perception, speech, and visual perceptions.

transition: Commonly used to refer to the change from secondary school to postsecondary programs, work, and independent living typical of young adults. Also used to describe other periods of major change such as from early childhood to school or from more specialized to mainstreamed settings.

white matter: Neural tissue, especially of the brain and spinal cord, that consists largely of myelinated nerve fibers bundled into tracts that help transmit signals between areas of the brain. It gets its name from the white color of the myelin.

Chapter 52

Directory of Resources Related to Learning Disabilities

General

American Speech-Language-Hearing Association (ASHA)
2200 Research Blvd.
Rockville, MD 20850-3289
Toll-Free: 800-638-8255
Phone: 301-296-5700
TTY: 301-296-5650
Fax: 301-296-8580
Website: www.asha.org
Email: actioncenter@asha.org

Association for Childhood Education International (ACEI)
17904 Georgia Ave.
Ste. 215
Olney, Maryland 20832
Toll-Free: 800-423-3563
Phone: 301-570-2111
Fax: 301-570-2212
Website: www.acei.org
Email: dwhitehead@acei.org

Centers for Disease Control and Prevention (CDC)
1600 Clifton Rd.
Atlanta, GA 30333
Toll-Free: 800-232-4636
Website: www.cdc.gov
Email: CDC-INFO@cdc.gov

Resources in this chapter were compiled from several sources deemed reliable; all contact information was verified and updated in June 2016.

Center for Parent Information and Resources (CPIR)
35 Halsey St., Fourth Fl.
Newark, NJ 07102
Website: parentcenterhub.org
Email: malizo@spannj.org

Council for Exceptional Children (CEC)
2900 Crystal Dr., Ste. 1000
Arlington, VA 22202-3557
Toll-Free: 888-232-7733
TTY: 866-915-5000
Website: www.cec.sped.org
Email: service@cec.sped.org

DO-IT (Disabilities, Opportunities, Internetworking, and Technology)
University of Washington
P.O. Box 354842
Seattle, WA 98195-4842
Toll-Free: 888-972-3648
Phone: 206-685-3648
TTY: 888-972-3648
Fax: 206-221-4171
Website: www.washington.edu
Email: doit@uw.edu

Eunice Kennedy Shriver *National Institute of Child Health and Human Development*
31 Center Dr.
Rm. 2A32 MSC 2425
Bethesda, MD 20892-2425
Toll-Free: 800-370-2943
Phone: 301-496-5133
TTY: 888-320-6942
Fax: 1-866-760-5947
Website: www.nichd.nih.gov
Email: NICHDInformation
ResourceCenter@mail.nih.gov

Genetic and Rare Diseases Information Center (GARD)
P.O. Box 8126
Gaithersburg, MD 20898-8126
Toll-Free: 888-205-2311
TTY: 888-205-3223
Fax: 301-251-4911
Website: www.rarediseases.info.nih.gov
Email: GARDinfo@nih.gov

GreatSchools
160 Spear St.
Ste. 1020
San Francisco, CA 94105
Website: www.greatschools.org

LD OnLine
WETA Public Television
2775 South Quincy Street
Arlington, VA 22206
Fax: 703-998-2060
Website: www.ldonline.org
Email: info@ldonline.org

Learning Disabilities Association of America (LDA)
4156 Library Rd.
Pittsburgh, PA 15234-1349
Phone: 412-341-1515
Fax: 412-344-0224
Website: www.ldaamerica.org
Email: info@ldaamerica.org

Learning Disabilities Worldwide (LDW)
P.O. Box 142
Weston, MA 02493
Phone: 978-897-5399
Fax: 978-897-5355
Email: info@ldworldwide.org

National Center for Education Statistics (NCES)
Potomac Center Plaza
550 12th St., S.W.
Washington, D.C. 20202
Phone: 202-245-7674
Website: www.nces.ed.gov
Email:daniel.goldenberg@ed.gov

National Center for Learning Disabilities (NCLD)
32 Laight St.
Second Floor
New York, NY 10016
Toll-Free: 888-575-7373
Phone: 703-476-4894
Fax: 202-842-1942
Website: www.ld.org
Email: info@ncld.org

National Council on Disability (NCD)
1331 F St.
Ste. 850, N.W.
Washington, DC 20004
Phone: 202-272-2004
TTY: 202-272-2074
Fax: 202-272-2022
Website: www.ncd.gov
Email: jdurocher@ncd.gov

National Institute of Mental Health (NIMH)
National Institutes of Health
6001 Executive Blvd.
Room 8184, MSC 9663
Bethesda, MD 20892-9663
Toll-Free: 866-615-6464
Phone: 301-443-4513
TTY: 301-443-8431
Fax: 301-443-4279
Website: www.nimh.nih.gov
Email: nimhinfo@nih.gov

National Institute of Neurological Disorders and Stroke (NINDS)
NIH Neurological Institute
P.O. Box 5801
Bethesda, MD 20824
Toll-Free: 800-352-9424
Phone: 301-496-5751
TTY: 301-468-5981
Website: www.ninds.nih.gov
Email: koroshetzw@ninds.nih.gov

National Institute on Alcohol Abuse and Alcoholism (NIAAA)
5635 Fishers Ln.
MSC 9304
Bethesda, MD 20892-9304
Phone: 301-443-3860
Website: www.niaaa.nih.gov
Email: niaaaweb-r@exchange.nih.gov

Orange County Learning Disabilities Association (OCLDA)
P.O. Box 25772
Santa Ana, CA 92799-5772
Website: www.oclda.org

PACER Center
8161 Normandale Blvd.
Bloomington, MN 55437
Toll-Free: 800-537-2237
Phone: 952-838-9000
TTY: 952-838-0190
Fax: 952-838-0199
Website: www.pacer.org
Email: pacer@pacer.org

Smart Kids with Learning Disabilities
Phone: 203-226-6831
Fax: 203-226-6708
Website: www.smartkidswithld.org
Email: info@smartkidswithld.org

U.S. Department of Education (ED)
400 Maryland Ave., S.W.
Washington, D.C. 20202
Toll-Free: 800-872-5327
Website: www2.ed.gov
Email: octae@ed.gov

Aphasia

Aphasia Hope Foundation
Website: www.aphasiahope.org
Email: theaphasiafamily@aol.com

National Aphasia Association
350 Seventh Ave.
Ste. 902
New York, NY 10001
Toll-Free: 800-922-4622
Phone: 212-267-2814
Fax: 212-267-2812
Website: www.aphasia.org
Email: naa@aphasia.org

Assistive Technology

Family Center on Technology and Disability (FCTD)
Academy for Educational Development (AED)
1825 Connecticut Ave., N.W.
7th Fl.
Washington, DC 20009-5721
Phone: 202-884-8068
Fax: 202-884-8441
Website: www.ctdinstitute.org
Email: fctd@aed.org

Attention Deficit Hyperactivity Disorder

Attention Deficit Disorder Association (ADDA)
P.O. Box 7557
Wilmington, DE 19083-9997
Toll-Free: 800-939-1019
Fax: 800-939-1019
Website: www.add.org
Email: info@add.org

*Children and Adults
with Attention-Deficit /
Hyperactivity Disorder
(CHADD)*
8181 Professional Pl., Ste. 150
Landover, MD 20785
Toll-Free: 800-233-4050
Phone: 301-306-7070
Fax: 301-306-7090
Website: www.chadd.org
Email: customer_service@chadd.
org

Autism and Pervasive Developmental Disorders

*Association for Science in
Autism Treatment (ASAT)*
PO Box 1447
Hoboken, NJ 07030
Website: www.asatonline.org
Email: info@asatonline.org

*Autism National Committee
(AUTCOM)*
Website: www.autcom.org

*Autism Network
International (ANI)*
P.O. Box 35448
Syracuse, NY 13235-5448
Website: www.autreat.com
Email: jisincla@syr.edu

*Autism Research Institute
(ARI)*
4182 Adams Ave.
San Diego, CA 92116
Toll-Free: 866-366-3361
Phone: 619-281-7165
Fax: 619-563-6840
Website: www.autism.com
Email: cme@autism.com

Autism Society
4340 E.-W. Hwy
Ste. 350
Bethesda, MD 20814
Toll-Free: 800-328-8476
Phone: 301-657-0881
Fax: 301-657-0869
Website: www.autism-society.
org
Email: info@autism-society.org

Autism Speaks, Inc.
1 East 33rd St.
4th Fl.
New York, NY 10016
Phone: 212-252-8584
Fax: 212-252-8676
Website: www.autismspeaks.org
Email: contactus@autismspeaks.
org

*MAAP Services for Autism,
Asperger Syndrome, and PDD*
P.O. Box 524
Crown Point, IN 46308
Phone: 219-662-1311
Fax: 219-662-1315
Website: www.
aspergersyndrome.org
Email: info@aspergersyndrome.
org

Chromosomal Disorders

Genetics Home Reference
Website: www.ghr.nlm.nih.gov

National Human Genome Research Institute (NHGRI)
National Institutes of Health
9000 Rockville Pike, Bldg. 31,
Rm. 4B09
31 Center Dr., MSC 2152
Bethesda, MD 20892-2152
Phone: 301-402-0911
Fax: 301-402-2218
Website: www.genome.gov
Email: Cristina.Kapustij@nih.gov

Dyslexia

International Dyslexia Association (IDA)
40 York Rd.
4th Fl.
Baltimore, MD 21204
Toll-Free: 800-222-3123
Phone: 410-296-0232
Fax: 410-321-5069
Website: www.eida.org
Email: info@interdys.org

Hearing Disorders

Children's Hearing Institute
380 Second Ave.
9th Fl.
New York, NY 10010
Phone: 646-438-7819
Fax: 646-438-7844
Website: www.childrenshearing.org
Email: cbohdan@nyee.edu

National Institute on Deafness and Other Communication Disorders (NIDCD)
NIDCD Information Clearinghouse
1 Communication Ave.
Bethesda, MD 20892-3456
Toll-Free: 800-241-1044
Phone: 301-496-7243
TTY: 800-241-1055
Fax: 301-480-0702
Website: www.nidcd.nih.gov
Email: nidcdinfo@nidcd.nih.gov

Vision Disorders

All About Vision
Access Media Group LLC
1010 Turquoise St.
Ste. 275
San Diego, CA 92109
Phone: 858-454-2145
Website: www.allaboutvision.com

Children's Vision Information Network
Website: www.childrensvisionwichita.com

National Eye Institute (NEI) Information Office
31 Center Dr.
MSC 2510
Bethesda, MD 20892-2510
Phone: 301-496-5248
Website: www.nei.nih.gov
Email: 2020@nei.nih.gov

Chapter 53

Sources of College Funding for Students with Disabilities

In addition to scholarships available to the general public, minorities, and people pursuing a particular field of study, there are many scholarships specifically for students with disabilities. Below are some examples:

General

Incight provides up to 100 scholarships to help students with disabilities pay for college, vocational school or Masters or Doctoral programs. Applicants must be residents of Oregon, Washington or California, although they don't have to attend a college or university in those states. (spring deadline)

111 S.W. Columbia St., Ste. 1170
Portland, OR 97201
Phone: 971-244-0305
Website: www.incight.org/education/scholarship
Email: scholarship@incight.org

Newcombe Scholarships for Students with Disabilities are grants paid directly to colleges or universities to help students with disabilities who demonstrate financial need.

This chapter includes text excerpted from "Are There Any Scholarships Specifically for Students with Disabilities?" Disability.gov, March 2, 2014. All contact information was verified and updated in June 2016.

The Charlotte W. Newcombe Foundation
35 Park Place
Princeton, NJ 08542-6918
Phone: 609-924-7022
Website: www.newcombefoundation.org/scholarship_swd.html
Email: info@newcombefoundation.org

The **American Association of Health & Disability (AAHD) Scholarship Program** is for students who are full-time undergraduates (freshman or greater status) or part-time or full-time graduate students. You must provide documentation of a disability.

Scholarship Committee
American Association on Health and Disability
110 N. Washington St., Ste. 328-J
Rockville, MD 20850
Phone: 301-545-6140
Fax: 301-545-6144
Website: www.aahd.us/initiatives/scholarship-program
Email: contact@aahd.us

The **Ability Center of Greater Toledo Scholarship** is for Greater Toledo, OH area residents with disabilities. (spring deadline)

5605 Monroe St.
Sylvania, OH 43560
Voice TTY: 419-885-5733
Fax: 419-882-4813
Website: www.abilitycenter.org/we-can-help/living-with-a-disability/center-resources/scholarship-application

The **Business Plan Scholarship for Students with Disabilities** is a $1,000 scholarship open to undergraduate or graduate students with disabilities who've written a business plan for a class, competition or to start a business. (spring and winter deadlines)

315 Madison Ave., 24th Fl.
New York, NY 10017
Website: www.fitsmallbusiness.com/learn-how-to-write-a-business-plan
Email: info@fitsmallbusiness.com

For Students Who Are Blind

American Foundation for the Blind awards scholarships from $500 to $3,500 to students who are blind or visually impaired (spring deadline).

American Foundation for the Blind
1000 Fifth Ave.
Ste. 350
Huntington, WV 25701
Toll Free: 800-232-5463
Website: www.afb.org/info/afb-2015-scholarship-application/5
Email: info@afb.net

The **American Council of the Blind** awards scholarships to students who are legally blind. A 3.3 cumulative point average is usually required (spring deadline).

American Council of the Blind
1703 N. Beauregard St., Ste. 420
Alexandria, VA 22201
Phone: 202-467-5081; 800-424-8666
Fax: 703-465-5085
Website: www.acb.org
Email: info@acb.org

The **Association of Blind Citizens** runs the Assistive Technology Fund, which covers 50 percent of the retail price of adaptive services or software for individuals who are legally blind (summer and winter deadlines).

Association of Blind Citizens
P.O. Box 246
Holbrook, MA 02343
Phone: 781-961-1023
Fax: 781-961-0004
Website: www.blindcitizens.org/assistive_tech.htm
Email: president@blindcitizens.org

Christian Record Services for the Blind offers partial scholarships to young people who are legally blind to obtain a college education (spring deadline).

National Camps for Blind Children
A 501(c)(3) nonprofit organization
Lincoln, NE 68506-0097
Phone: 402-488-0981
Website: www.christianrecord.org
Email: info@christianrecord.org

Learning Ally's Mary P. Oenslager Scholastic Achievement Awards are given to Learning Ally members who are blind or visually impaired and have received or will be receiving their bachelor's, master's or doctoral degree. The top three winners each receive a $6,000 scholarship and a chance to participate in a celebration in Washington, DC (spring deadline).

20 Roszel Rd.
Princeton, NJ 08540
Toll Free: 800-221-4792
Website: www.learningally.org/NAA.aspx

The **Lighthouse Guild scholarship program** offers scholarships of up to $10,000 to help high school students who are legally blind pay for college (spring deadline).

15 W. 65th St.
New York, NY 10023
Tollfree: 800-284-4422
Phone: 212-769-7801
Website: www.lighthouseguild.org

The **National Federation of the Blind Scholarship Program** offers many scholarships from $3,000 to $12,000 to college students who are blind, in recognition of their achievements (spring deadline).

National Federation of the Blind
200 E. Wells St.
Baltimore, MD 21230
Phone: 410-659-9314
Fax: 410-685-5653
Website: www.nfb.org

The **United States Association of Blind Athletes (USABA) Copeland Scholarship** is awarded to USABA members who are legally blind and enrolled at a two-year or four-year college, university or technical school as a full-time student (fall deadline).

1 Olympic Plaza
Colorado Springs, CO 80909
Website: www.usaba.org
Phone: 719-86-3224
Fax: 719-866-3400

For Students Who Are Deaf or Hard of Hearing

The **Alexander Graham Bell Scholarship Program** offers scholarships for students who have moderately severe to profound hearing loss and are getting a bachelor's, master's or doctoral degree (spring deadline).

Cochlear Americas has two scholarship programs—the **Graeme Clark Scholarship,** which is open to people who have the Nucleus ® Cochlear Implant, and the **Anders Tjellstrom Scholarship,** which is open to people who have the Baha® System (fall deadline).

Cochlear Americas
The Graeme Clark Scholarship
13059 E. Peakview Ave.
Centennial, CO 80111
Website: www.cochlear.com/wps/wcm/connect/us/recipients/baha-other-processors/baha-other-processors-support-and-community/scholarships

The **Gallaudet University Alumni Association** provides financial assistance to graduates of Gallaudet University and other accredited colleges and universities who are deaf and are getting their graduate degree at colleges and universities not specifically for deaf or hard of hearing people (spring deadline).

800 Florida Ave., N.E.
Washington, DC 20002-3695
Phone: 202-250-2590
TTY: 202-651-5060
Fax: 202-651-5062
Website: www.gallaudet.edu

The **Sertoma Hard of Hearing or Deaf Scholarship** helps undergraduate students with clinically significant bilateral hearing loss pay for college (spring deadline).

1912 E. Meyer Blvd.
Kansas City, MO 64132
Phone: 816-333-8300
Fax: 816-333-4320
Website: www.sertoma.org

For Students with Learning Disabilities

LD Resources Foundation Awards help college students with learning disabilities pay for testing and in some cases award specific types of assistive technologies, such as Dragon Naturally Speaking (fall deadline).

LD Resources Foundation, Inc
229 E 85th St.
P.O Box 1075
New York, NY 10028
Phone: 646-701-0000
Fax: 212-444-1061
Website: www.ldrfa.org/?portfolio=award-programs
Email: info@ldrfa.org

National Center for Learning Disabilities (NCLD) Scholarships are offered to high school seniors with documented learning disabilities who are getting a higher education (winter deadline). NCLD also offers a list of scholarships for students with learning disabilities or attention deficit hyperactivity disorder (ADHD).

32 Laight St., Second Fl.
New York, NY 10013
Website: www.ncld.org

Learning Ally offers the **Marion Huber Learning Through Listening Awards** for outstanding students with print or learning disabilities. The top three winners each receive a $6,000 scholarship and a chance to participate in a celebration in Washington, DC (spring deadline).

20 Roszel Rd.
Princeton, NJ 08540
Website: www.learningally.org/NAA.aspx

P. Buckley Moss Foundation Scholarships and Awards offer financial assistance to high school seniors with learning disabilities who are getting a higher education or are planning a career in the visual arts (spring deadline).

P. Buckley Moss Society
74 Poplar Grove Ln.
Mathews, VA 23109
Phone: 800-430-1320
Website: www.mosssociety.org/page.php?id=8
Email: society@pbuckleymoss.com

Rise Scholarships Foundation, Inc. offers scholarships for students who learn differently (winter deadline).

Website: www.risescholarshipfoundation.org
Email: risescholarshipfoundation@gmail.com

The **Western Illinois University Chad Stovall Memorial Scholarship** is a $500 scholarship for Western Illinois University students who have Tourette Syndrome, obsessive-compulsive disorder (OCD), or attention deficit disorder (spring deadline).

143 Memorial Hall
1 University Circle
Macomb, IL 61455 USA
Email: disability@wiu.edu
Phone: (309) 298-2512
Fax: (309) 298-2361

The **Learning Disabilities Association of Iowa** offers scholarships of $1,000 each to high school seniors planning to enroll in college or vocational programs (spring deadline).

5665 Greendale Rd., Ste. D
Johnston, IA 50131
Phone: 515-280-8558; 888-690-5324
Website: www.ldaiowa.org
Email: info@ldaiowa.org

The **Shire ADHD Scholarship Program** provides scholarships of $2,000 each to 50 students with ADHD (winter deadline).

Shire US Inc.
Wayne, PA 19087
Tollfree: 800-828-2088
Website: www.shireadhdscholarship.com

Index

Index

Page numbers followed by 'n' indicate a footnote. Page numbers in *italics* indicate a table or illustration.

brain, *continued*
 learning disabilities 33
 neurodevelopmental disorders 41
 neuroimaging studies 276
 nonverbal learning disability 119
 overview 4–19
 plasticity 13
 reading disorders 103
 Rett syndrome 262
 specific language impairment 268
 speech-language therapy 368
 Tourette syndrome 271
 see also traumatic brain injury
"Brain Basics: Know Your Brain"
 (NINDS) 4n
brain injury
 defined 503
 see also traumatic brain injury
brain plasticity
 response to stimulation 13
 speech and language
  development 28
brainstem, defined 504
Broca's area, depicted *5*
bulimia nervosa, defined 207
bullying
 conduct disorder 154
 homeschooling 385
 overview 427–30
 self-esteem 440
 social perception 432
"Bullying and Children and Youth
 with Disabilities and Special Health
 Needs" (StopBullying.gov) 427n

C

CAPD *see* central auditory processing
 disorder
captioning, assistive devices 241
caregivers
 autism medication caution 260
 child's early learning 24
 child's speech development 128
 fragile X syndrome diagnosis 178
 human sensitive periods 14
 special needs trust 497
 visual processing disorders
  treatment 138

"Caring for Siblings of Kids with
 Special Needs" (The Nemours
 Foundation/KidsHealth®) 414n
CASE *see* Conceptually Accurate
 Signed English
Cayler cardiofacial syndrome 199
CBT *see* cognitive behavioral therapy
CCDC40 gene, dyslexia research 108
cell body, depicted *9*
Center for Parent Information and
 Resources (CPIR)
 contact 510
 publications
  adult services 450n
  adulthood transition 450n
  children disability
   evaluation 62n
  early intervention 320n
  emotional disturbance 203n
  employment connections 460n
  epilepsy 211n
  independent living
   connections 462n
  learning disabilities 33n
  steps in special
   education 331n
  supports, modifications,
   and accommodations for
   students 343n
Centers for Disease Control and
 Prevention (CDC)
 contact 509
 publications
  attention deficit hyperactivity
   disorder 152n
  birth defects 170n
  consequences of traumatic
   brain injury 286n
  developmental
   disabilities 38n, 250n
  disability inclusion 431n
  fetal alcohol spectrum
   disorders 220n, 224n
  fragile X syndrome 177n
  hearing loss in
   children 238n, 243n
  Tourette syndrome 277n
  traumatic brain
   injury 284n, 286n

genital organs, Prader-Willi
syndrome 187
Gerstmann syndrome, overview 231–2
global aphasia, described 142
grand mal seizure, defined 212
Graves disease, 22q11.2 deletion
syndrome 198
gray matter, defined 505
GreatSchools, contact 510
guanfacine, Tourette syndrome 273
"Guide to Student Transition
Planning" (Disability.gov) 395n

H

haloperidol, Tourette syndrome 273
hearing aids
described 240
tools for hearing impairment 243
hearing disabilities
overview 234–47
see also auditory processing disorder
"Hearing Loss in Children" (CDC) 234n
heart murmur, Turner syndrome 196
hemiplegia
bullying 428
defined 163
heredity
emotional disturbance 204
executive function 16
learning disability 48
see also genetics
hindbrain
depicted 5
described 5
hip dislocation, Down syndrome 172
hippocampus
defined 505
depicted 8
Hirschsprung disease, down
syndrome 172
homeschooling, overview 380–9
homework
attention deficit hyperactivity
disorder (ADHD) 145
nonverbal learning disability 122
hormones
neurotransmitters 9
Prader-Willi syndrome 187

"How Are Learning Disabilities
Diagnosed?" (Omnigraphics) 58n
Huntington disease,
neurotransmitter 10
hyperactivity, defined 144
hypothalamus
depicted 8
described 7

I

IDEA *see* Individuals with Disabilities
Act
IEP *see* individualized education plan
independent educational evaluation
(IEE), described 72
independent living
overview 462–7
transition planning 395
transportation 446
"Independent Living Connections"
(CPIR) 462n
individualized education plan (IEP)
coping with learning disability 409
emotional disturbance 208
epilepsy 216
Klinefelter syndrome 184
nonverbal learning disability 121
overview 337–42
special education process 333
transition planning 399
visual processing disorders 138
"Individualized Education Programs
(IEPs)" (The Nemours Foundation/
KidsHealth®) 337n
individualized family services plan
(IFSP)
cerebral palsy 166
defined 165
early intervention strategies 326
epilepsy 215
Individuals with Disabilities Act
(IDEA)
adult transition services 450
cerebral palsy 163
described 306
early intervention strategies 323
emotional disturbance 203
epilepsy 214

special needs trusts,
  overview 497–500
"Special Needs Trusts"
  (Omnigraphics) 497n
specific language impairment (SLI)
  overview 265–8
  speech disorder 27
"Specific Language Impairment"
  (NIDCD) 265n
specific learning disability (SLD)
  defined 506
  evaluating learning disabilities 63
  Individualized Education
    Programs 339
spectrum disorders *see* autism
  spectrum disorder
"Speech and Language Developmental
  Milestones" (NIDCD) 26n
speech disorder
  apraxia 131
  speech and language therapy 366
speech-language therapy,
  overview 366–9
"Speech-Language Therapy"
  (The Nemours Foundation/
  KidsHealth®) 366n
SSDI *see* Social Security Disability
  Insurance
SSI *see* Supplemental Security Income
statistics
  homeschooling 380
  National Health Interview Survey
    (NHIS) 75
StopBullying.gov
  publication
    bullying disabled 427n
stress management, attention deficit
  hyperactivity disorder (ADHD) 150
stroke
  aphasia 141
  apraxia 132
  executive function disorder 17
  Gerstmann syndrome 231
  reading disorders 104
  Williams syndrome 200
students
  accommodations 343
  cerebral palsy (CP) 167
  choosing a tutor 390

students, *continued*
  diagnosing learning disabilities 58
  differentiated instruction 352
  dyscalculia 91
  dyslexia 103
  every student succeeds act
    (ESSA) 314
  gifted/learning disabled 113
  homeschooling 380
  job seekers 483
  nonverbal learning disability
    (NLD) 121
  response to intervention (RTI) 329
  Section 504 308
  social skills 431
  supportive technology for writing
    problems 356
  Tourette syndrome 275
  transition to college 401
"Students with Learning Disabilities
  in an Inclusive Writing Classroom"
  (ERIC) 365n
substance abuse
  attention deficit hyperactivity
    disorder (ADHD) 147
  coaching for attention deficit
    hyperactivity disorder
    (ADHD) 494
  Klinefelter syndrome (KS) 182
suicide
  ADHD 156
  Tourette syndrome 281
Supplemental Security Income (SSI)
  Social Security Administration
    (SSA) 457
  special needs trust 497
supports
  Job Coach 461
  overview 343–9
  Prader-Willi syndrome 186
  Supplementary Aids and
    Services 347
"Supports, Modifications, and
  Accommodations for Students"
  (CPIR) 343n
surgical procedures, attention deficit
  hyperactivity disorder (ADHD) 151
swallowing therapy, speech-language
  therapy 368